POPULATION
HEALTH IN CANADA

POPULATION HEALTH IN CANADA

ISSUES, RESEARCH, AND ACTION

EDITED BY

Ivy Lynn Bourgeault

Ronald Labonté

Corinne Packer

Vivien Runnels

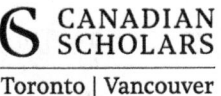

CANADIAN
SCHOLARS

Toronto | Vancouver

Population Health in Canada: Issues, Research, and Action
Edited by Ivy Lynn Bourgeault, Ronald Labonté, Corinne Packer, and Vivien Runnels

First published in 2017 by
Canadian Scholars
425 Adelaide Street West, Suite 200
Toronto, Ontario
M5V 3C1

www.canadianscholars.ca

Library and Archives Canada Cataloguing in Publication

Population health in Canada : issues, research, and action / edited by Ivy Lynn Bourgeault, Ronald Labonté, Corinne Packer, and Vivien Runnels.

Includes bibliographical references and index.
Issued in print and electronic formats.
ISBN 978-1-77338-009-4 (softcover).—ISBN 978-1-77338-010-0 (PDF).—
ISBN 978-1-77338-011-7 (EPUB)

1. Public health--Canada. I. Bourgeault, Ivy Lynn, 1967-, editor
II. Labonté, Ronald N., editor III. Packer, Corinne, 1967-, editor
IV. Runnels, Vivien, 1953-, editor

RA449.P67 2017   362.10971   C2017-906180-1
                                                                C2017-906181-X

Cover and text design by Elisabeth Springate
Cover image by mbbirdy
Typesetting by Brad Horning

17   18   19   20   21   5   4   3   2   1

Printed and bound in Canada by Webcom

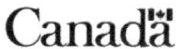

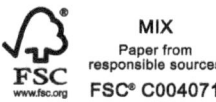

TABLE OF CONTENTS

SECTION IV ISSUES AND COMMENTARIES IN POPULATION HEALTH   245

LIST OF ACRONYMS

ACT – assertive community treatment

ACT UP – AIDS Coalition to Unleash Power

BMI – body mass index

CART – Classification Tree

CBC – Canadian Broadcasting Corporation

CCHS – Canadian Community Health Survey

CESCR – Committee on Economic, Social and Cultural Rights

COPD – chronic obstructive pulmonary disease

CIHI – Canadian Institute of Health Information

CIHR – Canadian Institute of Health Research

CMA – Canadian Medical Association

CMHA – Canadian Mental Health Association

CMHC – Canada Mortgage and Housing Corporation

CRPD – Convention on the Rights of Persons with Disabilities

CSDH – Commission on Social Determinants of Health

CVD – cerebral vascular disease

DAD – Discharge Abstract Database

DSM-IV – Diagnostic and Statistical Manual, Fourth Edition

EH – economic hardship

EIDM – evidence-informed decision making

EPL – employment protection legislation

ER – emergency room

FCTC –Framework Convention on Tobacco Control

HEST – healthy, equitable, and sustainable transportation

HIA – health impact assessment

HIV – human immunodeficiency virus

HUMA Committee – House of Commons Standing Committee on Human Resources,
   Skills and Social Development and the Status of Persons with Disabilities

IARC – International Agency for Research on Cancer

ICD-9 – International Classification of Diseases, Ninth Revision

ICES – Institute for Clinical Evaluative Studies

ICESCR – International Covenant on Economic, Social and Cultural Rights

ILO – International Labour Organization

LGBTQ – lesbian, gay, bisexual, transgender, and queer

LHIN – Local Health Integration Network

LIM – low-income measures

MCDD – multiple complex developmental disorder

MOHLTC – Ministry of Health and Long Term Care

NACRS – National Ambulatory Care Reporting System

NDP – New Democratic Party

NGO – non-governmental organization

NIHB – non-insured health benefits

NRCC – National Research Council of Canada

NSAID – nonsteroidal anti-inflammatory drug

NSRA – Non-Smokers' Rights Association

OCUL – Ontario Council of University Libraries

ODESI – an index/database access platform managed by the Ontario Council of University Libraries

OECD – Organisation for Economic Co-operation and Development

OHCHR – Office of the High Commissioner for Human Rights

OHIP – Ontario Health Insurance Plan

OHRC – Ontario Human Rights Commission

OMMAH – Ontario Ministry of Municipal Affairs and Housing

OPHID – Ontario Population Health Index of Databases

PHAC – Public Health Agency of Canada

PHIRIC – Population Health Intervention Research Initiative of Canada

PHIRN – Population Health Improvement Research Network

PHIRNET – Population Health Intervention Research

PROWRA – Personal Responsibility and Work Opportunity Reconciliation Act

PSC – Physicians for a Smoke-Free Canada

PTSD – post-traumatic stress disorder

RCTs – randomized controlled trials

RPDB – Registered Persons Database

SASS – Student Academic Success Service

SCID – Structured Clinical Interview for DSM-IV

SDH – social determinants of health

SE – social entrepreneurship

SES – Socioeconomic Status

SPSS – Statistical Package for Social Sciences

TAC – Treatment Action Campaign

TCPS – Tri-Council Policy Statement

UDHR – Universal Declaration of Human Rights

UN – United Nations

UNHRC – United Nations Human Rights Council

UNICEF – United Nations Children's Emergency Fund

UPR – Universal Periodic Review

WHO – World Health Organization

WMH-CIDI – World Mental Health–Composite International Diagnostic Interview

PREFACE

A Legacy of the Population Health Improvement Research Network

Ivy Lynn Bourgeault

This reader highlights some of the cutting-edge approaches and commentaries on population health research and focuses on two key issues: equity and interventions. It brings together a sample of the work undertaken by investigators funded by and affiliated with the innovative Population Health Improvement Research Network, or PHIRN for short.

THE POPULATION HEALTH IMPROVEMENT RESEARCH NETWORK

The Population Health Improvement Research Network, PHIRN, was a research network funded by the Ontario Ministry of Health and Long-Term Care from 2009 to 2014. Its mandate was to improve population health equity and strengthen population health interventions through high-quality applied population health research and knowledge exchange.

PHIRN's goals were threefold. The first was to create the necessary infrastructure to conduct more and better population health research with a focus on population-level interventions to improve health and address issues of health equity. The second was to enhance the capacity for population health research, in terms of both productive capacity and receptor capacity. Our third objective was to better inform policy and practice with state-of-the-art evidence. PHIRN was designed to provide research-based answers to questions about population health posed by governments, public health units, health promoters, health practitioners, and health organizations.

PHIRN's research and knowledge translation synthesis and exchange activities were organized into two main research programs: one on patterns and pathways of inequity, co-led by Carlos Quiñonez (University of Toronto) and Ronald Labonté (University of Ottawa), and one on population health interventions, co-led by Douglas G. Manuel (Ottawa Hospital Research Institute) and James Dunn (McMaster University). PHIRN was coordinated centrally at the University of Ottawa's Institute of Population Health, with Nancy Edwards as the scientific advisor and myself, Ivy Lynn Bourgeault, as the scientific director.

PATTERNS AND PATHWAYS OF INEQUITIES

The Patterns and Pathways of Inequities research program of PHIRN sought to expand the evidence base for policy interventions related to the social determinants of health. It acknowledged that a considerable base of research evidence already exists, but it needed to be enhanced, particularly with respect to policy influences on health inequities. The research strategies of this program went beyond the individual determinants of illness to examine:

- the intersections among different forms of social stratification (e.g., socioeconomic status, gender, and ethnocultural background);
- the connections between proximal and distal determinants of ill health;
- the institutions and processes that influence the allocation of health and social resources; and
- the global context affecting choices about resource allocation at national (Canada) and sub-national (Ontario, community) levels.

This program of research was collaborative, drawing on the expertise of Ontario health equity researchers. It emphasized a mixed-methods approach valuing both qualitative and quantitative research methods. It attended in particular to analyses of transferable policy interventions that have worked to reduce health inequities in other jurisdictions. The program also paid close attention to the difficult and contentious policy questions that surround health equity, and attempted to ground proposals for eliminating health inequity in Ontario using the best available scientific evidence and policy models from around the world.

Some of the key research priorities of this program of research were:

- to explore the impacts of closing the inequality gap on various outcomes, including health care utilization, social services utilization, and disease-preventing behaviours. This, we hoped, would aid in an assessment of what economic and social impacts can be expected through efforts such as poverty reduction strategies;
- to conduct retrospective and prospective analyses of governmental and non-governmental policies likely to have an influence on equity in health and the social determinants of health. This, we hoped, would aid in an assessment of the distributional impacts of various policies from the perspective of "health in all policies";
- to explore the nature of intersectionality, that is, how various social and cultural categories of discrimination interact on multiple and often simultaneous levels to influence health. This, we hoped, would aid in an assessment of where governments can concentrate efforts to have the greatest impacts;
- to explore citizen engagement and priority setting around health equity policies. This, we hoped, would aid in an assessment of what the public perceives as important, and what opportunities are available for change; and

- to both explore and engage in effective knowledge transfer and exchange activities (to both academic and public audiences) that we hoped would inform the public and policy dialogue on achieving greater health equity by "levelling up the bottom."

POPULATION HEALTH INTERVENTIONS

The Population Health Interventions research program of PHIRN sought to improve the overall health of Ontarians and reduce health inequities. It was anticipated that interventions would come in many forms. There would be those that target entire populations or groups of people who bear a disproportionally large amount of ill health, asking how we can mitigate risk among vulnerable populations. It was also anticipated that some interventions would address health opportunity structures (e.g., physical barriers, policies, norms) that shape health across whole populations. Other key questions included:

- What policy levers are most likely to optimize population health improvements and reduce health disparities?
- What have the population health impacts been of newly introduced policies and programs?
- How can we quickly adapt effective policies and programs from other jurisdictions to the Ontario context?

A key goal of the Population Health Interventions program was to build capacity to perform more and better intervention studies. We wanted to encourage the use of innovative evaluation methods that include real-life evaluation of new and existing programs. Similar to the Patterns and Pathways of Inequities program, this program encouraged the use of mixed methods to examine the health impacts of complex, multi-pronged interventions from a variety of policy sectors. In addition to the exploitation of existing and newly linked administrative datasets, other methodological approaches included systematic reviews, narrative syntheses, and realist syntheses of programs and policies from elsewhere.

Building partnerships was an explicit goal of this particular research program. It included organizations that make policy and delivery programs that influence health including many provincial government ministries, municipalities, public health departments, local health integration networks, and schools. We also partnered with the pan-Canadian Population Health Intervention Research Initiative of Canada (PHIRIC), which had as its mandate to coordinate national efforts and resources with the aim of increasing the quantity, quality, and use of population health intervention research. PHIRN hosted one of the training sites of the Canadian Institutes of Health Research–funded, pan-Canadian Strategic Training Program in Population Health Intervention Research (PHIRNET), with partnerships at the Université de Montréal, the University of Calgary, the University of Manitoba, the University of Toronto,

Dalhousie University, and the University of British Columbia. We also developed strategic partnerships with what was then called the Ontario Agency for Health Promotion and Protection, now Public Health Ontario.

PHIRN RESEARCH AND KNOWLEDGE EXCHANGE TOOLS

Beyond supporting these two research programs and its affiliated researchers, PHIRN centrally focused on creating a range of research and knowledge exchange tools to help achieve its research, capacity building, and knowledge exchanges goals. We undertook a series of consultations and created an advisory committee of key scientific and community representatives to delineate what activities we should undertake, particularly vis-à-vis other related organizations. We actively sought members to join us at PHIRN, and from this we created an online, searchable directory of population health expertise in the province. We undertook a scoping review to better understand our areas of strength and important gaps in our knowledge to inform our strategic plan, and from this we created an online platform for others to be able to search this literature (see Chapter 2). We partnered with other organizations like healthevidence.ca to appreciate the state of knowledge on some key equity and intervention topics (see Chapter 10). To liberate and make better use of available population health datasets, we created in partnership with the Ontario Council of University Libraries an online, searchable directory (see Chapter 4). In our knowledge exchange efforts, we built upon the pre-existing CHNET-Works webinar platform, which now boasts over 20,000 subscribers, and we have experimented with a peer-reviewed working paper series that includes innovative, bilingual, plain-language summaries with key messages for a range of knowledge users. Finally, we hosted a showcase event whereby the key results from the research PHIRN members have undertaken was presented in a series of panels with discussants from our advisory committee to a largely policy-decision-maker audience, culminating in a panel discussion with advice for how we could better connect evidence and policy to improve population health and reduce health inequities. These contributions and the extended versions of these analyses are archived on our bilingual website, www.rrasp-phirn.ca.

As noted by the subtitle of this preface, the knowledge created by the cutting-edge research our members undertook showcased in part in this volume represents a legacy of PHIRN. As so many promising initiatives developed across Canada, the activities undertaken by PHIRN have not been sustained through continued funding. It is our hope that we can nevertheless build upon the knowledge and resources developed during its four years of existence and move the field of population health equity and intervention research forward.

ACKNOWLEDGEMENTS

An edited book is neither a small nor a short undertaking. It is reliant on a lot of patience and good will on the part of its numerous contributors. This edited collection is no exception. We would like to acknowledge the funding provided for this and other work related to the Population Health Improvement Research Network, affectionately referred to as PHIRN, by the Ontario Ministry of Health and Long-Term Care. Additional funds were secured through a Knowledge Translation grant from the Canadian Institutes of Health Research.

Adept administrative support for the entire PHIRN initiative, as well as for the final stages of this book project, was provided by Lisa Childs. A number of other students working with Dr. Labonté and Dr. Bourgeault contributed to various elements, from the draft index to the list of acronyms and so on. A number of the papers were derived from the É/Exchange Working Paper series edited by Dr. Lynne Maclean, and we would like to acknowledge her input into the initial stages of those reports.

We would like to also acknowledge the cogent reviews we received by three anonymous reviewers. Their comments helped each of us to improve the accessibility and flow of the various contributions.

Finally, we would like to thank our PHIRN Advisory Committee members, on whose behalf Heather Manson provided our concluding commentary; other members included Arlene Bierman, Diane McArthur, Louise Potvin, and Penny Sutcliffe.

Ivy Lynn Bourgeault
Ron Labonté
Corinne Packer
Vivien Runnels

CHAPTER 1

Introduction

Ivy Lynn Bourgeault

The health of a population is influenced by a wide array of factors. What seems to be most salient to the public are genetic or biological factors, health practices or lifestyles, and to some extent one's immediate physical environment. But a broader population health perspective encourages us to look beyond these proximate factors to the social, political, economic, and cultural contexts that one experiences over the course of a life (Kindig & Stoddart, 2003). It is a unifying paradigm that links the biological to the social, political, and economic influences. A population health lens also encourages us to focus on the patterns of health and illness of a population, the distribution and systemic variations of health and illness, and how interventions that span the entire spectrum from health promotion and protection to illness prevention can improve the health and well-being not just of individuals but of populations more broadly (Public Health Agency of Canada, 2013).

This book centres on the conditions that influence, or contribute to, a population's health status, also referred to as social and economic determinants of health. These determine whether a population and its individuals are healthy or not, what can affect their health status, and what can improve it. Much thinking, writing, and media coverage about health generally makes reference to what takes place in the organized health care system and health care practices. This can lead to the impression that good health is a product of good health care. The focus of population health helps to make clear that health is more than health care, and in so doing makes the case for a focus on "health in all policies," in which policy- and decision-makers are encouraged to think about and plan for the health impacts of services not related to health care.

Critical to a population health perspective is a focus on the social determinants of health and a concern with health equity. First, the social determinants of health focus deals with the entire range of individual and collective factors, including but not limited to individual behaviour, along with components of the social (e.g., income, education, employment, culture) and physical (e.g., urban design, clean air, water) environments, or what some refer to as the conditions of living. As Dennis Raphael notes in Chapter 8, the social determinants of health "refer to the economic and social conditions that shape health and create health inequities." Because of these broad, all-encompassing definitions, some have critiqued the population health perspective as being so broad as to include everything—and therefore not very useful in guiding specific research or policy. But there is value in its broad focus in that it enables the integration of knowledge that cuts across the many factors that influence health and health outcomes and therefore the various disciplines that bring this into focus (Kindig & Stoddart, 2003).

Related to this social determinants of health approach is a concern with health equity. Health equity, according to the popular definition by Margaret Whitehead (1992), refers to "differences in health which are unnecessary and avoidable but, in addition, are also considered unfair and unjust." Three key criteria of health inequities are that they are:

1. Systematic: these inequities follow a particular pattern.
2. Socially produced: these patterns of inequities can be traced back to the social determinants of health.
3. Unfair: these patterns of inequities embody a sense of injustice (Whitehead & Dahlgren, 2006).

It is this latter criteria of fairness (or lack thereof) that most keenly distinguishes health inequities from a focus on health equality; there is a social justice element, and therefore cause for action.

Health equity as an achievable social goal has gained new policy relevance. Internationally, the WHO Commission on Social Determinants of Health (CSDH, 2008) focused attention on disparities in health that are avoidable by reasonable action, and therefore inequitable. Its commissioners argued forcefully that "social injustice is killing people on a grand scale" (WHO, 2008). Nationally, Canada's first Chief Public Health Officer targeted health inequalities in his agency's first annual report (2008), noting the importance of policy intervention in improving health outcomes. He stated, "Health inequalities are fundamentally societal inequalities that we can overcome through public policy, and individual and collective action" (p. iii). Provincially, the Government of Ontario's Poverty Reduction Strategy (2008) has recognized social inequalities as important to health, with a particular focus on children: "Providing for the health and wellbeing of children is a moral responsibility and essential to poverty reduction efforts." There is clearly a growing need and demand for strategic short- and long-range policy evidence in order to inform action on reducing health inequity by way of the social determinants of health.

Another key strand of a population health perspective is a focus on interventions—that is, once one identifies systematic variations in patterns of health and illness, it is imperative to apply the resulting knowledge to develop and implement policies and actions to improve the health and well-being of those populations. Population health interventions are a particular type of intervention reflecting an equally broad focus. According to the Population Health Intervention Research Initiative for Canada (CIHR, 2012), they include policies, programs and resource distribution approaches that impact a number of people by changing the underlying conditions of risk and reducing health inequities. Examples of such interventions include introduction of organizational changes in workplace design, housing policies to reduce homelessness, immunization programs and new taxes on products such as tobacco.

These interventions may come in many forms that may target entire populations or groups of people who bear a disproportionately large amount of ill health.

OVERVIEW OF THE SCOPE, CONTENT, AND METHODOLOGIES USED IN THE READER

This reader highlights some of the cutting-edge approaches in this broader population health perspective, focusing on key findings from population health equity and intervention research and commentaries on critical issues. It brings together a sample of the innovative work undertaken by investigators with the Population Health Improvement Research Network (PHIRN). Although a few chapters are focused on the Ontario context, much of the content centres more broadly on the conditions that influence or otherwise contribute to a population's health status.

We begin with some important background information and tools for the neophyte reader of population health research, particularly of a methodological nature. The complexity of the range of social, political, and economic factors influencing population health and their interaction necessitates a multi-dimensional methodological approach. To this end, we include an introduction to how one would use a range of qualitative and quantitative approaches to study population health. We include chapters on the use of administrative datasets that address various layers of influences on population health, as this is an underutilized area. Uncovering where these datasets are and what variables of interest they include is the focus of the chapter on the creation of the Ontario Population Health Index of Databases (OPHID), a resource that also points to important and often untapped sources of Canadian data. The information in the qualitative chapters were seen to be of particular value to community representatives we partnered with during our tenure at PHIRN. Having this background enables the reader to better understand and appreciate the approach to and findings emerging from the chapters that follow, which report on empirical research.

As noted at the outset, one of our core concerns is the social determinants of health and population health equity. The chapters address such topics as what we eat, where we live, what kind of work we have available, and how the environmental determinants of health affect us inequitably. The chapters in Section 2 address health equity issues experienced locally, such as the population health impacts of wildfires in northern Ontario, at the pan-Canadian level, such as inequities in housing for recent immigrants, and globally. It is here that we see how the local is truly connected to the global where the social determinants of health and health equity are concerned.

We then turn our attention to some wide-ranging population health interventions and descriptions of community action on the social determinants of health. These approaches take an intersectoral approach that includes areas a reader would not necessarily intuitively connect to health: building codes, regulations on media advertising, tax policy, and international human rights laws. Chapters in this section cause us to question how activities such as walking can be linked to health disparities, and present us with innovative ideas of how entrepreneurial communities can and have organized local food charters and services for marginalized groups, including youth. If a health equity lens reveals disparities that are unjust, a population health intervention approach can surely be seen as an instrument of social justice.

A unique set of contributions in our reader include weblog commentaries that cut across health equity and intervention issues, addressing a number of key population health topics in short, accessible, yet thought-provoking formats by scholars and practitioners. It is intended that these commentaries will encourage readers to think even more critically about some of the taken-for-granted assumptions about health prevalent in Canadian society.

Although our reader addresses a range of topics in population health, with some in particular depth, it does not cover all of the research and knowledge exchange activities undertaken by PHIRN researchers. For these, we refer readers to various reports and bilingual plain-language summaries on our archived website, www.rrasp-phirn.ca. Beyond these omissions, there are some notable gaps. We do not, for example, cover in depth issues related to how sex and gender are critical determinants of health, beyond the methodological piece offered on intersectionality in administrative datasets. Similarly, our chapters have not focused extensively on the experiences of inequity of Indigenous Canadians. These omissions on our part reflected the wealth of existing resources already available through Canadian Scholars' Press, most notably *Women's Health: Intersections of Policy, Research, and Practice* (Armstrong & Pederson, 2015) and *Determinants of Indigenous Peoples' Health in Canada: Beyond the Social* (Greenwood, de Leeuw, Lindsay, & Reading, 2015). It is also clear that there have been a number of recent political and economic events, such as the global refugee crisis, a new federal government, and increasing concerns over climate change, that are not fully reflected in the reader. All books are incomplete, but this text can be drawn upon as a framework through which a reader can begin to address these emerging issues.

REFERENCES

Armstrong, P., & Pederson, A. (2015). *Women's health: Intersections of policy, research and practice*. Toronto: Canadian Scholars' Press.

Canadian Institutes of Health Research (CIHR). (2012). *Population health intervention research initiative for Canada*. Retrieved from http://www.cihr-irsc.gc.ca/e/38731.html

Chief Public Health Officer of Canada. (2008). *The chief public health officer's report on the state of public health in Canada*. Retrieved from http://www.phac-aspc.gc.ca/cphorsphc-respcacsp/2008/fr-rc/pdf/CPHO-Report-e.pdf

Commission on Social Determinants of Health (CSDH). (2008). *Closing the gap in a generation: health equity through action on the social determinants of health*. Geneva: World Health Organization.

Government of Ontario. (2008). *Realizing our potential: Ontario's poverty reduction strategy (2014-2019)*. Retrieved from https://www.ontario.ca/page/realizing-our-potential-ontarios-poverty-reduction-strategy-2014-2019-all

Greenwood, M., de Leeuw, S. Lindsay, M. N., & Reading, C. (2015). *Determinants of indigenous peoples' health in Canada: Beyond the social*. Toronto: Canadian Scholars' Press.

Kindig, D. A., & Stoddart, G. (2003). What is population health? *American Journal of Public Health, 93*, 366–369.

Public Health Agency of Canada. (2013). *What is the population health approach?* Retrieved from http://www.phac-aspc.gc.ca/ph-sp/approach-approche/appr-eng.php

Whitehead, M. (1992). *The concepts and principles of equity and health*. Copenhagen: World Health Organization.

Whitehead, M., & Dahlgren, G. (2006). *Levelling up (part 1): A discussion paper on concepts and principles for tackling social inequities in health*. Liverpool: WHO Collaborating Centre for Policy Research on Social Determinants of Health.

World Health Organization (WHO). (2008, August 28). *Inequities are killing people on grand scale, reports WHO's Commission* [Press release]. Retrieved from http://www.who.int/mediacentre/news/releases/2008/pr29/en

SECTION I

METHODOLOGICAL TOOLS FOR POPULATION HEALTH

CHAPTER 2

Population Health Equity and Intervention Research: A Scoping Review of the Published and Grey Literature in Ontario, 2005–2011

Hasu Ghosh and Ivy Lynn Bourgeault

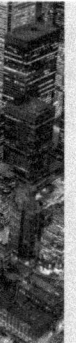

TAKE-HOME MESSAGE

- The literature tends to focus on quantitative research in large urban settings in Ontario, leaving a number of key knowledge gaps.
- Key populations of concern are low-income and immigrant populations.
- Action on health equity requires a sustainable path for interdisciplinary research capacity-building that embraces multiple methods of inquiry, with additional attention directed to the regions of Ontario with underdeveloped research strengths.

INTRODUCTION

Over the past decade, a growing body of national and international studies have encouraged population health equity and intervention research to focus more broadly on the contextual determinants of health within which health and illness behaviours are embedded and perpetuated (Canadian Public Health Association, 2008; Macintyre, 2007; Marmot, 2010; National Collaborating Centre for Determinants of Health [NCCDH], 2010; Östlin et al., 2009; Public Health Association of Australia, 2009; Standing Senate Committee on Social Affairs, Science and Technology, Subcommittee on Population Health, 2009). Interventions should not only focus on determinants in isolation, but also address the intersections among these different determinants and their cumulative impacts on health, given that they tend to cluster for disadvantaged populations (NCCDH, 2010; Östlin et al., 2009). Calls are also for interventions through policy and program initiatives that reside not only within but also outside of the health care domain. Because of this broad orientation, population health equity and intervention research requires multiple methods of inquiry from experts from a range of disciplinary backgrounds.

A comprehensive state of the knowledge of the broad areas of population health inquiry was not available at the time we were developing our strategic plan for the Population Health Improvement Research Network (PHIRN). It was instructive, therefore, for us to undertake a scoping review of the literature to locate and describe the population health equity and intervention research in Ontario. We opted to focus on the province of Ontario largely to inform the work of PHIRN, but many of the resources we found also covered other Canadian jurisdictions. Evidence around the strength of population health equity and intervention research, especially by the disciplinary, thematic, and geographic focus of that research, was our orientation. The specific goals of our scoping review were to:

- locate the primary areas of population health research undertaken in the province;
- identify researchers involved and the geographic location of research undertaken; and
- determine critical knowledge gaps to inform our research program.

METHODS

Our scoping review followed the typical methodological framework outlined by Arksey and O'Malley (2005). Table 2.1 outlines the six stages from that approach (columns 1 and 2) and how we applied that to our area of inquiry (column 3). To capture emerging published and grey literature in French and English, we searched for, retrieved, and analyzed original scholarly research sourced primarily from electronic databases (PubMed, Health Star, PsychInfo, Google Scholar, and Embase) and grey literature through the websites of various population health organizations and community groups (see Ghosh et al., 2011, for websites and keywords used). We began with literature published from 2005 to 2009 (which resulted in the working paper by Ghosh et al., 2011); this was subsequently updated with sources published in 2010 and 2011.

Selecting the Research Studies: Inclusion and Exclusion Criteria

The inclusion and exclusion criteria helped us to eliminate studies that did not meet our study selection parameters. In both phases of the search (2005–2009 and 2010–2011), we included studies that had a clear focus on health equity, social determinants of health, or population health interventions, and that had relevance to the province of Ontario. We included Canadian studies provided those studies included Ontario data. We excluded sources that had no data or that focused exclusively on medical care or strategies without a population health intervention or an equity lens. A total of 232 academic and 306 grey literature documents published in English or French during the publication period of 2005 to 2011 were identified.

Table 2.1: Scoping Review Framework: Stages and Results

Stage	Description	Results
• Identifying the research questions or locating the review topic	Provide a roadmap for subsequent stages. Research questions are generally broad in nature as they are focused on providing breadth of coverage.	• What are the primary areas of population health research undertaken in the province? • Who is primarily undertaking this research and where? • What are the gaps insofar as they relate to population health equity and interventions research?
• Identifying the relevant studies from both academic and grey literature sources	Develop a decision plan for selecting the keywords/search terms; sources include electronic databases, contact lists, organizations' web pages, etc. This also includes planning for practical limitations including resources, time, and personnel available.	• Over 2100 academic articles • Over 100 websites reviewed for grey literature • 706 academic articles selected as potential cases for full-text review • 701 grey literature documents selected as potential cases for full-text review
• Selecting the research studies through the development of inclusion and exclusion criteria	Select articles based on inclusion and exclusion criteria that build upon the specific research questions and research foci by familiarizing oneself with the subject matter and reading through the studies.	• 232 confirmed academic articles selected for scoping review analysis (all English publications) • 306 confirmed grey literature documents selected for scoping review analysis (111 English and 3 French documents)
• Extracting data	Extract and collate qualitative and quantitative data from each study according to descriptive variables agreed upon by the research team. A descriptive analytical review method is used to extract information from the studies.	• Data were extracted and summarized using two separate but identical Excel databases for academic and grey literature • These extracted data were a mixture of general information about the study and specific information relating to, for example, the sub-population experiencing inequities, explicit health focus, key methods, etc.
• Collating, summarizing, and reporting the results	Present a descriptive analysis of the extent and nature of the studies reviewed by using tables and charts.	• For the 232 (173+59) academic and 306 (114+192) grey literature sources, a series of charts and bar graphs were created from the categories coded in the respective Excel databases.
• Consultation (optional)	Provides opportunity to consult among the stakeholders, which includes people inside and outside the review team.	• Continuous consultation and communication among the PHIRN executive and reviewers resolved the uncertainties (if any).

1. Inter-Quintile rate ratio between poorest and wealthiest = (Q1-Poorest)/Q5-Wealthiest)
2. % Excess deaths due to differences between wealthy and all other Canadians = [100*(Total-Q5)/Total]

Source: Adapted from Tjepkema, M., R. Wilkins, & A. Long. (2013). Cause-Specific Mortality by Income Adequacy in Canada: A 16-Year Follow-Up Study. Health Reports, 24(7), 14–22: Tables 2 and 3, pp. 17–18.

Extraction and Analysis of the Data

Data from selected articles were extracted and summarized using two separate but identical Excel templates for the academic and grey literatures. First, the bibliographic details of selected articles were imported into the Excel databases. The next stage of the review process involved extracting key data from the academic and grey literature selected. We applied a thematic coding scheme developed both deductively (a priori) and inductively following the review of each article; this required some recoding of articles that had been coded earlier. The data extracted from these Excel files included a mixture of information relating to, for example, research funding sources, types of research, explicit health focus, key methods and types of documents, the subpopulation experiencing inequities, social determinants of health, other determinants of health, policy implications, and recommendations. Each of the categories was coded either 0 (no) or 1 (yes) for subsequent descriptive quantitative analysis. Descriptive statistics, including frequency and cross-tabulations, were prepared and presented in chart form.

RESULTS

Location of Research

The locations where the academic and grey literature research was conducted or the locations from where the samples were drawn are presented in Figure 2.1. A majority of the academic articles (41 percent) report on research that took place in urban Ontario settings, particularly in Toronto (28 percent). In contrast, only a small percentage of studies were conducted in rural Ontario (4 percent) or northern Ontario (7 percent). Similar to the academic literature, the majority (31 percent) of the research published in grey literature was conducted in urban Ontario settings, again largely in Toronto (24 percent). Only 6 percent and 4 percent of research published in grey literature was carried out in rural and northern Ontario locations, respectively. Noticeably, a considerable percentage (36 percent and 34 percent) of research published in grey literature took place in various locations across the province of Ontario (Ontario—All category) and across the country (Canada—All category), respectively. Many areas of Ontario remained understudied.

Methodological Approaches

Figure 2.2 demonstrates the different types of research methodologies employed in the articles we reviewed. Epidemiological studies appear to be most prevalent (47 percent) in the academic literature, followed by experiential studies, whereas experiential (27 percent), conceptual (25 percent), and policy-oriented research (24 percent) had more of a balance in the grey literature. Policy-oriented research constituted only 9 percent of the total academic studies, in spite of their already recognized importance in the field

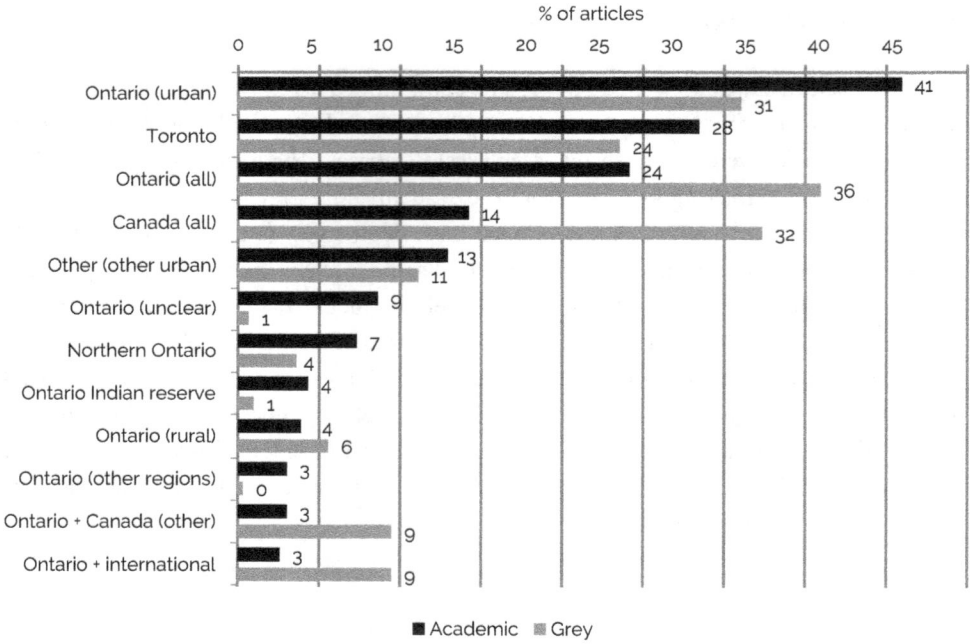

Figure 2.1: Distribution of Research Locations in Academic (n=232) and Grey (n=306) Literature Ω¹

of population health by researchers and health advocates (Raphael, 2003; Marmot and Wilkinson, 2006). The higher share of policy research captured in grey literature review could be due to the larger amount of policy and strategic reports published by federal, provincial, or territorial government departments, research institutes, and policy think tanks. Interestingly, intervention research was more prevalent in the academic literature, and although its share was small, this may reflect its being a newly emerging field of research.

Populations of Focus

Figure 2.3 presents the populations of focus in the academic and grey literature. A focus on those with low socioeconomic status (SES) is most frequently represented in both academic (36 percent) and grey (37 percent) articles, but in the grey literature, immigrants/newcomers/refugees also appear to be another commonly studied population (37 percent); this was the second most commonly studied population in academic literature (27 percent). Women (35 percent), infants, children, and youth (33 percent), and Aboriginal peoples (29 percent) are the remaining most commonly studied populations in the grey literature. Notably, these population subgroups are not mutually exclusive, as many of these people belong to multiple subpopulation groups. For example, immigrant women of colour tend to belong to the low-SES group, and could be simultaneously facing housing and financial insecurities.

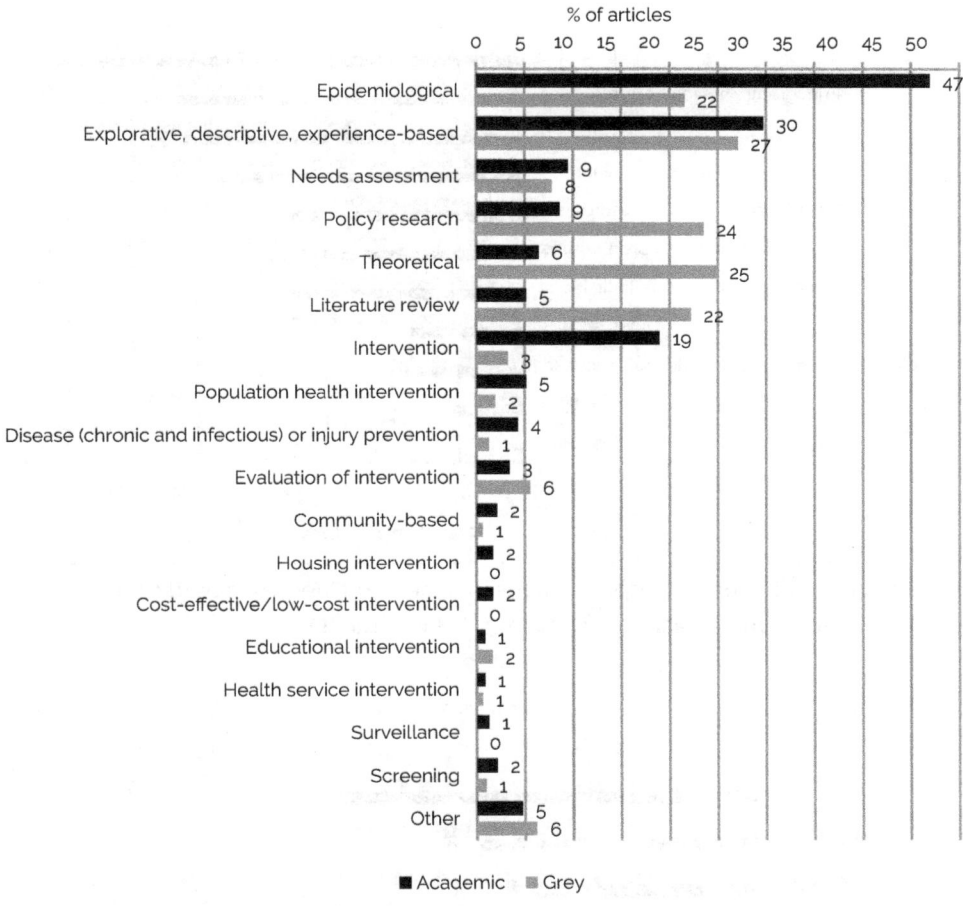

Figure 2.2: Distribution of SDH Studied in Academic (n=232) and Grey (n=306) Literature Ω

Social Determinants of Health

Figure 2.4 outlines the relative appearance of various social determinants of health (SDH) in the literature coded for this review. First, in the academic literature, income was the main determinant of health that was focused on (46 percent). Immigrant status (30 percent) and gender (28 percent) were the next most frequently examined determinants of health in the academic literature. Income was even more prominent in the grey literature (67 percent). This was followed by gender (63 percent) and access to health service (60 percent). The grey literature also reveals a stronger emphasis on employment (57 percent), age (57 percent), education and literacy (56 percent), SES (56 percent), and housing (52 percent) than the academic literature. These differences between the two pools of literature may reflect a time trend, meaning the content of these reports has not yet made its way into academic articles, or they may be reflective of truly differential research foci of organizations producing grey literature.

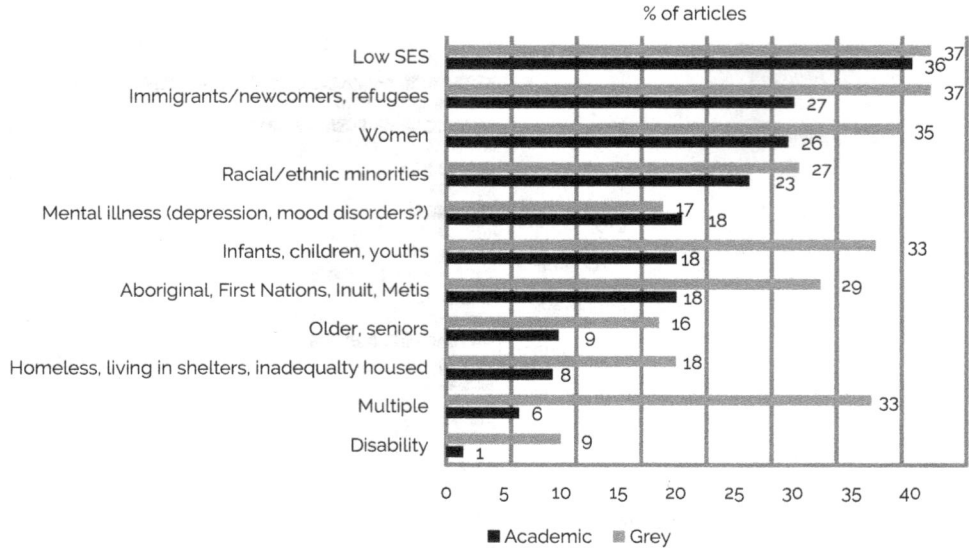

Figure 2.3: Distribution of Subpopulations Experiencing Inequities Studied in Academic (n=232) and Grey (n=306) Literature Ω

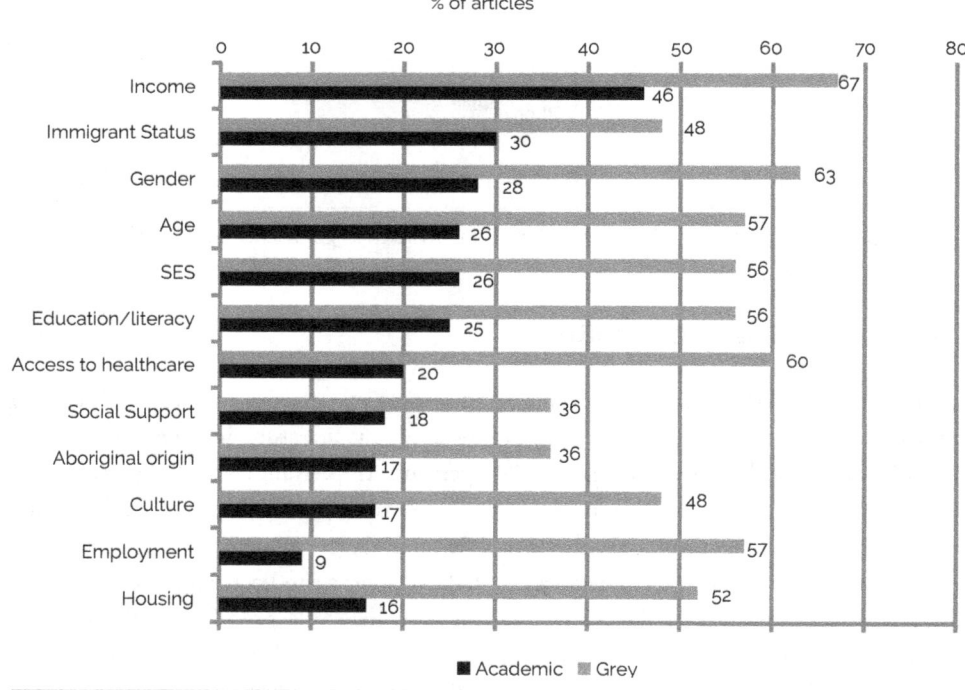

Figure 2.4: Distribution of SDH Studied in Academic (n=232) and Grey (n=306) Literature Ω

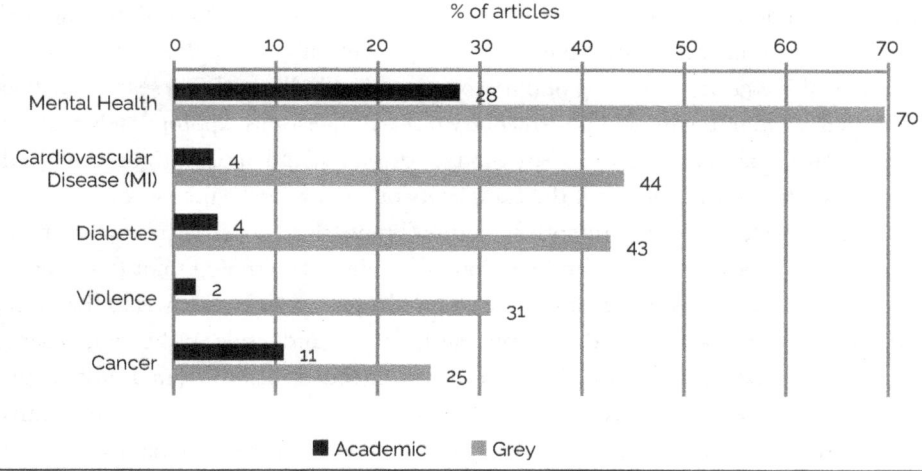

% of articles

Figure 2.5: Distribution of Population Health Outcomes in Academic (n=232) and Grey (n=306) Literature Ω

Population Health Outcomes

Figure 2.5 presents data on the population health outcomes studied in the academic and grey literature. Mental health outcomes is the most frequently studied category in the academic (28 percent) and grey (70 percent) literature. Cancer is the second most studied health issue or outcome that emerged from this review of academic (11 percent) and grey (25 percent) literature. Diabetes (4 percent in academic and 43 percent in grey literature), violence (2 percent in academic and 31 percent in grey literature), and cardiovascular disease (4 percent in academic and 44 percent in grey literature) constitute other frequently studied categories of health outcomes.

DISCUSSION

Our review suggests that both academic and grey literature privilege large urban areas, with far fewer studies undertaken in rural and northern Ontario. This trend indicates the need for a more distributed focus across the province. Much of this pattern could be explained by the location and size of the academic faculties and facilities and by the institutional support and encouragement for collaborative inter-institutional research. Cost, required resources, and population size in many small areas may present barriers to research. Given that different geographic areas in Ontario have unique characteristics and factors contributing to health inequity, further research undertaken in un- and under-researched locations must be encouraged.

Studies grounded in quantitative research paradigms predominate, particularly in the academic literature. Quantitative research was also prevalent in the grey literature, but it included more qualitatively oriented policy-focused studies. Because population health equity is a complex and multi-faceted issue, utilizing only one portion of our methodological toolbox (i.e., quantitative methods) will present only incomplete pictures of the root causes of inequities. Findings of our scoping review indicate that research designed to address a range of population health equity research questions, appropriately matched to quantitative, qualitative, or mixed-methods approaches, and applied rigorously would allow for a better understanding of the complexity of population health issues.

Key subgroups of concern in both literatures emphasized those with low income or SES, but there was also special consideration of immigrants, ethnic minorities, women, and Aboriginal peoples. The grey literature revealed a particular concern as to how social determinants affected access to health care/health services and service utilization, whereas the academic literature addressed the social determinants of health from a broader perspective. Both academic and grey literatures emphasize the overlap among a broad range of the social determinants of health, as well as an emphasis on their interactive or collective impact and influence on the health outcomes of the above-mentioned subpopulations.

Since population health outcomes are not exclusively influenced by a single determinant, but rather result from various determinants affecting and interacting with each other at various levels, the influence of multiple determinants on population health outcomes is important to consider. Individuals' social lives are complex, and dimensions of social life cannot be easily separated into measurable elements. As Simien (2007) argued in reference to women, "diverse life experiences [of] stereotyping, silencing and marginalization do not lend themselves to simple, categorical analysis based solely on gender" (p. 267). From an intersectional perspective, social categories such as ethnicity, gender, geographic location, and so on are dynamic, socially constructed, simultaneous, and mutually different, and work at both micro and macro levels (Weber & Parra-Medina, 2003). Thus, social categories that intersect to create unique social locations for population groups are critical to understand for policy and program development.

Findings of this scoping review resonate with those emerging from other local, national, and international reviews (Marmot, 2010; NCCDH, 2010; Östlin et at., 2009; Public Health Association of Australia, 2009; Standing Senate Committee on Social Affairs, Science and Technology, Subcommittee on Population Health, 2009; Canadian Public Health Association, 2008; World Health Organization Commission on Social Determinants of Health, 2008; Toronto Central LHIN, 2008; MacIntyre, 2007; Wilkinson and Marmot, 2003). As these reviews note, there is a clear need to move beyond a focus on health and illness behaviours. We must address the other determinants of illness, as the majority of the factors that influence health are not related to the health care system (Standing Senate Committee on Social Affairs, Science and Technology, Subcommittee on Population Health, 2009). In light of this, action on health equity requires research and activities across the range of intersecting social determinants of health so as to reduce inequalities in life circumstances (Marmot, 2010; Macintyre, 2007). Although the literature in Ontario, like that of other jurisdictions, tends to focus on the most disadvantaged, focusing on this alone, as Marmot (2010) argues, will not reduce health inequalities sufficiently. At the same time, however, we must recognise the need, as Macintyre (2007) notes, for more intensive support among more socially disadvantaged groups that experience multiple forms of deprivation (Public Health Association of Australia, 2009).

Involving affected populations in the design and conduct of research is becoming increasingly essential (Östlin et al., 2009). In this regard, more emphasis will need to be placed on studies grounded in community-based research approaches that generate local knowledge of diverse lived experiences. This kind of community-based research will help inform and guide policies and service delivery that speak to the needs of local people to enhance health equity at the local level (Toronto Central LHIN, 2008). With the increasing diversity of the Ontario population, further examination and identification of the full range of factors that bear on the health status of these subpopulations is necessary. Future collaborative and interdisciplinary research may provide more comprehensive explanations for the differences in health outcomes among these subpopulations of various geographic locations.

ADDITIONAL RESOURCES

For the complete list of articles included in this scoping review, please visit the following:

- PHIRN Library at http://www.rrasp-phirn.ca/index.php?option=com_content &view=article&id=224&Itemid=66
- PHIRN Scoping Review: Ghosh, H., Donovan, S., Bourgeault, I. L., Packer, C., Estable, A., & Meyer, M. (2011). *Scoping review of the population health equity and intervention literature in Ontario.* É/Exchange Working Paper Series. Available at http://www.rrasp-phirn.ca/images/stories/docs/workingpaperseries/wps_report_ Sep_2011.pdf

GLOSSARY

Academic literature: Peer-reviewed (reviewed by more than one anonymous subject matter expert) publications in scholarly journals, books, and monographs.

Grey literature: Publications in non-peer-reviewed journals, books, and magazines, or on the agency websites produced by organizations including government departments, non-governmental organizations, for-profit organizations, and web-based communities.

Health equity research: Population health equity research is concerned with the unjust and unfair systemic differences that precipitate health inequalities within and between subpopulations occupying unequal social positions.

Intervention research: Intervention research undertakes interdisciplinary methods of inquiry by developing policies and programs to influence upstream determinants that reside within and outside the health care domain in order to reduce inequalities and improve equity in health outcomes at the population level.

Scoping review: Refers to "mapping," a process of summarizing evidences in order to convey the breadth and depth of a field. Scoping reviews differ from systematic reviews as the quality of included studies is usually not assessed. Additionally, scoping reviews differ from narrative or literature reviews because the scoping process requires analytical reinterpretation of the literature.

DISCUSSION QUESTIONS

1. Mental health has been the most frequently studied population health outcome in both academic and grey literature. What are your thoughts on how to address this health issue to reduce health inequities among Ontario populations?
2. How do you think we could address the gaps in our knowledge of population health issues, not only in Ontario but across Canada?
3. Do you think the findings of this chapter would differ if a systematic versus a scoping review methodology were undertaken? How?

NOTE

1. This symbol (Ω) signifies multiple coding. That is, the categories listed are not exclusive: a study may be epidemiological in nature as well as needs assessment, and can also have a policy focus.

REFERENCES

Arksey, H., & O'Malley, L. (2005). Scoping studies: Towards a methodological framework. *International Journal of Social Research Methodology, 8*, 19–32.

Canadian Public Health Association. (2008). *Canadian Public Health Association response to the World Health Organization (WHO) report on the Commission on the Social Determinants of Health.* Retrieved from http://www.rrasp-phirn.ca/index.php?option=com_content&view=article&id=291%3Ascoping-reviewof-Itemid=49&lang=en

Ghosh, H., Donovan, S., Bourgeault, I. L., Packer, C., Estable, A., & Meyer, M. (2011). *Scoping review of the population health equity and intervention literature in Ontario.* É/Exchange Working Paper Series. Retrieved from http://www.rrasp-phirn.ca/images/stories/docs/workingpaperseries/wps_report_Sep_2011.pdf

Macintyre, S. (2007). *Inequalities in health in Scotland: What are they and what can we do about them?* Glasgow: MRC Social & Public Health Sciences Unit.

Marmot, M. (2010). Fair society, healthy lives: A strategic review of health inequalities in England post-2010. *The Marmot Review.* Retrieved from http://www.instituteofhealthequity.org/resources-reports/fair-society-healthy-lives-the-marmot-review

Marmot, M., & Wilkinson, R. (2006). *Social determinants of health* (2nd ed.). Oxford: Oxford University Press.

National Collaborating Centre for Determinants of Health (NCCDH). (2010). *Integrating social determinants of health and health equity into Canadian public health practice: Environmental scan 2010*. Antigonish, NS: National Collaborating Centre for Determinants of Health, St. Francis Xavier University.

Östlin, P., Schrecker, T., Sadana, R., Bonnefoy, J., Gilson, L., Hertzman, C., ... Vaghri, Z. (2009). *Priorities for research on equity and health: Implications for global and national priority setting and the role of WHO to take the health equity research agenda forward*. Retrieved from http://www.globalhealthequity.ca/electronic%20library/Priorities%20for%20research%20on%20equity%20and%20health.pdf

Public Health Association of Australia. (2009). *Health inequities policy*. Retrieved from http://www.phaa.net.au/documents/policy/20091028HealthInequitiesPolicy.pdf

Raphael, D. (2003). When social policy is health policy: Why increasing poverty and low income threatens Canadians' health and health care system. *Canadian Review of Social Policy, 51*, 9–29.

Simien, E. M. (2007). Doing intersectionality research: From conceptual issues to practical examples. *Politics & Gender, 3*(2), 264–271.

Standing Senate Committee on Social Affairs, Science and Technology, Subcommittee on Population Health. (2009). *A healthy productive canada: A determinant of health approach*. Retrieved from http://www.parl.gc.ca/Content/SEN/Committee/402/popu/rep/rephealth1jun09-e.pdf

Toronto Central LHIN. (2008). Environmental scan of research by community-based organizations within the Toronto Central LHIN. Retrieved from http://www.torontocentrallhin.on.ca/uploadedFiles/Home_Page/Report_and_Publications/TCBRNReportfinal.pdf

Weber, L., & Parra-Medina, D. (2003). Intersectionality and women's health: Charting a path to eliminating health disparities. In M. T. Segal & V. Demos, *Gender perspectives on health and medicine: Key themes, advances in gender research* (vol. 7, pp. 18–230). Oxford: Elsevier.

Wilkinson, R., & Marmot, M. (eds.). (2003). *Social determinants of health: The solid facts* (2nd ed.). Copenhagen, Denmark: World Health Organization.

World Health Organization Commission on Social Determinants of Health. (2008). *Closing the gap in a generation: Health equity through action on the social determinants of health*. Final Report of the Commission on Social Determinants of Health. Geneva: World Health Organization.

CHAPTER 3

An Overview of Qualitative Methods and Design: Tools and Resources for Population Health Research

Vivien Runnels, Ivy Lynn Bourgeault, and Danielle Rolfe

TAKE-HOME MESSAGE

- Qualitative research can be used to explore people's experiences and perceptions, the contexts in which they live, work, play, and grow, which are fundamental components of knowledge that can be used to improve population health.
- In choosing qualitative methods, public health practitioners can conduct research that informs their practice and decision making and contributes to improved health among the populations and communities that they serve.

INTRODUCTION

Quantitative research dominates the population health literature in Ontario (see Chapter 2 by Ghosh & Bourgeault, this volume), and public health practitioners seem particularly familiar with quantitative evidence found in epidemiological studies and systematic reviews. These studies may not always explain the life contexts or experiences of people who are members of populations of interest or communities of concern to public health practitioners. Public health practitioners often have important health research questions related to local communities that better lend themselves to more qualitative methodologies. Some health practitioners may have received little to no formal training in qualitative research, and may not be aware that qualitative research can be very useful for developing theory, informing practice, and building knowledge.

Qualitative methods are well suited to some of the research questions that practitioners have; they are particularly effective for engaging community members and useful for helping them explore the knowledge of their own lives and contexts, in turn helping to explain the social patterning of health and illness in contemporary society (Popay & Williams, 1996; Popay, Williams, Thomas, & Gatrell, 1998). As noted by Evans (2002):

> Qualitative research has an important role in evidence-based health care, in that it represents the human dimensions and experiences of the consumers of health care…. It also provides a means of giving consumers a voice in the decision-making process through the documentation of their experiences, preferences, and priorities. (p. 290)

Importantly, qualitative research can help to inform evidence-based practice (Grypdonck, 2006). This chapter provides a brief overview of qualitative research and links to a more in-depth qualitative population health research manual (Runnels, Rolfe, & Bourgeault, 2013).

The chapter comes with an important caveat: we advise researchers and readers that qualitative research is theoretically driven; its data collection and analysis require great care and the findings are often very rich and highly nuanced. What is presented here is a brief introduction and is not sufficient in itself for public health practitioners to carry out rigorous and ethical research. Our hope is that interest is piqued, but enthusiasm be carefully channelled.

Box 3.1: Understanding Context through Local Knowledge

In the following example, listening in the real-world context provided practitioners with local knowledge that could be used to inform interventions that were otherwise failing in the case of diabetes treatments. In an email addressing patient experiences of living in poverty and "non-compliance" with diabetes treatments posted to the Social Determinants of Health listserv (SDH at York University, February 8, 2013), nurse Frances Desjarlais wrote:

> I base our interactions with our population which [are] all First Nation with a focus on "relationships." Part of our assessment was acknowledging to ourselves that the client may not be focused on diabetes at that moment, but was very concerned with having enough money to buy groceries, or to run lunch to the school because they didn't [have] the food to send as lunch earlier in the day, etc.
>
> Just because we were there to do screening—[we] did not solve their everyday issues. Instead we would put down the paper and pen and listened [sic]. We geared ourselves with strategies and resources especially within the community, i.e., special funding for affordable food for those with health conditions, community freezers, community cupboards, etc.… our workplan "sucked"—in other words, we didn't do our job in promoting self-management.

This example shows the complexity of local contexts, and the importance of understanding people's lives within that context. For the nurses, developing relationships and gaining local knowledge of people's lives assisted them to understand the difficulties and barriers that clients/patients experienced and tailor their responses accordingly.

QUALITATIVE AND QUANTITATIVE RESEARCH: WHAT ARE THE DIFFERENCES?

Qualitative and quantitative research studies are embedded in different research paradigms (Veenstra, 1999; Labonte et al., 2005; Bourgeault, Dingwall, & DeVries, 2010). A paradigm is fundamentally a way of knowing about the world (Kuhn, 1962). This "worldview" colours, shapes, and organizes the ways that researchers approach their research. Quantitative research and associated descriptive and statistical analysis are based on certain assumptions about the ways to gather and present data and learnings about the world, often referred to as the positivist paradigm. The researcher's role in this paradigm, for example, is seen as objective, neutral, and non-influential. Quantitative researchers study, measure, and analyze populations. Quantitative analysis of data allows researchers to quantify a problem, describe a distribution of the problem—such as a disease—across whole populations using samples of the same population, and extrapolate and deduce or come directly to conclusions from the findings. Differences or "outliers" are singled out and treated differently in order to generate a picture—to give one example—of a representative or normal distribution of a disease in a population.

Qualitative research examines phenomena in depth to address the questions of "Why?" or "How?", as well as "What?", "Where?", and "When?" Thus, qualitative research is not just "not about numbers." Qualitative research can be descriptive, but it is also theoretical, used to observe and explore phenomena and develop understanding of many realities. Qualitative research investigates the lives and views of people from their perspective, and the contexts in which they live, learn, play, and grow. Some of the research paradigms more closely associated with qualitative research include the interpretive, critical, and constructivist paradigms (see Veenstra, 1999; Guba & Lincoln, 1994). Qualitative data emphasize "people's 'lived experience' [and] are fundamentally well suited for locating the meanings people place on the events, processes and structures of their lives ... and for connecting these meanings to the social world around them" (Miles & Huberman, 1994, p. 10). Qualitative data tend to include differences in participants' perceptions, experiences, and behaviours, rather than excluding them or treating them as outliers.

Despite multiple paradigms associated with qualitative research, and many theoretical approaches, there are a number of commonalities between them. For example, the researcher's roles and contributions are deliberately considered, the researcher's position or stance is publicly declared (referred to as *positionality*), and the researcher thinks carefully about how her or his involvement might affect the research findings (descriptive bias), and how it affects her or him personally (reflexivity and subjectivity). It is said that, in these paradigms, the researcher is the instrument (Lofland, Snow, Anderson, & Lofland, 2006).

As in quantitative research, qualitative research includes a number of steps that are systematically undertaken: problem identification, sampling, data collection, data analysis and data display, writing, reporting, and transferring knowledge (Morse, 1995; Miles & Huberman, 1994). Qualitative research, however, uses the "real world" or natural settings as opposed to controlled settings to collect data. Data are collected directly from people, either a sample of a population or the whole population itself. Collected data are treated and analyzed systematically. Analyzed data are then often repeatedly viewed and interpreted. Although qualitative research processes are often depicted as linear, they are more likely to be iterative, meaning that some parts of the process might be repeated. Collated and analyzed qualitative data are then assessed for "fit"—meaning how well the findings and theory generated from the findings fit within the specific context for the population under study.

Box 3.2: General Resources for Qualitative Research

Bourgeault, I., Dingwall, R., de Vries, R. (eds.). (2010). *The Sage handbook of qualitative methods in health research*. London: Sage Publications.

Denzin, N. K., & Lincoln, Y. S. (2008). *The landscape of qualitative research* (3rd ed.). Thousand Oaks, CA: Sage.

Flick, U., von Kardorff, E., & Steinke, I. (2004). *A companion to qualitative research*. London: Sage Publications.

Oakes, J. M., & Kaufman, J. S. (eds.). (2006). *Methods in social epidemiology* (pp. 239–266). San Francisco: Jossey-Bass.

Sandelowski, M., & Barroso, J. (2007). *Handbook for synthesizing qualitative research*. New York: Springer Publishing Company.

QUALITATIVE RESEARCH APPROACHES

Qualitative research approaches—in other words, the methods and tools suitable for these approaches—include (but are not limited to): grounded theory, ethnography, phenomenology, biography, and case study. By way of introduction to qualitative research approaches, we highlight two commonly used approaches in health research: grounded theory and case study. We also include a brief section on community-based research, which is a very common approach to research in public and population health studies. Community-based research can employ a variety of data collection methods and analytic approaches, such as grounded theory, case study, and phenomenology.

Grounded Theory

Grounded theory provides tools for data collection, data analysis, and synthesis (Morse et al., 2009). It uses the organization of the data themselves and constant comparison and analysis as methods of creating theory. Constant comparison or constant comparative method or analysis means that the researcher compares incidents to others that are similarly coded. She or he notes differences or similarities, relating them to each other (or not) (Dye, Schatz,

Rosenberg, & Coleman, 2000; Gasson, 2003; Locke & Golden-Biddle, 1997). Greenhalgh (2006) describes the constant comparative method as follows: "Each new piece of data is compared with the emerging summary of all the previous items, allowing step-by-step refinement of an emerging theory" (p. 174). Grounded theory does not emerge from the data, but through the interaction with the data and interpretation of the data by the analyst. It is in this way that the theory is inductive, grounded in the data, rather than deductive.

Box 3.3: A Key Resource on Grounded Theory

Charmaz, K. (2009). Shifting the grounds: Constructivist grounded theory methods. In J. M. Morse, P. Noerager Stern, J. Corbin, B. Bowers, K. Charmaz, & A. E. Clarke (eds.), *Developing grounded theory: The second generation* (pp. 127–154). Walnut Creek, CA: Left Coast Press Inc.

Case Study

Case study research focuses on a specific case, which could be a program or policy or group. According to Denzin (2001), a case study has depth, in contrast to the breadth of a grounded-theory-oriented study. As Stake (1994) notes, "Case study is defined by individual cases, not by the methods of inquiry used" (p. 236). Case study emphasizes relationships and processes instead of results and products, and offers a general, qualitative, and systematic way of looking at a specific phenomenon. Case study uses different methods for data collection. Commonly used qualitative research methods for conducting case studies include interviews, observation (which can involve participation), and the collection of artifacts and texts such as institutional documents and meeting minutes. It is also possible to collect descriptive quantitative data for a case study.

Box 3.4: Key Resources on Case Study

Stake, R. E. (1994). Case studies. In N. K. Denzin & Y. S. Lincoln (eds.), *Handbook of qualitative research* (pp. 236–247). Thousand Oaks, CA: Sage Publications.

Stake, R. E. (1995). *The art of case study research.* Thousand Oaks, CA: Sage Publications.

Yin, R. K. (1989). *Case study research: Design and methods* (2nd ed.). Newbury Park, CA: Sage Publications.

Community-Based Research

Community-based research is rarely presented in the literature as a specific research method, but rather as an approach or orientation to research (Minkler & Wallerstein,

2008). In the health domain, community-based research is largely taken as an intentional approach to research, having an end goal of addressing health inequalities and improving the health of communities, using the knowledge of community participants (Lantz, Israel, Schulz, & Reyes, 2006; Wallerstein & Duran, 2006). In light of this, community-based research has been defined as:

> A collaborative approach to research that engages partners from a community—geographic or otherwise defined—in all phases of the research process, with a shared goal of producing knowledge that will be translated into action or positive change for the community. (Lantz et al., 2006, p. 239)

> Research conducted in partnership between civil society groups and academics. It seeks to democratize knowledge creation by validating multiple sources of knowledge and promoting the use of multiple methods of discovery and dissemination. The goal of participatory research is social innovation and action. (Gall, Millot, & Neubauer, 2009, p. 23)

The significant and intentional orientation of community-based research towards the needs of community members have led Israel et al. (2003) to develop a set of principles designed to define and guide its conduct (see Box 3.5 below). The use of the term *participatory* denotes the active engagement of community members in the research.

Box 3.5: Summary of Israel et al.'s (2003) Principles of Community-Based Participatory Research

- Recognizes community as a unit of identity (p. 55)
- Builds on strengths and resources within the community (pp. 55–56)
- Facilitates a collaborative, equitable partnership in all phases of the research, involving an empowering and power-sharing process that attends to social inequalities (p. 56)
- Promotes co-learning and capacity-building among all partners (p. 56)
- Integrates and achieves a balance between research and action for the mutual benefit of all partners (pp. 56–57)
- Emphasizes local relevance of public health problems and ecological perspectives that recognize and attend to the multiple determinants of health and disease (p. 57)
- Involves systems development through a cyclical and iterative process (p. 57)
- Disseminates findings and knowledge gained to all partners and involves all partners in the dissemination process (p. 57)
- Involves a long-term process and commitment (p. 58)

Box 3.6: Key Resources on Community-Based Research

Israel, B. A., Eng, E., Schulz, A. J., & Parker, E. A. (2005). *Methods in community-based participatory research for health.* San Francisco, CA: Jossey-Bass.

Lutz, J., & Neis, B. (eds.). (2008). *Making and moving knowledge: Interdisciplinary and community-based research in a world on the edge.* Montreal and Kingston: McGill-Queen's University Press.

Minkler, M. (ed.). (2004). *Community organizing and community building for health* (2nd ed.). New Brunswick, NJ: Rutgers University Press.

Reid, C., Brief, E., & LeDrew, R. (2009). *Our common ground: Cultivating women's health through community based research. A primer.* Vancouver: Women's Health Research Network. Retrieved from http://www.bccewh.bc.ca/publications-resources/documents/OurCommonGroundcultivatingwomenshealththroughcommunitybasedresearch.pdf

---

A note on mixing quantitative and qualitative research data: Qualitative data may be used to complement quantitative data and vice versa, but the different paradigms and the different assumptions that underlie quantitative and qualitative research mean data may be neither interpreted nor displayed similarly. Caution is required when researchers combine different types of data.

COLLECTING QUALITATIVE DATA

Qualitative researchers typically rely on a number of methods for gathering data, including observation, the conduct of individual or group interviews, and the analysis of documents or other archival materials. In all cases, the collection of qualitative data needs to be systematic but flexible to best respond to the given circumstances. For example, individual or group interviews are typically guided by a semi-structured set of questions (i.e., an interview guide). The structured questions ensure that key topics are addressed, but the interview is also open to the inclusion of questions that arise from the interview process itself. As more and more interviews are conducted, these emergent questions can be included as structured questions in later interviews. As well as being one example of where the researcher as instrument plays a role in plumbing the depths of an informant's knowledge, this approach demonstrates the flexibility and adaptability of qualitative research designs.

In some cases, audio or visual materials are created through the research process, or are used to elicit responses. Photovoice is a participatory approach in which participants take photographs that represent or influence their experiences. These could be photographs of their environment and how they perceive it influencing their health. The photographs are then annotated, or given voice, with words, phrases, or stories that provide explanations of what is happening in the photograph. In other cases, a set of photographs or video segments can be used to spark a group discussion or responses from an individual participant in an interview.

However qualitative data are collected, what is collected needs to be organized for systematic analysis. Interviews are often transcribed, and photos or documents digitized. Qualitative data software is used not only for the systematic management of data, but also to aid in the process of analysis.

Computer-aided qualitative data analysis is available widely through different softwares (e.g., Quirkos; NVivo; ATLAS.ti; MAXQDA; QDA Miner; Dedoose; HyperRESEARCH). "Computer-aided" means that the software helps the analyst, but it is critical to note that qualitative data analysis software does not do the thinking behind the performance of the analysis.

ANALYZING QUALITATIVE DATA

The process of analyzing qualitative research, like other topics related to qualitative research, takes time to master. It is also important to stress the iterative nature of qualitative analysis that co-occurs with data collection. The "how-to" of qualitative data analysis also depends on the qualitative research approach being taken. One of the most typical approaches is content analysis, whereby the researcher examines a group of qualitative data—such as a transcribed interview or a section of a written document—and highlights the key themes that reflect the content of the excerpt. The constant comparative approach described above for grounded theory involves reducing the data in a similar manner to content analysis: identifying the key themes in the data, integrating these codes into larger categories, and refining the relationship between themes into a grounded theory. There are several books and articles that can assist in qualitative data analysis.

Box 3.7: Key Resources on Qualitative Data Analysis

Bernard, G. R., & Ryan, G. W. (2009) *Analyzing qualitative data: Systematic approaches.* Thousand Oaks, CA: Sage Publications.

Corbin, J., & Strauss, A. (2015). *Basics of qualitative research: Techniques and procedures for developing grounded theory* (4th ed.). Thousand Oaks, CA: Sage Publications.

Saldana, J. (2013). *The coding manual for qualitative researchers* (2nd ed.) Los Angeles: SAGE.

Spiggle, S. (1994). Analysis and interpretation of qualitative data in consumer research. *Journal of Consumer Research, 21*, 491–503. Retrieved from https://noppa.aalto.fi/noppa/kurssi/23e88001/harjoitustyot/23E88001_spiggle_1994.pdf

ISSUES OF QUALITY IN THE CONDUCT OF QUALITATIVE RESEARCH

Because qualitative research is set in different research paradigms from quantitative research, terminologies used for quantitative research are not transferable to qualitative research. Rigour is defined as "the checks and balances built into qualitative research to ensure that it is credible, trustworthy and transferable" (Sandelowski, 1986). To avoid confusion, it is preferable not to use quantitative methods' terminology for qualitative research.

Generalizability versus Transferability

Qualitative research approaches (strictly speaking, those that are based in the interpretive/ constructivist research paradigm) are not intended to be generalizable (i.e., applying research findings derived from a study sample to an entire population). Sandelowski (1986) explains, "From the qualitative perspective, generalizability is based on the reification of a context-free structure that does not exist and the assumption that the multiple realities in any given situation can be controlled to illuminate the effects of a few variables" (p. 31). As generalizability is for quantitative research, transferability, a form of external validity meaning that research findings have applicability in other contexts, is for qualitative research (Lincoln & Guba, 1985).

Validity

Validity in qualitative research is challenging because it incorporates rigour as well as subjectivity and creativity into the scientific process (Whittemore, Chase, & Mandle, 2001, p. 522). Concepts of external validity appropriate for quantitative research are not applicable to qualitative research because "[qualitative research] emphasizes the study of phenomena in their natural settings and with few controlling conditions" (Sandelowski, 1986, p. 31).

Other terms used in qualitative research include *dependability*, which is a form of reliability; *confirmability*, which refers to the extent to which the results can be confirmed by others; and *credibility*, a type of internal validity. *Verification* refers to methods for testing interpretations for plausibility, "sturdiness," or confirmability. Other terms include *authenticity*, *criticality*, and *integrity* (Whittemore et al., 2001).

As public health professionals or population health researchers engage in qualitative research to inform or guide their work, certain practices can be easily implemented to help ensure quality. For example, member checking and triangulation of data help to establish credibility; rich or "thick" description helps to establish transferability— that is, providing sufficient detailed description of the context in which the research was conducted to enable the findings to be useful to others facing similar situations in similar contexts. Member checking, or asking a subset of participants whether the findings from the research aptly reflect their experience, will also help to ensure that findings are credible and grounded in the experiences of the participants.

Box 3.8: Key Resources for Understanding Quality and Rigour in Qualitative Research

Caelli, K., Ray, L., & Mill, J. (2003). "Clear as mud": Toward greater clarity in generic qualitative research. *International Journal of Qualitative Methods*, *2*, 1–24. Retrieved from https://ejournals.library.ualberta.ca/index.php/IJQM/article/viewArticle/4521

Graneheim, U. H., & Lundman, B. (2004). Qualitative content analysis in nursing research: Concepts, procedures and measures to achieve trustworthiness. *Nurse Education Today*, *24*, 105–112.

Tracy, S. J. (2010). Qualitative quality: Eight "big-tent" criteria for excellent qualitative research. *Qualitative Inquiry*, *16*, 837–851. Retrieved from http://chelt.anu.edu.au/sites/default/files/hero/Qualitative%20Inquiry-2010-Tracy-837-51.pdf

Trochim, W. (2006). *Qualitative validity*. Research Methods Knowledge Base. Retrieved from http://www.socialresearchmethods.net/kb/qualval.php

Whittemore, R., Chase, S. K., & Mandle, C. L. (2001). Validity in qualitative research. *Qualitative Health Research*, *11*, 522–537.

ETHICAL, INCLUSIVE, AND EQUITABLE QUALITATIVE HEALTH RESEARCH

Inclusive and equitable qualitative health research sets out to ensure that research does not exclude those that should be included. To give one historical example, women and girls were often excluded from much clinical research, and adult males were assumed to be the standard. Nowadays, researchers know that excluding women and girls means that research findings cannot be applied to them. Other forms of social categorization, including sex, gender (see Canadian Institutes of Health Research [CIHR], 2016), racial and ethnic origins, disability, and sexuality, should also be considered to ensure that qualitative research is conducted inclusively, ethically, and equitably.

Box 3.9: The Tri-Council Policy Statement

In Canada, the Tri-Council Policy Statement: Ethical Conduct for Research Involving Humans (or the TCPS 2) is the official human research ethics policy of Canada's publicly funded research agencies (Canadian Institutes of Health Research, the Social Sciences and Humanities Research Council, and the Natural Science and Engineering Research Council of Canada). The policy statement is not only helpful for its ethical guidelines, but it also has chapters that guide research involving First Nations, Métis, and Inuit peoples of Canada (Canadian Institutes of Health Research, Natural Sciences and Engineering Research Council of Canada, and Social Sciences and Humanities Research Council of Canada, 2014).

Box 3.10: A Research Model for Participation in Research and Governance of Research

Models that incorporate a range of participation by non-specialists in research, such as members of the public, include Callon's Model 3, which "actively involve[s] lay people in the creation of knowledge concerning them" (Callon, 1999, p. 89). In this model, research participation is collaborative and interactive, and members participate on an equal footing (Callon, 1999). Community members' involvement or participation in the governance of community-based research has had less attention in the literature, but is becoming more of a topic of study in its own right, and is something that researchers need to consider carefully (Runnels & Andrew, 2013).

COLLABORATIVE RESEARCH

To ensure that qualitative research is rigorous, ethical, and relevant, collaboration with members of the public, community organizations, and university and college researchers is recommended. Indeed, there is an increasing trend for applied health research to have "knowledge users" involved from the outset. Collaboration in research includes participation in decision making and governance of the research. This may be referred to as *community-based research* or *collaborative research*, but note that not all collaborative research is necessarily community-based research, and vice versa.

CONCLUSION

People's experiences and perceptions, the contexts in which they live, work, play, and grow, are fundamental components of knowledge that can be used to improve population health and public health interventions. Qualitative research can be used to explore these issues. With training and practice in qualitative research, public health practitioners are well positioned to conduct research that can inform their practice and decision making and contribute to improved health among the populations and communities that they serve.

GLOSSARY

Constructivist paradigm: A paradigm that emphasizes the subjective position of the researcher; their values and assumptions are an intricate part of their research process instead of them being objective observers. Meaning emerges from the relationships between the researcher and the participant (Guba & Lincoln, 1994).

Descriptive bias: How a researcher's involvement might affect the research findings.

"Fit" assessment: How well the findings and theory generated from the findings fit within the specific context for the population under study.

Grounded theory: A theory that provides tools for data collection, data analysis, and synthesis where theory emerges inductively from the data, through interaction between the data and its interpretation by the analyst.

Iterative: This signifies a process in which steps are repeated.

Paradigm: A way of knowing about the world (Kuhn, 1962).

Photovoice: A participatory approach whereby participants take photographs of associations and influences on their experiences.

Positionality: The researcher's position or stance, which is publicly declared.

Positivist paradigm: In this paradigm, reality is considered to be objectively measurable and the researcher's role to be objective, neutral, and non-influential.

Reflexivity/subjectivity: These terms refer to how a researcher's involvement affects her or him personally.

Rigour: Checks and balances built into qualitative research to ensure that it is credible, trustworthy, and transferable (Sandelowski, 1986).

Transferability: A form of external validity in which research findings have applicability in other contexts (Lincoln & Guba, 1985).

DISCUSSION QUESTIONS

1. Why would health practitioners favour qualitative methods over quantitative methods in research related to public health issues?
2. What is meant by "the researcher is the instrument" in qualitative methods?
3. How can both qualitative and quantitative methods be used in the research process without compromising the quality of the research?

REFERENCES

Bourgeault, I. L., Dingwall, R., & DeVries, R. (eds.) (2010). *Handbook of qualitative health research.* London: Sage.

Callon, M. (1999). The role of lay people in the production and dissemination of scientific knowledge. *Science, Technology and Society, 4,* 81–94.

Canadian Institutes of Health Research (CIHR). (2016). *Sex, gender and health research guide: A tool for CIHR applicants.* Retrieved from http://www.cihr-irsc.gc.ca/e/32019.html

Canadian Institutes of Health Research, Natural Sciences and Engineering Research Council of Canada, and Social Sciences and Humanities Research Council of Canada. (2014). *Tri-council policy statement: Ethical conduct for research involving humans.* Retrieved from http://www.pre.ethics.gc.ca/pdf/eng/tcps2-2014/TCPS_2_FINAL_Web.pdf

Denzin, N. K. (2001). *Interpretive interactionism* (2nd ed.). Thousand Oaks, CA: Sage Publications.

Dye, J. F., Schatz, I. M., Rosenberg, B. A., & Coleman, S. T. (2000). Constant comparison method: A kaleidoscope of data. *The Qualitative Report* (online serial), *4.* Retrieved from http://www.nova.edu/ssss/QR/QR3-4/dye.html

Evans, D. (2002, July). Database searches for qualitative research. *Journal of the Medical Library Association, 90*(3), 290–293. Retrieved from http://www.ncbi.nlm.nih.gov/pmc/articles/PMC116400/

Gall, É., Millot, G., & Neubauer, C. (2009). *Participation of civil society organisations in research.* Science, Technology and Civil Society project (STACS). Paris: Fondation Sciences Citoyennes.

Gasson, S. (2003). Rigor in grounded theory research: An interpretive perspective on generating theory from qualitative field studies. In M. Whitman & A. Woszczynski (eds.), *Handbook for information systems research* (pp. 79–102). Hershey, PA: Idea Group Publishing.

Greenhalgh, T. (2006). *How to read a paper: The basics of evidence-based medicine* (3rd ed.). Oxford: Blackwell Publishing Limited.

Grypdonck, M. H. F. (2006). Qualitative health research in the era of evidence-based practice. *Qualitative Health Research, 16,* 1371–1385.

Guba, E., & Lincoln, Y. (1994). Competing paradigms in qualitative research. In N. K. Denzin & Y. S. Lincoln (eds.), *Handbook of qualitative research* (pp. 105–117). Thousand Oaks, CA: Sage Publications.

Israel, B. A., Schulz, A. J., Parker, E. A., Becker, A. B., Allen III, A. J., & Guzman, J. R. (2003). Critical issues in developing and following community-based participatory research principles. In M. Minkler & N. Wallerstein (eds.), *Community-based participatory research for health* (pp. 53–76). San Francisco: Jossey-Bass.

Kuhn, T. S. (1962). The structure of scientific revolutions. *International Encyclopedia of Unified Science,* II.

Labonte R., Polanyi, M., Muhajarine, N., McIntosh, T., & Williams, A. (2005). Beyond the divides: Towards critical population health research. *Critical Public Health, 15,* 5–17.

Lantz, P. M., Israel, B. A., Schulz, A. J., & Reyes, A. (2006). Community-based participatory research: Rationale and relevance for social epidemiology. In J. M. Oakes & J. S. Kaufman (eds.), *Methods in social epidemiology* (pp. 239–266). San Francisco: Jossey-Bass.

Lincoln, Y. S., & Guba, E. G. (1985). *Naturalistic inquiry.* Newbury Park, CA: Sage Publications.

Locke, K., & Golden-Biddle, K. (1997). Constructing opportunities for contribution: Structuring intertextual coherence and "problematizing" in organizational studies. *The Academy of Management Journal, 40,* 1023–1062.

Lofland, J., Snow, D., Anderson, L., & Lofland, L. (2006). *Analyzing social settings: A guide to qualitative observation and analysis* (4th ed.). Boston: Wadsworth.

Miles, M. B., & Huberman, A. M. (1994). *Qualitative data analysis: An expanded sourcebook.* Thousand Oaks, CA: SAGE Publications, Inc.

Minkler, M., & Wallerstein, N. (2008). *Community-based participatory research for health: From process to outcomes* (2nd ed.). San Francisco: Jossey-Bass.

Morse, J. (1995). The significance of saturation. *Qualitative Health Research, 5,* 147–149.

Morse, J. M., Noerager Stern, P., Corbin, J., Bowers, B., Charmaz, K., & Clarke, A. E. (2009). *Developing grounded theory: The second generation.* Walnut Creek, CA: Left Coast Press Inc.

Popay, J., & Williams, G. (1996). Public health research and lay knowledge. *Social Science & Medicine, 42,* 759–768.

Popay, J., Williams, G., Thomas, C., & Gatrell, T. (1998). Theorizing inequalities in health: The place of lay knowledge. *Sociology of Health & Illness, 20*, 619–644.

Runnels, V., & Andrew, C. (2013). Community-based research decision-making: Experiences and factors affecting participation. *Gateways: International Journal of Community Research and Engagement, 6*(1), 22–37.

Runnels, V., Rolfe, D., & Bourgeault, I. (2013). *Resource manual on qualitative research.* Ottawa: Institute of Population Health: Population Health Improvement Research Network. Retrieved from http://www.rrasp-phirn.ca/images/stories/Resource_Manual_on_Qualitative_Research.pdf

Sandelowski, M. (1986). The problem of rigor in qualitative research. *Advances in Nursing Science, 8*(3), 27–27.

Stake, R. E. (1994). Case studies. In N. K. Denzin & Y. S. Lincoln (eds.), *Handbook of qualitative research* (pp. 236–247). Thousand Oaks, CA: Sage Publications.

Veenstra, G. (1999). Different wor(l)ds: Three approaches to health research. *Canadian Journal of Public Health, 90*, S18–S21.

Wallerstein, N., & Duran, B. (2006). Using community-based participatory research to address health disparities. *Health Promotion Practice, 7*, 313–323.

Whittemore, R., Chase, S. K., & Mandle, C. L. (2001). Validity in qualitative research. *Qualitative Health Research, 11*, 522–537.

CHAPTER 4

Giving Voice: Practical Approaches to Qualitative Multilingual Health Research

Mechthild Meyer and Alma Estable

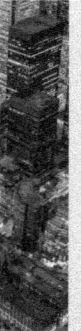

TAKE-HOME MESSAGE

- Researchers need to think about the language of participants when planning, designing, and analyzing their study, particularly in a multilingual country like Canada.
- Qualitative health researchers need to carefully weigh the benefits and challenges of working across languages and ensure sufficient resources to capture the diverse experiences of minority language populations, their varied situations, and unique experiences.

INTRODUCTION

Few researchers think about the language of participants when planning, designing, or analyzing their study, unless they are asking questions that can be answered only by people who speak a language they don't share. And yet, many Canadian residents' mother tongue is neither English nor French. Rather, their first language may be an Aboriginal language or one of the many immigrant languages. Some residents do not speak English or French at all, while many use their first language not only at home but also at work. In the Canadian context, it is essential to consider language in qualitative health research, given the linguistic diversity of the Canadian population, and the legal and ethical commitment to provide equitable health access to all (Bowen, Gibbens, Roy, & Edwards, 2010; Pottie et al., 2008).

Why Is This an Issue?

Linguistic minority populations may have a different perspective or lived experience than members of dominant language groups that could provide important insights into health issues. If there are experiences that are unique to specific populations that speak non-dominant languages, these questions are best answered by those populations in their own languages.

Members of these populations may be more confident and comfortable describing their thoughts, feelings, and experiences in their first language, and may be able to do so in greater depth and with their own cultural nuances. This may be particularly the case if they are talking about the personal, intimate, complex, stressful, or painful experiences that are sometimes investigated through qualitative research (Wallin & Ahlström, 2006).

This chapter provides practical suggestions (based on our experiences and those of others) for qualitative health researchers who are considering developing multilingual tools and collecting multilingual data. What follows is a step-by-step guide to incorporating a cross-language dimension in qualitative health research, from choosing a multilingual design to reporting.

Should You Embark on a Multilingual Health Research Project?

Qualitative health researchers should carefully weigh the benefits and challenges of working across languages, given the resources required to do it with sufficient rigour. With limited resources, you may be unable to capture the diverse experiences of minority language populations, their varied situations, and unique experiences.

Any type of qualitative research across languages will require translation at some point in the study process. Once you decide on multilingual research, think about when the "language crossing" should occur (e.g., at the point of tool development, transcription, data analysis, or findings; see Figure 4.1).

In part, this may be influenced by your overall research approach. In projects with participatory methodologies, translation back and forth may be an ongoing process during all research phases. For other research designs, there are many considerations that will guide decisions about when it is most effective, economical, opportune, or aligned with the desired research outcomes to "cross the language bridge." From a very practical perspective, the choice of methods depends on the language skills of the research team and the investigators that conceptualize and carry out the research (see also van Nes, Abma, Jonsson & Deeg, 2010).

Whatever your choice (unilingual or multilingual), explain your decision. If you choose a unilingual project, communicate the limitations of health research conducted in only one language. Make your reasons clear, as you would when research involves only one gender, for example. Noting the limitations to transferability may highlight the need to adequately resource cross-language research on that topic. You may recommend conducting follow-up research with minority language groups.

FINDING, REVIEWING, AND USING MULTILINGUAL LITERATURE

Languages in their cultural contexts create unique conceptual maps, which give rise to diverse representations of experience, human relations, and world views (Moser, 2000;

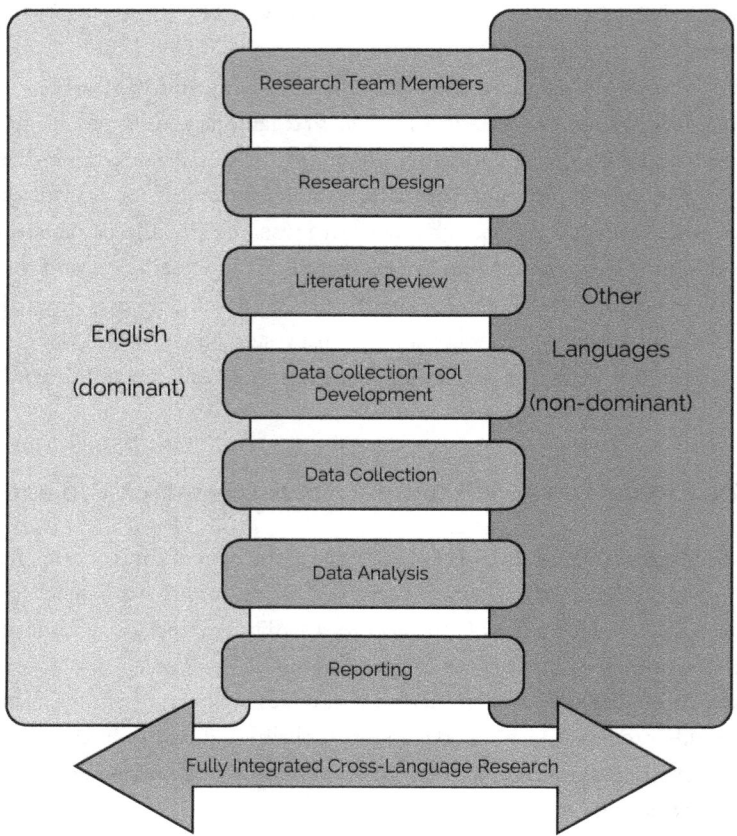

Figure 4.1: When to Cross the Language Bridge

Source: Authors

Schmitt, 2005)—all important considerations when reviewing literature for qualitative research. A multilingual literature search process to access published knowledge created by
others who work in the minority language can take into account health-related concepts,
theories, or terms arising from research conducted in the target language.

Reviewing fundamental concepts at an early stage can also help you work around
ideas and terms that may not be understood in a different context, even if translated accurately. This can save time and avoid costly misunderstandings later on.

Expand the Search

Make use of the linguistic capacity of your research team to identify publications in minority languages that may open doors to evidence otherwise not available.

Table 4.1: Decision-Making Tree: When Do We Cross Languages?

RESEARCH STAGE	CHOICES FOR BILINGUAL RE-SEARCHERS	CHOICES FOR UNILINGUAL RESEARCHERS
	When do we cross languages? (internal and external)	When do we cross languages? (external)
Research Questions, Conceptual Frameworks	1. Internal language crossing (translating yourself) 2. External if working with others	1. Develop unilingual framework 2. Cross to other researchers and/or validate with target language population
Tool Development	1. Develop new tool in target language 2. Translate existing tool Consider: Being bilingual is insufficient for translation of tools; it must involve others to increase reliability	1. Translate data collection tools: translation, back translation, and pilot 2. Cross to other language through interpreters
	Test data collection tools with target group	
Recruitment, Sampling, Consents	1. Self or other bilinguals 2. Use unilingual researchers and translator • Requires development of recruitment material and consent in target language • Direct recruitment by bilingual researcher not necessarily the only or best way (possible coercion)	1. Assess degree of source language/target language fluency of population sought 2. Interpretation is required if participants are unilingual in target language • Requires translation of recruitment materials and consents (see above: translate, back translate, and pilot)
	Consider: Language is not the same as community or culture • Develop sampling frame for language(s) (i.e., number of participants using target language versus dominant language)	
Data Collection	1. Self 2. Self and/or other bilinguals 3. Self and/or other unilinguals (source language or target language): cross languages externally	1. Self and interpreter 2. Self and bilingual research assistant 3. Bilingual research assistant • If participants are unilingual, need to cross languages externally
	Consider: Type of data collection (verbal or observational data)	

Seek Out Translated Documents

Consult international sources (e.g., WHO, European Research Council) for key documents published in several languages, and identify key terms, frameworks, summaries, and citations that could be used to compare and verify how terms are translated by others.

Identify journals (e.g., *Canadian Medical Association Journal*, *Canadian Journal of Program Evaluation*, *Forum: Qualitative Social Research*) that translate articles or abstracts into several languages.

Translate

Translate abstracts (less costly than entire articles) to identify concepts and terminology in target languages.

Consult and Review

Finally, consult with minority language speakers (including colleagues or students with minority language mother tongues). They may be able to tell you if a particular phrase, concept, or metaphor is easily understood and has a similar meaning in their language, or alert you to other ways of addressing the issues that may yield useful material as you search the literature.

DEVELOPING MULTILINGUAL TOOLS TO COLLECT DATA (INTERVIEWS, CONSULTATIONS, FOCUS GROUPS)

A great challenge in any cross-language data collection is ensuring that the same meaning is attributed to questions that are asked in different languages. Translation and independent back translation are recommended for quantitative interview tools, but seldom mentioned as a practice for the development of qualitative interviews (Chen & Boore, 2009). Since qualitative schedules often permit greater flexibility in wording and order, it can be challenging to translate these adequately ahead of time. Interviewers may vary questions to ensure understanding. They may use probes to elicit detail or depth, or spontaneously ask supplementary questions to follow emerging information.

In practice, we have found that tool translation often occurs ad hoc in the data collection process. For example, a participant displays less language knowledge than anticipated, so a community interpreter is brought in to translate questions. In other cases, a bilingual interviewer may switch to the other language to make sure the informant really understands the question, or may spontaneously include terms when speaking with a participant. In these cases, there is less opportunity to carefully consider the wording of the questions ahead of time, or to select among different ways of phrasing equivalent meanings (see, for example, Meyer, Estable, MacLean, & Peterson, 2010).

Option 1: Adapt or Work with Existing Target Language Tools

Identify instruments that have been validated in the other language as a starting point, but ensure that they suit the Canadian context, considering regional variations in language use, and differences in terminology that reflect health system variations across countries.

Pilot the adapted tools with assistance from translators, interpreters, or target language speakers. Although this step can be time-consuming and requires resources, it ensures maximum consistency in tools across languages (Arriaza, Nedjat-Haiem, Lee, & Martin, 2015; Estable, Meyer, & MacLean, 2004).

Option 2: Develop Tools in the Minority Target Language

You might consider this option for empowerment-focused or participatory research. Developing tools in a minority language can enhance empowerment, as there is shared control about how an issue is going to be explored with those who speak that language. Existing knowledge from community members thus enters the research at the tool development stage. By developing tools in the target language, you may find it easier to incorporate conceptual maps and communication patterns that are inherent to that language, rather than trying to make the translated tools "fit" the dominant language communication patterns and conceptual maps (Sidhu et al., 2016)

Work with the target language population
Although this approach is used less frequently, it offers the possibility of working more closely with members of the target language population. Together you can explore how they might understand the issue being researched, how they would approach the topic, and what concepts are commonly used when speaking of it.

Validate and pilot
Take into account validation and ways to ensure conceptual equivalence, if developing new tools.

Decide ahead of time when you will cross back to the dominant language
Remember you will have to "return" to the source (dominant) language(s). If you develop tools in the target language, you need to consider when and how you will cross back to the dominant languages and plan accordingly. This also includes deciding ahead of time whether data collected with multilingual tools will be analyzed in the source languages or the target languages, and how findings will be shared and back-translated with participants (see also Santos, Black, & Sandelowski, 2015).

Option 3: Translate Dominant Language Tools into Target Language

Translate tools prior to data collection, even if you plan to involve interpreters. At a minimum, ensure interpreters have the interview schedule ahead of time, and ask them to provide a translation of questions, to avoid ad hoc interpretation. This will give the interpreter the opportunity to review any terms with which they are not familiar, or which may have ambiguous meanings. If you cannot translate the entire tool, providing the interpreter with a list of key terms, and those terms' translations, also helps avoid interpretation errors, especially if you will be using a very open interview style, with supplementary spontaneous questions or probes.

Control Quality of Translation

If tools are to be translated, plan how to assess the skills of translators in both languages; how you will know that translations are accurate and comparable in style and tone; and how translated tools will be modified after piloting.

Involve translators as part of the research team

In multilingual research projects, translators can become an important part of the research team. As well as translating an interview guide, they can participate in the piloting of the translated guide. Many future misunderstandings can be avoided at this stage by asking translators to listen to pilot or early interview recordings and reflect on the type of responses that are being generated. Translators should also be involved in the revisions of any tools after piloting to ensure that the revisions work.

Provide translators with in-depth knowledge about research context and objectives. This will help translators use the appropriate vocabulary and style of language, and may help them select among different expressions; translate jargon, technical terms, and metaphorical language more accurately; and use appropriate probes to pick up nuances and get to a deeper level with questions asked (van Nes, Abma, Jonsson, & Deeg, 2010).

Develop a translation lexicon

A translation lexicon, evolving with the research process and in analysis, can also contribute to conceptual equivalence at the analysis stage (Squires, 2009).

Use qualified and skilled mother-tongue speakers for translation and back translation. It is ideal to have translations validated by a qualified bilingual individual not directly involved with data collection or the initial translation.

Be clear about the aim of the translation: conceptual equivalence or word-for-word translation. In general, we suggest that translators emphasize the interpretation of meaning (conceptual equivalence) over word-for-word translations that preserve form. In some cases, however, you may want to have the translator provide both types of translation for selected passages (for example, if you are using metaphor analysis). Communicate your preference to the translator, and discuss what may be gained or lost with each approach.

Match the style and level of formality in the translation to the intent of the original. Regional expressions, gender, age, and many other factors are associated with usage within any single language. We generally aim for a neutral tone in translated content, but this depends on the purpose of the research and on the target population.

ANALYZING DATA

As with any qualitative research, the qualitative analyst is the most important research tool in multilingual projects (Denzin & Lincoln, 2005). A number of different approaches to cross-language analysis are possible. Your choice will be influenced by the language capacity of the analysts. Each option has advantages and disadvantages (see also Fersch, 2013):

- *Data analysis in dominant language only.* This option is used when all data records are created in the dominant language or if all data are translated into the dominant language prior to analysis.
- *Data analysis primarily in dominant language; transcripts remain in original language, with only quotes translated.* This approach requires one or more analysts able to understand both the dominant and the minority language. The analysis will mainly be carried out in the dominant language; quotes from transcripts in other languages will be included to illustrate findings.
- *Simultaneous data analysis in more than one language.* Multiple languages are used for data collection. Bilingual analysts analyze data in the language in which they were originally collected. This option shares some features of a "multiple case study" in which each language group becomes one case. Analysts discuss findings in the common language, but continue the analysis in the original language, until the determined integration point. At that time, findings are translated into the common language. For example, node reports in French and Spanish generated through a computer-assisted coding process might be translated; a joint analysis would then continue in a selected common language (such as English).
- *Parallel data analysis.* Original data and translated data are used, and analysis compared. The same set of data are analyzed in the original language and in the translated dominant language version. Once the analyses are completed, findings from the analysis done on original language data are translated and compared to analysis of those data that were translated into the dominant language for analysis. This approach increases the reliability and trustworthiness of the analysis of data generated in another language because the interpretation of both the originally generated data and the translated versions can be compared. However, it is very time consuming and costly.

Other suggestions that improve multilingual analysis include:

- *Work in a multidisciplinary team.* Input from different disciplines is particularly enriching for multilingual qualitative analysis. If your research team is not multidisciplinary, you may want to consult with experts from other disciplines when issues surface that might benefit from a different theoretical lens.
- *Use interpreters' skills and knowledge in data analysis.* Try to work with translators trained in qualitative data analysis. If this is not possible, allocate resources so that they can at least participate in the discussion of findings.
- *Use multiple coders for interview transcripts.* If you are coding interviews in the target languages, involve at least two people with the same language background. Ensure that they systematically take note of differences when analyzing text segments. It is expected that there will be variations in interpretation of meaning, as in any qualitative analysis; it also will be useful to

discuss any differences that arise from divergent interpretations of the language itself.

- Try to distinguish language from other analytic categories (nationality, ethnicity, religion, birth country, immigrant status) or levels of aggregation. Many of these categories are socially constructed and overlap.
- Avoid cultural bias by considering alternative critical interpretations. During the analysis process we have the tendency to explain differences between linguistic groups as arising from cultural factors. Triangulation and searching for negative examples of phenomena, careful comparisons across languages, and tentative assertions (rather than conclusions) may be more appropriate ways of understanding differences (Arriaza, Nedjat-Haiem, Lee, & Martin, 2015).

REPORTING FINDINGS START HERE

A key issue is that participants who provided access to their lives and experiences may be unable to read reports that are written about them. Therefore, they may be unable to participate in debates about recommendations arising from the research. We believe this puts a special onus on multilingual researchers to seek alternative ways of ensuring that reported findings reach minority language populations.

Some suggestions to improve reporting of multilingual qualitative research include:

- If full reports cannot be translated, provide summaries of research findings and recommendations in the minority language.
- Acknowledge the limitations of cross-language work. Note how your findings may have been affected by interpretation and translation, working across languages, and analyzing data in a language not of the researchers.
- Provide as much detail as possible in method sections about the researcher's linguistic capacities (mother tongue, language learned, number of years living in the country, written or spoken language knowledge, etc.), as well as when translation occurred in the data collection and analysis process.

BUDGETING AND COST

It has been our experience that the cost of ensuring trustworthy multilingual research is often underestimated and seldom reported. There is also a cost to not conducting sound research with conclusions that can be trusted. Hyman (2009) reports a similar situation in relation to the lack of provision of interpretation services in health care, in the context of the ethical and legal obligation to address health inequities and ensure that language barriers do not contribute to inequities for Canada's non-official-language speakers. We suggest a similar approach to costing multilingual research, which should be seen as an essential component of qualitative health research.

HOW TO SUPPORT DEVELOPMENT OF CROSS-LANGUAGE QUALITATIVE RESEARCHERS

From our review, it seems that there is little guidance for qualitative researchers who want to conduct cross-language projects in the published literature and standard texts. We do not know to what extent specific skills are taught, or issues discussed, in qualitative research curricula, but suspect that there may be important gaps. We hope that this chapter will serve to encourage educators to emphasize the importance of cross-language and multi-lingual dimensions in qualitative health research, and stimulate them to apply, and improve on, some of the suggestions we provide.

GLOSSARY

Dominant and non-dominant language: The dominant language refers to the language that is spoken by most people in a specific geographic region (e.g., a province, a country), in contrast to other languages spoken by fewer people (non-dominant).

Interpreters/interpretation: "Interpreters are professional communicators who orally transmit a spoken message from one language to another. As with translation, there are different types of interpretation, the best known of which are conference interpretation and court interpretation" (Canadian Translators, Terminologists and Interpreters Council, n.d.). *Community interpreting* has emerged as a recognized category for interpretation in recent decades. It is defined as "bidirectional oral translation or sign language interpreting used in Canada by professionals in public settings such as healthcare and social services to deliver services to limited-English and limited-French speakers" (Canadian Translators, Terminologists and Interpreters Council, 2013).

Linguistic minority: People belong to a linguistic minority if they speak a non-dominant language (see above).

Mother tongue: As defined by Statistics Canada, this refers to the first language learned at home in childhood and still understood by the individual on the date of the most recent Census (Statistics Canada, 2011).

Source language and target language: We use the terms *source language* and *target language(s)* to distinguish between the language in which a text is originally created and the language or languages into which these words are transformed (interpreted, translated). Depending on the context, the same language may be either source or target.

Translators: "Translators are professional communicators who transpose a written text from one language into another and convey its content as faithfully as possible. They must have an excellent knowledge of the source language and a mastery of the target language. Translators generally translate from their second or third language into their mother tongue. [...] There are several types of translation – administrative, legal, literary, promotional or commercial, scientific, technical, etc." (Canadian Translators, Terminologists and Interpreters Council, n.d.).

DISCUSSION QUESTIONS

1. What are the benefits and challenges of conducting qualitative research in multiple languages? Why do researchers need to collect data from participants who do not speak their language?
2. How can unilingual researchers competently conduct qualitative health research in a language not their own? On the other hand, perhaps less frequently asked but perhaps implied, how can bilingual researchers conduct research rigorously and fairly in both languages?
3. Why is it important that different concepts, metaphors, theories, and terminology from the minority language be taken into account? And how can the socio-political linguistic context, including possible relations between interpreters/participants, affect multilingual health research?
4. What are some of the limitations of language crossing at different steps in the analytic process? What type of translation is needed for different types of data (e.g., interview transcripts, observation notes, photographic images)?
5. What is lost and what is gained through the language choices made about reporting research findings?

REFERENCES

Arriaza, P., Nedjat-Haiem, F., Lee, H. Y., & Martin, S. S. (2015). Guidelines for conducting rigorous health care psychosocial cross-cultural/language qualitative research. *Social Work in Public Health, 30*(1), 75–87. Retrieved from http://dx.doi.org/10.1080/19371918.2014.938394

Bowen, S., Gibbens, M., Roy, J., & Edwards, J. (2010). From 'multicultural health' to 'knowledge translation'—rethinking strategies to promote language access within a risk management framework. *The Journal of Specialised Translation, 14*, 145–164.

Canadian Translators, Terminologists and Interpreters Council. (2013, June 12). *A milestone reached for community interpreting in Canada* [Press release]. Retrieved from http://www.cttic.org/pressreleases/1213/FOR%20IMMEDIATE%20RELEASE_CCCI.pdf

Canadian Translators, Terminologists and Interpreters Council. (n.d.). *Language professions.* Retrieved from http://www.cttic.org/Professions.asp

Chen, H., & Boore, J. R. P. (2009). Translation and back-translation in qualitative nursing research: Methodological review. *Journal of Clinical Nursing, 19*, 234–239.

Denzin, N. K., & Lincoln, Y. S. (2005). Introduction: The discipline and practice of qualitative research. In Denzin, N. K., & Lincoln, Y. S. (eds.), *Qualitative Research* (3rd ed., pp. 1–32). Thousand Oaks, CA: Sage.

Estable, A., Meyer, M., & MacLean, L. (2004). *Newcomer infant care survey - piloting an approach and a tool.* Ottawa: Community Health Research Unit.

Fersch, B. (2013). Meaning: lost, found or 'made' in translation? A hermeneutical approach to cross-language interview research. *Qualitative Studies, 4*(2), 86–99.

Hyman, I. (2009). *Literature review: Costs of not providing interpretation in health care.* Toronto: Access Alliance. Retrieved from http://accessalliance.ca/Cost_of_Not_Providing_Interpretation

Meyer, M., Estable, A., MacLean, L., & Peterson, W. (2010). Family home visitors: Increasing minority women's access to health services. Jour*nal of Health Disparities Research and Practice, 3*(3), 1–20.

Moser, K. S. (2000). Metaphor analysis in psychology—method, theory, and fields of application. *Forum: Qualitative Social Research, 1*(2). Retrieved from http://www.qualitative-research. net/index.php/fqs/article/view/1090

Pottie, K., Ng., E., Spitzer, D., Mohammed, A., Glazier, R. (2008). Language proficiency, gender and self-reported health: An analysis of the first two waves of the Longitudinal Survey of Immigrants to Canada. *Canadian Journal of Public Health, 99*(6), 505–510.

Santos, H. P., Jr., Black, A. M., & Sandelowski, M. (2015). Timing of translation in cross-language qualitative research. *Qualitative Health Research, 25*(1), 134–144. Retrieved from http://dx.doi. org/10.1177/1049732314549603

Schmitt, R. (2005). Systematic metaphor analysis as a method of qualitative research. *The Qualitative Report, 10*(2), 358–394. Retrieved from http://www.nova.edu/ssss/QR/QR10-2/ schmitt.pdf

Sidhu, M. S., Kokab, F., Jolly, K., Marshall, T., Gale, N. K., & Gill, P. (2016). Methodological challenges of cross-language qualitative research with South Asian communities living in the UK. *Family Medicine and Community Health, 4*(2), 16–28.

Squires, A. (2009). Methodological challenges in cross-language qualitative research: A research review. *International Journal of Nursing Studies, 46*(2), 277–287.

Statistics Canada. (2011). *Census dictionary.* Catalogue no. 92-301-X 2011. Ottawa: Statistics Canada.

van Nes, F., Abma, T, Jonsson, H. & Deeg, D. (2010). Language differences in qualitative research: Is meaning lost in translation? *European Journal of Ageing, 7*(4), 313–316.

Wallin, A., & Ahlström, G. (2006). Cross-cultural interview studies using interpreters: Systematic literature review. *Journal of Advanced Nursing, 55*(6), 723–735.

CHAPTER 5

An Index of Population Health Databases: Addressing the Challenge of Finding Evidence for Population Health Research and Decision Making

David N. Williams, Corinne Packer, Leanne Trimble, and Ivy Lynn Bourgeault

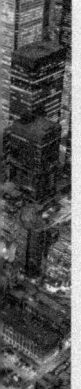

TAKE-HOME MESSAGE

- There are a number of datasets that could be exploited to enhance population health research and decision making; the challenge is in finding and accessing them.
- Reducing the barriers between researchers, decision- and policy-makers, and the data and/or evidence they both require to carry out their work can help enhance population health.
- The Population Health Improvement Research Network (PHIRN) created the Ontario Population Health Index of Databases (OPHID) to address these gaps. It is a resource not only for Ontario-based researchers but for those across Canada.

INTRODUCTION

The volume of research using population health both as a paradigm and health policy discourse has expanded over the past decade, but it is still only scratching the surface (Chow et al., 2009; Ghosh & Bourgeault, Chapter 2, this volume; Krewski et al., 2007; Raphael, 2008). Different reviews of this research present three reoccurring themes: much more research is needed using a population health approach (Chow et al., 2009; Curtis, Setia, & Quesnel-Vallee, 2009; Edwards & Di Ruggiero, 2011; Krewski et al., 2007; Wigle et al., 2008); there is a lack of data or other evidence to support this research (Chow et al., 2009; Craig et al., 2008; Guyer et al., 2009; Hruschka, 2009; Wigle et al., 2008); and evidence and data generated will not be useful unless it is effectively made available to policy-makers and practitioners (Bhala, Patterson, Johnman, & Bhopal, 2012; Krewski et al., 2007; Wigle et al., 2008). Robust evidence needs to be translated into practice (Bhala, Patterson, Johnman, & Bhopal, 2012), but finding evidence in a field new to decision- and policy-makers can be a daunting task (Hunink et al., 2001; Muir Gray, 2004).

Practitioners in new fields of study, as well as those applying a new paradigm in decision- and policy-making in relatively novel cross-disciplinary research, often face shortages of data (Edwards & Di Ruggiero, 2011; Guyer et al., 2009; Hruschka, 2009; Wigle et al., 2008). There appear to be two different informal camps for explaining the relative dearth of evidence on which to base population health–based research and decision making. One is the "pioneer" philosophy—the idea that trailblazers rarely have roads built ahead of them (Guyer et al., 2009; Hruschka, 2009). The other is the bridge dilemma: researchers attempting to bridge two (or more) disciplines will rarely have expertise in what lies on the other side (Kumanyika & Morssink, 2006).

A key objective of the Population Health Improvement Research Network (PHIRN) was to enhance the capacity to undertake and to use population health research. This involved, in part, reducing the barriers between researchers, decision- and policy-makers, and the data and/or evidence they both require to carry out their work. A step towards this objective was the creation of an online, comprehensive, searchable index of population health databases: the Ontario Population Health Index of Databases (OPHID). In addition to addressing the broader issues raised above, a more proximate instigator for the creation of the index was the scoping review we conducted to inform the work undertaken at PHIRN (Ghosh & Bourgeault, Chapter 2, this volume). It became clear from the scoping review that there were critical gaps in our knowledge of population health equity and intervention research that an index of available databases could begin to address. Specifically, an overall goal of this project was to do the legwork to uncover and liberate existing datasets that could be more fully exploited by a range of users to address these critical knowledge gaps. To achieve this goal, the index had two specific objectives:

1. to serve as a guide to the array of databases available to potential users, and to inform on their contents and the actions required to access them; and
2. to serve as a medium for data custodians to make their databases known, and to attract users.

In short, OPHID was created to enable more researcher pull and data holder push with increased utilization overall. The following paper describes the steps taken and guidelines followed to design, develop, and bring online this index.

METHODS

Guidelines

The initial scope of OPHID and our design guidelines were established through a series of interviews with researchers from a wide variety of disciplines that use a population health paradigm, many of whom were affiliated with PHIRN. First, while limited to the population(s) of Ontario, no other boundaries were set. Thirteen different subject areas were identified, reflecting in part the key themes emerging from the scoping review we conducted (Ghosh & Bourgeault, Chapter 2, this volume):

1. Aboriginal health
2. Aging
3. Built environment
4. Crime
5. Education
6. Financial security and employment
7. General health and morbidities
8. Health behaviours
9. Infant and youth
10. Mental health and addictions
11. Natural environment
12. Immigration
13. Reproductive health

These subject areas served both as search terms around which explorations for datasets were conducted and categories to organize the gathered datasets. Second, the design guidelines that emerged from our consultations were that the index should be:

- inclusive of all disciplines working with and utilizing all applications of a broad population health paradigm;
- free and openly accessible to all users; and
- growth oriented, meaning that the index must continue to grow, be updated, and expanded in order to be most useful.

The Search for Databases

"Well, it depends on what you mean by 'database'...."
—Administrator, Environment Canada

An operational definition of *database* was necessary before a search could get underway. We found that a strict definition of database—"a systematized collection of data that can be accessed immediately by a data processing system" (Database, 2003)—would unnecessarily limit our offerings on a number of grounds. A more flexible and inclusive definition was created: any large store of information, raw, aggregated, or presentation ready, irrespective of time frame, sampling method, or other limitations. Basically, by database we refer to any organized collection of data, whether aggregated or in individual (Database, 2011).

Two key guidelines were established to facilitate our search for databases and determine whether they should be included or not:

1. Stay flexible: Many different names are applied to databases available for use, including datasets, data records, databases, indexes of data, and statistics. Each may contain information that could be of value to users; all were reviewed and added (or not) based on the value that they might add to population health research and/ or decision making.
2. Err towards inclusion: Recognize that data may not be important to research at present, but may be of use in future.

The search took place across a number of contexts:

- Library resources, including academic and public sources. This included existing online databases, search platforms for databases, as well as "offline" databases.
- Government agencies within each subject area, including federal, provincial, regional, and municipal.
- Non-governmental agencies within each subject area.
- Morbidity specialty organizations, such as cancer, heart disease, and diabetes.
- Government information agencies, such as census and statistics, trade, immigration, finance, employment, and education at both federal and provincial levels.
- Organizations responsible for summarizing and reporting activities, such as police and enforcement services, welfare agencies, municipal financial offices, health service agencies, social service agencies, school districts, and health care regions.
- Private industry, including companies and agencies within each subject area that make data available.

The majority of "leads" were established through a web-based search augmented with a review of public and academic library resources.

Once discovered, the content of each database was reviewed to ensure that the information presented was current, sufficient, and in a format serviceable to possible users. In addition, the means of data access was carefully verified through either contact with the data custodian or actual hands-on access to the database. Only a minority of the databases referenced in OPHID allow for direct access to the data. Contact with the data custodian was made principally to verify requirements for a researcher to gain access to the data, contact information, and sources of additional information if available. Several lessons were learned from the experience:

- Never take the word of a website. We learned early that information presented on websites was often wrong or out of date.

- Direct confirmation is essential. Each database was confirmed by direct contact with a person or through access to the database. Dropped links, dated email addresses, reorganizations, personnel attrition, and complex organization charts were all impediments to verifying the existence and current status of a database.
- Keep trying. Databases are invisible; often relatively few people, sometimes as few as one, might know of a database, what is in it, who is responsible for it, and the steps necessary to gain access to it. It often took several tries to find that person.
- Don't take no for an answer, at least not the first time. People would often say no before understanding that we were not asking for open access to their database. Usually, after deference was paid to confidentiality and due process, and assurances were made that all we wanted to know was the required steps if someone did want access to the data, we were given the needed access information.
- Know when to quit trying. We discovered that some leads were a mirage; there may have been a database there at some point, but it did not exist any longer. Information on some of the most enticing databases seemed to be just another email or phone call away.

Once "discovered," the content of each database was reviewed to ensure that the information was current, sufficient, and in a format accessible and of value to possible users. Metadata about the database was collected; this often required additional contact with the data custodian and source management. The metadata gathered for OPHID includes:

- Database name
- Source agency (custodian or partial custodian)
- Method used in collecting the data, such as sample survey, administrative data, clinical research, environmental testing sites, academic reports, or financial reports filed
- Initial purpose for collecting the data
- Limitations on the data, including sample, scope, time frame, and content limitations
- Descriptive information such as scope, time span, size, etc.
- Highlights, such as an example of information contained in the database
- Access requirements and procedures, including contact information if available
- Contents description, such as a data dictionary or description of the data
- Previous users and uses, including work that had been done with the data in the database, who did it, and examples of the results (if available)
- Keywords for the search engine

Establishing the Access Platform

As noted above, it was critical to make the index as readily available in as user-friendly a platform as possible. Fundamental to establishing the access platform were two guidelines:

1. No matter how good the content, if it is perceived as difficult to access or as an inconvenience to work with, people will not use it.
2. Someone (likely) has done this before and already knows how to do it better than you, so it does not make sense to reinvent the wheel.

We did a non-exhaustive survey and evaluation of index platforms to assess what did and did not work. Approximately 12 indexes were identified and evaluated. They ranged from academic library resources to government agencies. Each was assessed for:

- ease of index access
- ease of use, including self-directed, intuitive instructions where and when needed
- ease of information access, including navigation and directions
- general visual appeal
- instructions and explanations in plain language

There were wide disparities between the various platforms reviewed.

One of our PHIRN scientists, Terry Wade, referred us to ODESI, an index/database access platform managed by the Ontario Council of University Libraries (OCUL) through the Scholars Portal program. A review of their index service scored high against our criteria. This service has indexed and allows access to over 3,000 data files that are hosted at Scholars Portal as well as an additional (approximately) 9,000 metadata records that link to externally hosted data files. The service is available as an online resource through academic libraries. The OCUL staff had the expertise needed to build an index, and their management was willing to work with us.

Partnering with OCUL gave us access to their software development and metadata expertise, developed using their experience with creating and maintaining technical infrastructure and collections shared by the 21 Ontario university libraries. It also gave us access to their expertise in dataset documentation standards, such as the Data Documentation Initiative (DDI) metadata standard, to ensure that detailed documentation is available. Widely used within the data repository community, this standard allows for easy sharing of information about data collections.

Scholars Portal developers were able to create the OPHID database index by customizing existing ODESI code to suit the unique features of OPHID. This allowed us to create the OPHID index with few of the glitches inherent to the design of a new system. Modifications primarily included the information displayed. Important quality control steps were applied in partnership with OCUL staff. Ongoing quality checks and updates will be managed by Scholars Portal. The Ontario Population Health Index of Databases (OPHID) launched in September 2012.

FUTURE DIRECTIONS

The third design goal, growth, is a journey rather than a goal. There are four "planks" to our growth plan:

1. Build end-users. Just because the index is operational doesn't mean that it will be used. An extensive and continuous marketing effort is needed to establish and build user knowledge of and access to the index. In addition, effective measurements, such as tracking the number of hits to the OPHID website, will be reported on an ongoing basis.
2. Build partnerships with data custodians to use OPHID as a resource for getting their databases known and used. An online database submission form is available that will allow any agency, data custodian or otherwise, to propose their database for addition to OPHID.
3. Build cross-Canada partnerships. OPHID is an index of databases that represent, at least in part, population health within Ontario. Other provinces have built comparable indexes; we hope to form links with them in order to expand the databases represented across Canada.
4. Build the index. While it is hard to know, we estimate that less than half of relevant databases are captured in OPHID. Offline databases should be included in the next survey. By building partnerships, inviting agencies to add databases, and continuing our own search, OPHID will continue to grow.

CONCLUSION

There is recognition that more research based on valid, accurate data is needed in population health research. Researchers, decision-makers, and policy-makers are limited by a perceived lack of data, or lack of access to data, but a substantial portion of these perceptions may be incorrect. The relative newness of the field and the cross-disciplinary nature of population health are, in part, responsible for these perceptions; people do not know what is available in disciplines within which they have not worked before. The OPHID database index is a partial solution or a first step in responding to this challenge. It makes available a fully searchable index of databases from a wide range of disciplines and stakeholders. Key to its success will be growth of two user groups: end-users of population health data, and partner agencies that will use the index as a medium for making their databases known to larger audiences. To remain relevant it must be kept current and continue to grow, but most importantly, it must be used.

GLOSSARY

Database (in population health research): Any large store of information, raw, aggregated, or presentation ready, irrespective of time frame, sampling method, or other limitations; any organized collection of data, whether aggregated or in individual form (Database, 2011).

Data custodian: The person (or people) who has control or is responsible for enabling access to an agency's or organization's data.

Data dictionary: Information describing the contents (e.g., questions or variables), format, and structure of a dataset.

Metadata: Data that describe and provide information about a set of data, including the data custodian, data collection process, and different data elements.

DISCUSSION QUESTIONS

1. Discuss the pros and cons of accessing different sets of data to answer population health research questions—from a researcher's perspective, from a research user's perspective, and from a data custodian's perspective.
2. Why do we need to have a broader definition of the term *database* (or be more inclusive when gathering datasets), in contrast to a more traditional and narrower definition, when working with the population health paradigm?

REFERENCES

Bhala, N., Patterson, D., Johnman, C., & Bhopal, R. (2012). Epidemiology Congresses XIX, XX and beyond: Back to the future of population health. *Public Health, 126*(3), 271–273.

Chow, C. K., Lock, K., Teo, K., Subramanian S. V., McKee, M., & Yusuf, S. (2009). Environmental and societal influences acting on cardiovascular risk factors and disease at a population level: A review. *International Journal of Epidemiology, 38*, 1580–1594.

Craig, L., Brook, J. R., Chiotti, Q., Croes, B., Gower, S., Hedley, A., & Williams, M. (2008). Air pollution and public health: A guidance document for risk managers. *Journal of Toxicology and Environmental Health, 71*, 588–698.

Curtis, A., Setia, M., & Quesnel-Vallee, A. (2009). Socio-geographic mobility and health status: A longitudinal analysis using the National Population Health Survey of Canada. *Social Science & Medicine, 69*, 1845–1853.

Database. (2003). In *Collins english dictionary pro* (5th ed.). New York: HarperCollins Publishers.

Database. (2011). *Wikipedia.* Retrieved from http://en.wikipedia.org/wiki/Database

Edwards, N., & Di Ruggiero, E. (2011). Exploring which context matters in the study of health inequities and their mitigation. *Scandinavian Journal of Public Health, 39*, 43–49.

Guyer, B., Ma, S., Grason, H., Frick, K. D., Perry, D. F., Sharkey, A., & McIntosh J. (2009). Early childhood health promotion and its life course health consequences. *Academic Pediatrics, 9*, 142–149.

Hruschka, D. J. (2009). Culture as an explanation in population health. *Annals of Human Biology, 36*, 235–247.

Hunink, M., Glasziou, P., Siegel, J., Weeks, J., Pliskin, J., Elstein, A., & Weinstein, M. (2001). *Decision-making in health and medicine: Integrating evidence and values* (1st ed.). Cambridge: Cambridge University Press.

Krewski, D., Hogan, V., Turner, M. C., Zeman, P. L., McDowell, I., Edwards, N., & Losos, J. (2007). An integrated framework for risk management and population health. *Human and Ecological Risk Assessment: An International Journal, 13*, 1288–1312.

Kumanyika, S., & Morssink, C. (2006). Bridging domains in efforts to reduce disparities in health and health care. *Health Education & Behavior, 33*(4), 440–458.

Muir Gray, J. A. (2004). Evidence based policy making: Is about taking decisions based on evidence and the needs and values of the population. *BMJ, 329*(7473), 988–989.

Raphael, D. (2008). Grasping at straws: A recent history of health promotion in Canada. *Critical Public Health, 18*, 483–495.

Wigle, D. T., Arbuckle, T., Turner, M. C., Bérubé, A., Yang, Q., Liu, S., & Krewski, D. (2008). Epidemiologic evidence of relationships between reproductive and child health outcomes and environmental chemical contaminants. *Journal of Toxicology and Environmental Health, 11*, 373–517.

CHAPTER 6

Multiple Chronic Diseases in Canada: Using Health Administrative Data to Address Research Gaps

Elizabeth Muggah, Erin Graves, Carol Bennett, and Douglas G. Manuel

TAKE-HOME MESSAGE

- There is growing recognition that chronic diseases do not occur in isolation and that many people are suffering from more than one chronic condition. The co-occurrence of chronic conditions, or multimorbidity, provides new challenges to the clinician, health system, and researcher that have traditionally focused on individual diseases. And, despite the common occurrence of multiple chronic disease in clinical practice, research efforts have been slow to develop consensus about how to define multimorbidity and often focus on index diseases and associated comorbidity.
- Accurate and timely measurement of the burden of chronic diseases is the cornerstone of sound evidence-based health care planning. Increasingly, population-based health administrative data are being used for disease surveillance. This administrative data has proven to be valuable for chronic disease surveillance because it is relatively easy to access and process, can be used to monitor a variety of diseases and outcomes simultaneously, and can provide both cross-sectional and longitudinal information about disease prevalence and incidence for entire populations.
- The Multiple Chronic Disease Database (MCDD) pools administrative disease definitions, providing an important addition to the information available to researchers, decision-makers, and health care providers on multiple chronic diseases. We present, for the first time, estimates of the prevalence and incidence of disease burden across time for nine chronic illnesses.

INTRODUCTION

Chronic diseases are the leading cause of death and disability worldwide (WHO, 2005). In Canada these diseases result in a substantial burden contributing to morbidity, mortality, and economic costs. Close to 60 percent of Canadians have at least one chronic disease (Statistics Canada, 2010). In 2007, cancer and heart disease, the two leading causes of death for Canadians, were responsible for over one-half of all deaths (Statistics Canada, 2007). There is a growing recognition that chronic diseases do not occur in isolation and that many people, particularly the elderly, are suffering from more than one chronic condition. A recent chronic disease report from the Canadian Institute for Health Information found that one-third of adults and one-half of seniors with a chronic disease reported at least one additional condition (Data Quality Documentation, Discharge Abstract Database, 2011).

The co-occurrence of chronic conditions, or multimorbidity, provides new challenges to the clinician, health system, and researcher that have traditionally focused on individual diseases. For the clinician, some co-occurring conditions may have few interactions and be effectively managed synergistically, but other conditions are discordant, and treatment and symptoms may interfere with each other. From a health system perspective, patients with multimorbidity often receive individual disease-oriented services that can result in fragmented and inefficient care (Boyd & Fortin, 2010). While multiple chronic disease is common in clinical practice, research approaches have been lagging. There is no consensus about how to define multimorbidity, and research efforts often focus on index diseases and associated comorbidity.

This project was developed to fill knowledge gaps about individuals living with multiple chronic conditions—including a more detailed characterization of the population and the impact of this disease on the individual, the population as a whole, and the health care system. This research uses linked health administrative data to provide information that will support clinicians and policy-makers to coordinate and manage care for this population and improve health care system strategies to best serve this population.

Using Health Administrative Data for Multiple Chronic Disease Surveillance

Accurate and timely measurement of the burden of chronic diseases is the cornerstone of sound evidence-based health care planning. Increasingly, population-based health administrative data—such as health insurance registry, physician billing, and hospital admission databases—are being used for disease surveillance. These administrative databases have proven to be valuable tools for chronic disease surveillance because they are relatively easy to access and process, can be used to monitor a variety of diseases and outcomes simultaneously, and can provide both cross-sectional and longitudinal information about disease prevalence and incidence for entire populations.

In Canada, there are a number of disease-specific surveillance initiatives at the federal and provincial levels that use health administrative data, such as the Canadian Cancer Registry and the National Diabetes Surveillance System. Provincially, many jurisdictions (including Nova Scotia, Quebec, Ontario, Manitoba, and British Columbia) use health administrative data to collect information on disease burden. In 2009, the Public Health

Agency of Canada established the Canadian Chronic Disease Surveillance System, a network of provincial and territorial surveillance systems, to build a comprehensive national picture of multiple chronic diseases (Public Health Agency of Canada, 2007).

Health administrative data is collected for purposes other than research. As a result, using these data for research presents challenges for the accurate and valid estimation of disease (Benchimol et al., 2010; Manuel, Rosella, & Stukel, 2010). The key step in disease ascertainment using health administrative data is to develop a disease definition that uses the diagnostic and treatment codes from physician billing and hospital discharge databases to identify individuals with the disease. The combined input of clinical experts and people knowledgeable about the data and coding standards is used to ensure validity of the definition. This step can often involve several iterations of a given methodology, and developing a single case ascertainment definition can be a sizable research project on its own. The case definition should then be validated using chart review or population health surveys that are considered the *reference standard*. Some chronic diseases have been shown to be more accurately identified in hospital and physician billing data than others (Benchimol et al., 2010). Thus, the accuracy of health administrative data depends not only on the quality of the data but also the specific condition being identified and the validity of the codes in the patient group (Benchimol et al., 2010).

In response to the identified need for more rigorous assessments of the quality of administrative data, the Institute for Clinical Evaluative Sciences developed the Quality Assessment of Administrative Data Model (Iron & Manuel, 2007). This model applies typically used indicators of data quality (Box 6.1) to administrative data across four dimensions: accuracy, reliability, completeness, and usability. Accuracy is most commonly evaluated by comparing disease ascertainment using administrative data to a reference-standard source of information—most often the medical chart review—and is reported using measures such as sensitivity and specificity. Validity of the data can be measured through comparison of disease counts across datasets using measures of inter-rater reliability such as a kappa statistic or percent difference in the data (Iron & Manuel, 2007). Completeness and coverage of the data needs to be described and a comparison between datasets can uncover missing data or gaps in the populations covered. Finally, a complete description of the data should be presented including collection methods, population sampled, database structure, timelines, and linkages in order to assess how the data can be used and interpreted.

Population-Based Chronic Disease Cohorts in Ontario, Canada

This project used health administrative data from Ontario, Canada, housed at the Institute for Clinical Evaluative Sciences (ICES) to calculate the chronic disease burden. The individual-level provincial databases available to us are annually updated and can be individually linked to health care and other data. All of the data is de-identified and individually linked using an anonymous, unique identifier number.

Box 6.1: Indicators of Data Quality Grouped into Four Broad Categories

1. Are the data correct?
   Accuracy: Do the data reflect the truth?

2. Are the data reliable?
   Reliability: Are the data reproducible?
   Validity: Do the data make sense?

3. Are the data complete?
   Completeness: Do the data include all records that are collected?
   Comprehensiveness and coverage: Do the data cover 100 percent of the intended population?

4. Are the data usable?
   Anonymity: Do the data adhere to jurisdictional privacy laws, procedures, and practices?
   Linkability: Can the data be connected to other data to reflect health care system complexity?
   Timeliness: Is there a short lag between data collection and use?
   Usability: Are the data organized, accessible, and provided in a format that can be easily used?
   Temporal consistency: Are the data elements standardized to evaluate change over time?

Source: Iron & Manuel, 2007

Over the past decade, population-based disease cohorts for Ontario have been created using the linked databases at the ICES. The individual databases used to create these cohorts include: the Registered Persons Database (RPD), the Ontario Health Insurance Plan (OHIP), the Discharge Abstract Database (DAD), the National Ambulatory Care Reporting System (NACRS), and the Canadian Census. Information about the completeness and coverage of the databases used in this study are reported elsewhere (Canadian Institute for Health Information, 2011; Data Quality Documentation, Discharge Abstract Database, 2011; Institute for Clinical Evaluative Sciences, 2005; Statistics Canada, 2010). This project includes nine disease cohorts. Details of these case ascertainment methodologies, cohort-specific exclusion criteria, and the accuracy of each case ascertainment strategy are listed in Appendix 6.1. For the majority of these diseases, peer-reviewed validation studies have been conducted reporting the sensitivity and specificity of the strategies. Although the data in Ontario is available, in many cases from 1991 onwards a "wash-out" period of a few years is established to minimize the possibility of overestimating incidence rates in the initial years. More detailed technical information on the disease definitions is included in Appendix 6.2. This information is useful for the assessment of data quality and comparisons with other studies.

Multiple Chronic Disease Database Development

To address the growing need for information on the burden of multiple chronic conditions we developed a new database to identify persons with more than one chronic disease. To do this, we combined the existing disease cohorts into a single database with a structure that was computationally efficient and easy to use. The initial Multiple Chronic Disease Database began with the combination of six validated disease cohorts—asthma, hypertension, congestive heart failure, chronic obstructive pulmonary disease, acute myocardial infarction, and diabetes (Iron et al., 2011). These existing datasets were combined (Statistical Analysis Software (SAS) 9.2, SUN OS Unix environment) without adding any exclusion criteria to the cohorts beyond those contained in their case ascertainment methodologies (see Appendix 6.2). This initial Multiple Chronic Disease Database allowed for individual disease ascertainment algorithms to be used together to identify co-occurring and multiple diseases in patients, as well as to estimate the prevalence of different combinations of diseases, total and type of health care use, and sociodemographic risk factors for disease (Iron, Gerson, Lu, & Manuel, 2011).

To allow for the addition of new diseases while minimizing computing resource requirements, the database was structured with two relational tables indexed on the unique encoded personal identifier. The first, or Disease Table, is used to ascertain disease status and has three data elements: the unique encoded personal identifier, the disease status, and the date of diagnosis for the disease. The Disease Table has multiple rows for a single person, and each time a person is identified as having a new disease, a row is added to the table. The second, or Dates Table, includes (in addition to the unique identifier) the date of onset of disease, birth date, death date, and date of last contact with the health care system; each person in the Multiple Chronic Disease Database has only a single row in the Dates Table. To calculate disease prevalence and incidence, a standardized program was created to merge the two database tables using the unique identifier and produce a final table. That final table includes the unique identifier, the number of diseases (in order based on diagnosis date) and the status (incidence, prevalence, or death) in a separate data element for each year of interest. This program has the flexibility to be looked at either by specific disease (or disease combination) or by number of diseases in a given individual.

Three additional chronic diseases were added to the initial Multiple Chronic Disease Database: peripheral vascular disease, stroke, and end-stage renal disease. While these three diseases have not been validated in peer-reviewed studies, there is sufficient information about the disease cohort definition that a high degree of validity and reliability can be assured (Manuel et al., 2008). Using the unique identifier, the updated database was linked to Census data. Estimates of the incidence and prevalence of multiple chronic diseases in Ontario from 1999 to 2009, as well as information on sociodemographic profile, were produced using SAS.

METHODS

Study Population

The study cohort included all persons, aged 20 years and older, identified in the Ontario provincial Registered Persons Database, who were alive and eligible for provincial health insurance on April 1st of the year for estimates being calculated (Figure 6.1). To minimize the possibility of including deceased or out-of-province persons in our calculations, we excluded individuals who had no contact with the health care system in the past 5 years. In all other respects, the Multiple Chronic Disease Database cohort was prepared as outlined above, using the DAD and physician service claims from the Ontario Health Insurance Plan database to identify all persons with at least one of the nine chronic diseases.

Data Analysis

Incidence and prevalence rates were calculated for each individual disease as well as by the number of diseases for the Ontario population. All rates were standardized by age and sex to the 1991 Canadian Population for trending comparisons across years. Incidence rates for the number of chronic diseases were calculated using a 10 percent sample of the Multiple Chronic Disease Database, while all other rates were calculated using the full database.

We used the Registered Persons Database to calculate the disease incidence and prevalence rates, as well as to estimate the number of people with none of the diseases in our database. This database can overestimate the number of people living in Ontario, as it includes some individuals who are deceased or no longer living in the province (Glazier, Creatore, Agha, & Steele, 2003). To address this limitation, the ICES prepares an augmented database that uses other administrative data sources to improve address and death information; this augmented database was incorporated into the Registered Persons Database to improve the accuracy of our estimates (Iron, Zagorski, Sykora, & Manuel, 2008).

Sociodemographic Profile Variable Definitions

We derived neighbourhood income quintiles by linking our Multiple Chronic Disease Database to the 2006 Census data using the patients' residential postal code. Statistics Canada adjusts income for household size and community size such that each community would be expected to have 20 percent of its population in each income quintile. Those in quintile 1 had the lowest income and those in quintile 5 had the highest. The estimation of socioeconomic status from neighbourhood income has been previously reported by different authors (Creatore et al., 2007). We examined the characteristics of population stratified by geographic location according to the Rurality Index of Ontario (Kralj, 2005). The strata used were major urban (index 0–9), non-major urban (10–44), and rural (≥ 45) (Jaakkimainen et al., 2011).

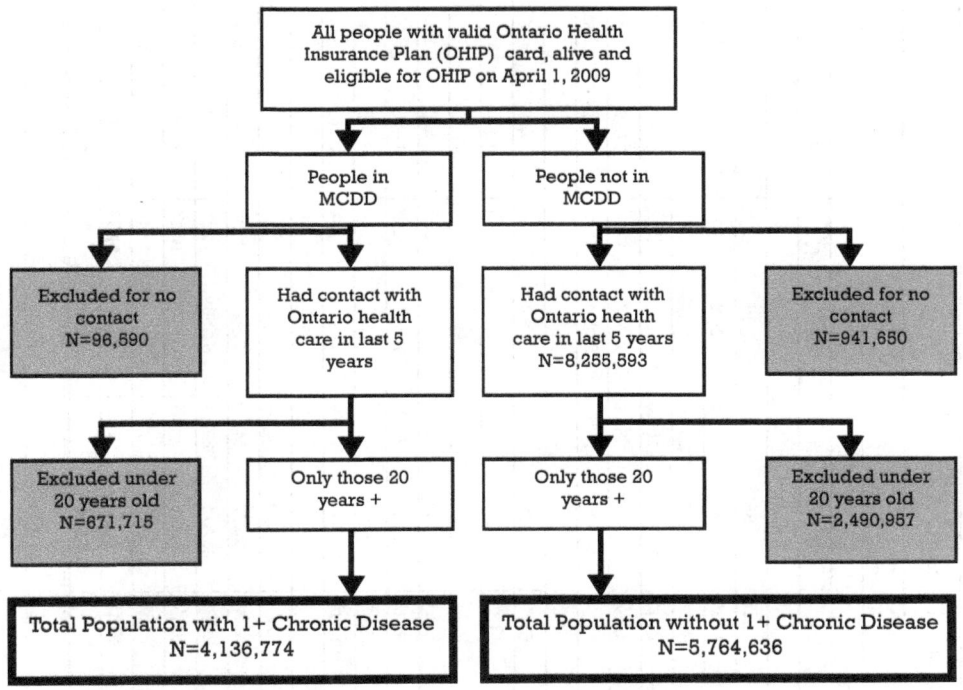

Figure 6.1: Study Population by Inclusion Criteria, Multiple Chronic Disease Database (MCDD), 2009

RESULTS

A total of 4,136,774 persons in 2009 met our inclusion criteria for the Multiple Chronic Disease Database (Figure 6.1). Of these, 58.1 percent had at least one of the nine diseases, 26.3 percent had two or more, and 15.8 percent had three or more (Table 6.1).

Prevalence of multiple chronic conditions increased with age. Persons 65 and older made up two thirds, or 62.4 percent, of those with three diseases, compared with 24.7 percent of those with one condition, and 46.8 percent of those with two conditions. There were more women with one, two, or three conditions (52.5 percent versus 47.5 percent for men), but more men with four or more conditions (51.4 percent versus 48.6 percent for women). People from the lowest income quintile had disproportionally higher numbers of chronic diseases. For the majority of chronic disease categories there was a consistent gradient across income quintiles: the proportion of individuals with fewer than two conditions increased by income, whereas the inverse relationship was noted with three or more chronic conditions (Table 6.1).

Standardized estimates of incidence and prevalence for both number of chronic conditions and by individual condition are presented in Figures 6.2 to 6.5. Hypertension and asthma were consistently the most prevalent diseases from 1999 through 2009 (Figure 6.2), followed by diabetes and chronic obstructive pulmonary disease. Incidence of these four diseases during this same time period has dropped or leveled off (Figure 6.3).

Table 6.1: Characteristics of Ontario Eligible Population by Number of Chronic Diseases, 2009

	Number of Chronic Diseases													
	0		1		2		3		4		5		6+	
	N	%	N	%	N	%	N	%	N	%	N	%	N	%
Age Group														
20–44	3,573,233	62.4%	842,274	32.4%	95,201	9.5%	11,975	3.4%	1,588	1.3%	348	0.9%	77	0.5%
45–64	1,859,619	32.5%	1,113,925	42.9%	437,577	43.7%	120,931	34.2%	31,796	25.1%	8,098	19.9%	3,081	20.8%
65–74	211,503	3.7%	355,553	13.7%	231,281	23.1%	91,928	26.0%	33,997	26.9%	10,897	26.8%	4,179	28.2%
75–79	45,324	0.8%	126,161	4.9%	98,566	9.8%	47,458	13.4%	20,328	16.1%	7,393	18.2%	2,792	18.8%
80–84	24,734	0.4%	88,650	3.4%	74,652	7.5%	41,071	11.6%	19,145	15.1%	6,977	17.2%	2,550	17.2%
85+	15,276	0.3%	72,634	2.8%	64,885	6.5%	39,980	11.3%	19,726	15.6%	6,960	17.1%	2,142	14.5%
Sex														
F	2,944,831	51.4%	1,370,947	52.8%	522,422	52.1%	182,800	51.7%	63,006	49.8%	19,082	46.9%	6,423	43.3%
M	2,784,858	48.6%	1,228,250	47.3%	479,740	47.9%	170,543	48.3%	63,574	50.2%	21,591	53.1%	8,396	56.7%
Rurality*														
Missing	497,762	8.7%	49,322	1.9%	16,632	1.7%	5,685	1.6%	2,143	1.7%	727	1.8%	243	1.6%
0 to 9	3,529,524	61.6%	1,585,531	61.0%	604,902	60.4%	205,927	58.3%	71,937	56.8%	22,658	55.7%	8,598	58.0%
10 to 44	1,124,894	19.6%	641,420	24.7%	247,850	24.7%	91,052	25.8%	33,611	26.6%	11,186	27.5%	3,915	26.4%
45+	577,509	10.1%	322,924	12.4%	132,778	13.3%	50,679	14.3%	18,889	14.9%	6,102	15.0%	2,063	13.9%
Income Quintile†														
Missing	119,483	2.1%	31,241	1.2%	8,467	0.8%	2,674	0.8%	970	0.8%	301	0.7%	118	0.8%
1	1,062,670	18.6%	476,645	18.3%	205,983	20.6%	80,517	22.8%	31,279	24.7%	10,591	26.0%	3,983	26.9%
2	1,095,088	19.1%	511,318	19.7%	210,762	21.0%	76,980	21.8%	28,270	22.3%	8,968	22.1%	3,293	22.2%
3	1,115,660	19.5%	514,893	19.8%	199,966	20.0%	69,603	19.7%	24,448	19.3%	7,809	19.2%	2,730	18.4%
4	1,171,110	20.4%	536,227	20.6%	195,894	19.6%	65,563	18.6%	22,379	17.7%	7,069	17.4%	2,618	17.7%
5	1,165,678	20.3%	528,873	20.4%	181,090	18.1%	58,006	16.4%	19,234	15.2%	5,935	14.6%	2,077	14.0%
Total	**5,729,689**		**2,599,197**		**1,002,162**		**353,343**		**126,580**		**40,673**		**14,819**	

* RIO2008 from the Ministry of Finance (2008 version)

† Income Quintile from the Postal Code Conversion File, Statistics Canada (2006 version)

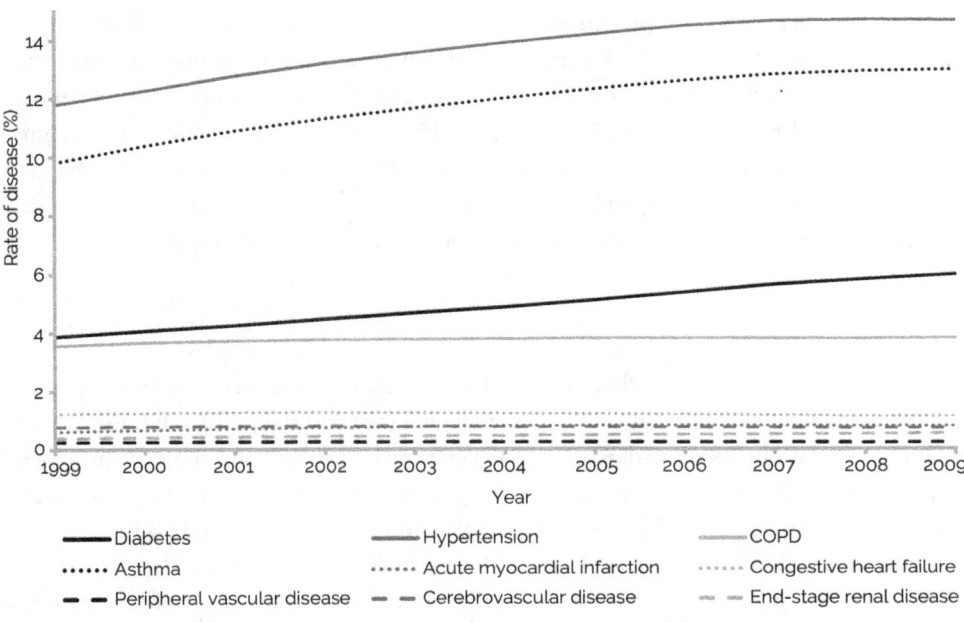

Figure 6.2: Age and Sex-Adjusted Prevalence of Nine Chronic Diseases, Ontario, 1999 to 2009

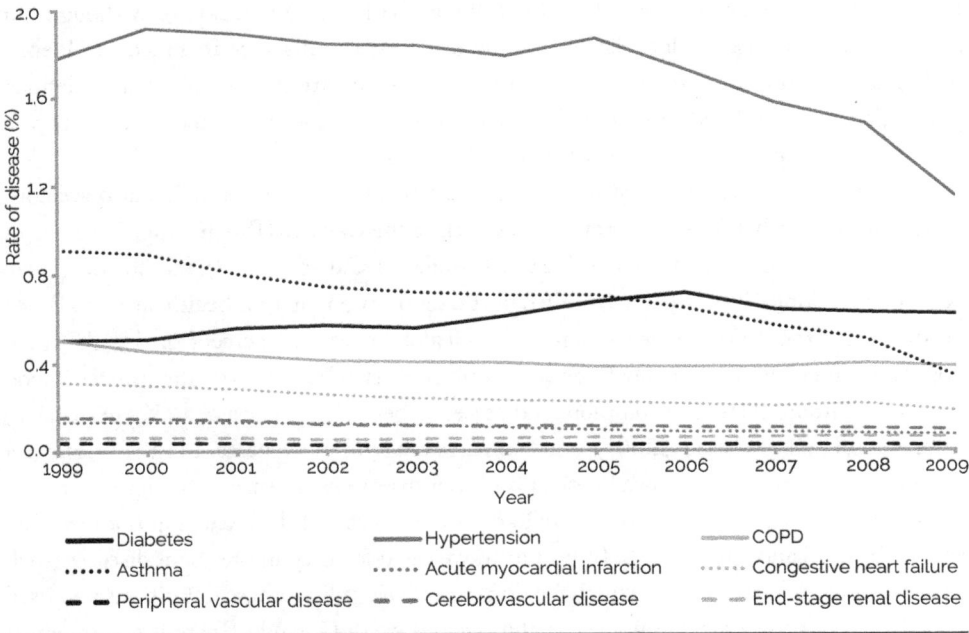

Figure 6.3: Age and Sex-Adjusted Incidence of Nine Chronic Diseases, Ontario, 1999 to 2009

The prevalence of multiple chronic diseases by number of conditions is depicted in Figure 6.4. From 1999 to 2009, the prevalence of having any one condition increased from 17.5 percent to 20.5 percent; of having two conditions, from 2.8 percent to 34.9 percent; and of having three or more conditions, from 0.84 percent to 0.95 percent. The incidence of multiple chronic conditions decreased between 1999 and 2009 (Figure 6.5). The incidence of any one disease dropped from 3.0 percent to 1.8 percent, of two diseases from 1.0 percent to 0.6 percent, and of three diseases from 0.34 percent to 0.20 percent.

DISCUSSION

Estimates of multiple chronic disease burden can differ widely depending on the population studied, source of data, and diagnoses included (Fortin et al., 2010). For example, in a Quebec study, the 2005 unadjusted prevalence of two or more conditions in the general population was 10 percent in men and 13 percent in women (based on self-report from a list of seven diseases) and 52 percent in men and 46 percent in women in a primary care practice population (using medical chart abstraction) (Fortin et al., 2010). This variation highlights the importance of reporting the data characteristics as well as the precise multiple chronic disease definition used to allow for comparisons across studies. While there has been no consensus about what diseases to include in a multiple chronic disease definition, a number of studies have used a combination of disease prevalence and disease impact to develop lists of key conditions (Broemeling, Watson, & Prebtani, 2008; Diederrichs, Berger, & Bartels, 2010; O'Halloran, Miller, & Britt, 2004). Although our study did not use a complete list of chronic diseases, the diseases included are identified for inclusion in the literature. Strengths of this study are the use of a clearly defined population and validated disease definitions that permit reproducibility of the data and meaningful comparison of the results with other studies.

Our population estimates of multiple chronic disease prevalence in Ontario are consistent but somewhat lower to previous research from Canada (Broemeling, Watson, & Prebtani, 2008; Fortin et al., 2010; Health Council of Canada, 2007) and abroad (Uijen & van de Lisdonk, 2008) that used self-report data from population health surveys. Based on data from the 2005 Canada Community Health Survey, 12 percent of the Canadian population reported two or more conditions from a list of seven (arthritis, cancer, mood disorders, chronic obstructive pulmonary disease, diabetes, heart disease, and hypertension) (Health Council of Canada, 2007), and estimates ranged from 6 percent in the Northwest Territories to 17 percent in Nova Scotia. Our lower disease prevalence estimates may reflect a real difference in prevalence, but more likely are the result of differences in both the disease definitions and data sources. Importantly, we excluded certain prevalent diseases (such as depression and arthritis) for which we do not yet have valid disease definitions and used very disease-specific case definitions for the diseases we did include. There is no consensus about the accuracy of self-report compared to record-based (chart or health administrative) estimations of disease, and the direction of bias may go either way depending on the

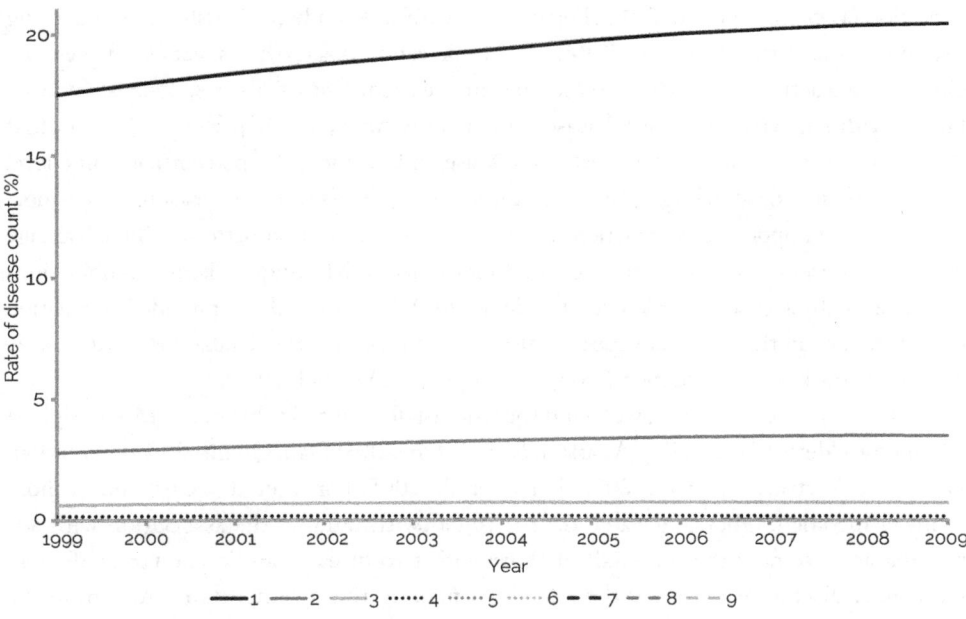

Figure 6.4: Age and Sex-Adjusted Prevalence of Multiple Chronic Diseases, Ontario, 1999 to 2009

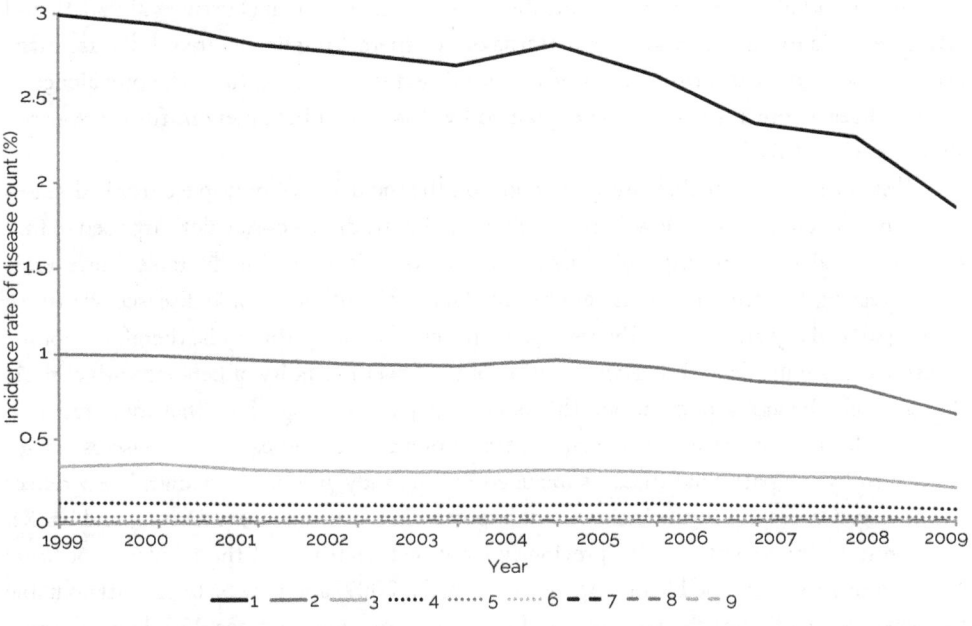

Figure 6.5: Age and Sex-Adjusted Incidence of Multiple Chronic Diseases, Ontario, 1999 to 2009

condition (Benchimol et al., 2010; Fortin et al., 2010). A study in British Columbia using health administrative data and a list of 11 chronic conditions (arthritis, cancer, depression, chronic obstructive pulmonary disease, diabetes, ischemic heart disease, congestive heart failure, asthma, cerebrovascular disease, cardiac arhythmia, and hypertension) found that 35 percent of individuals had at least one disease and, of those, 91 percent had some level of co-morbidity (Broemeling, Watson, & Black, 2005). The summary measures of co-morbidity provide important information about health care utilization patterns. The advantage of using disease-specific definitions of multimorbidity is that unique disease combinations associated with a greater burden can be identified. While we did not provide information for this report on the burden of specific disease combinations, the database structure easily allows for this kind of evaluation (Iron, Gerson, Lu, & Manuel, 2011).

Similar to other research, we found that the risk for multiple chronic disease is highest among the elderly (Broemeling, Watson, & Prebtani, 2008; Data Quality Documentation, Discharge Abstract Database, 2011; Fortin et al., 2005; Fortin et al., 2010) and in those of lower income (Agborsangaya et al., 2012). Notwithstanding the association with advancing age, we note that one half of those with two diseases and one quarter of those with three diseases were under the age of 65, making this an important problem in the younger adult population as well. While female sex has been identified as a risk factor for multiple chronic conditions in population-based studies (Diederrichs, Berger, & Bartels, 2010), in our population more women had one, two, or three diseases, but more men had four or more. A study of multiple chronic disease in a primary care practice population similarly found higher multiple chronic disease prevalence in men (Fortin et al., 2010) and attributed this to differences in the patterns of health-seeking behavior and disease diagnoses between men and women. As health administrative data captures the prevalence of treated disease, our results may be explained by this same phenomenon; future research should explore this further.

This is the first Canadian study to report on the incidence of multiple chronic diseases over time. Given what we know from other population studies, we were not surprised to find that the prevalence of multiple diseases by disease count is increasing. Notable, however, is the decreasing incidence of a number of individual and multiple chronic diseases by disease count, particularly after 2005. The rising prevalence of multimorbidity is, therefore, not increasing disease incidence but a combination of the lower mortality of persons with chronic diseases and the aging population. This is an important finding given that most research on multiple chronic diseases has been limited to prevalence studies. Our disease estimates are driven by the particular diseases included in our study and, in particular, likely reflect the observed decreases in the incidence of hypertension, asthma, heart disease, and stroke. These results are consistent with previously identified decreases in the incidence of heart disease and stroke (Public Health Agency of Canada, 2009) and may be in part attributable to increasing public health awareness and prevention of these diseases. While we found a significant decrease in the incidence of hypertension and asthma, particularly after 2005, previous reports from Ontario (Tu, Zhongliang, & Lipscombe, 2008) found the incidence of hypertension to be increasing and that of asthma to be stable from 1995 through to 2005 (Gershon, Guan, Wang, & To, 2010). It is hard to say if these discrepancies reflect a difference in measurement or a change in disease burden in the population.

Lessons Learned and Future Opportunities

The amount of data included in the Multiple Chronic Disease Database was computational-intensive for the computer systems at ICES, particularly when more complex calculations were required. For example, the calculation of annual disease prevalence by total number of diseases took several days of computing time, and the calculation of incidence by total number of diseases was not possible on the whole data sample. One solution would be to use a random sample, and future efforts will compare the accuracy of this approach and minimum sample sizes required to determine estimates with sufficient power.

Presently our study excludes some important chronic conditions that add significant burden to the patient and health care system, most notably joint disease and depression. Our results should thus be interpreted with this limitation in mind. Efforts to validate definitions for additional diseases are ongoing at ICES, and the database structure is flexible enough that diseases can easily be added or disease definitions altered depending on the research question of interest. While this report looked at multimorbidity by total number of diseases, it will be important to explore the impact of particular disease combinations. For example, a researcher may be interested to know what the timing and total burden of disease accrual is in a patient with newly diagnosed diabetes, or the incidence of a particular disease combination in all patients with diabetes over time.

In the future, we can link the database to additional health administrative datasets to provide information on patterns of health care utilization. Specifically, hospitalizations, family physician visits, specialist visits, emergency department visits, and medication use can be examined. This database is set up in such a way that it is possible to look at different time periods, depending on specific research interest and policy questions. Furthermore, linkages to national population health surveys will reveal the individual impact of multiple chronic diseases, as these surveys have measures of health-related quality of life and self-reported health as well as information on specific health-related behaviours. Finally, all of the data can be explored by geographic region and subpopulation to better identify populations at risk.

CONCLUSION

The strength of this study is the use of clearly defined and validated definitions to ascertain chronic diseases in a large population. These results are an important contribution to what we know in Canada and provide some of the most accurate estimates we have internationally of multiple chronic disease using administrative data.

The Multiple Chronic Disease Database provides an important addition to the information available to researchers, decision-makers, and health care providers on multiple chronic diseases. Our initial study has presented, for the first time, estimates of the prevalence and incidence of disease burden across time for nine chronic illnesses. By continuing to add newly defined diseases to this database, we will continue to expand our understanding of multimorbidity in Canada and to further elucidate the impact that this is having on our health care system. We also hope to be able to distribute the database to make this information on multimorbidity available to those interested in the topic. Furthermore, by continuing to pool administrative disease definitions and making the aggregated data available, we are hoping to begin a dialogue that will allow researchers, decision-makers, and health care providers to better understand this aspect of health and health care in Ontario.

GLOSSARY

Burden: The impact or size of a health problem in an area, measured by cost, mortality, morbidity, or other indicators.

Comorbidity: Disease(s) that coexist in a study participant in addition to the index condition that is the subject of study.

Data quality: The quality of data measured according to its reliability and validity; the completeness and accuracy of a dataset. It is usually measured by comparing the dataset to another one identified as the "gold standard," and assessing the level of agreement.

Health administrative data: Data that is generated through routine administration of health care programs. This information is collected, usually by the government, for some administrative purpose, but not primarily for research or surveillance purposes.

Health-related quality of life: A concept that includes a person's level of functioning, activities of daily living, and ability to participate in society.

Multimorbidity: Co-occurrence of two or more chronic medical conditions in one person.

DISCUSSION QUESTIONS

1. Describe the importance of the validation of identification methods of cohorts derived from health administrative data (see also Benchimol et al., 2010; Manuel, Rosella, & Stunkel, 2010).
2. Define *incidence* and *prevalence*; describe how definitions of incidence and prevalence can differ between clinical studies and studies using health administrative data.
3. Why is it important to identify multimorbidity in populations (see also Boyd & Fortin, 2010)?

REFERENCES

Agborsangaya, C.B., Lau, D., Lahtinen, M., Cooke, T., & Johnson, J.A. (2012). Multimorbidity prevalence and patterns across socioeconomic determinants: A cross-sectional survey. *BMC Public Health, 12*(201).

Benchimol, E., Manuel, D., To, T., Griffiths, A. M., Rabeneck, L., & Guttmann, A. (2010). Development and use of reporting guidelines for assessing the quality of validation studies of health administrative data. *Journal of Clinical Epidemiology, 64*, 821–829.

Boyd, C. M., & Fortin, M. (2010). Future of multimorbidity research: How should understanding of multimorbidity inform health system design? *Public Health Reviews, 32*, 451–474.

Broemeling, A.-M., Watson, D. E., & Black, C. (2005). *Chronic conditions and co-morbidity among residents of British Columbia*. Vancouver: Centre for Health Services and Policy Research, University of British Columbia.

Broemeling, A.-M., Watson, D. E., & Prebtani, F. (2008). Population patterns of chronic health conditions, co-morbidity and healthcare use in Canada: Implications for policy and practice. *Healthcare Quarterly, 11*(3), 70–76.

Canadian Institute for Health Information. (2011). *Data Quality Documentation, National Ambulatory Care Reporting System*. Ottawa: CIHI.

Creatore, M.I., Gozdyra, P., Booth, G. L., Ross, K., & Glazier, R. H. (2007). Socioeconomic status and diabetes. In R. H. Glazier, G. L. Booth, P. Gozdyra, M. I. Creatore, M. Tynan (eds.), *Neighbourhood environments and resources for healthy living—A focus on diabetes in Toronto: ICES atlas* (pp. 35–56). Toronto: Institute for Clinical Evaluative Sciences.

Data Quality Documentation, Discharge Abstract Database. (2011). *2009–2010 executive summary*. Ottawa: CIHI.

Diederrichs, C., Berger, K., & Bartels, D. B. (2010). The measurement of multiple chronic diseases—A systematic review of existing multimorbidity indices. *Journal of Gerontology, Series A, Biological Sciences and Medical Sciences, 66*, 301–311.

Fortin, M., Bravo, G., Hudon, C., Vanasse, A., & Lapointe, L. (2005). Prevalence of multimorbidity among adults seen in family practice. *The Annals of Family Medicine, 3*, 223–228.

Fortin, M., Hudon, C., Haggerty, J., van den Akker, M., & Almirall, J. (2010). Prevalence estimates of multimorbidity: A comparative study of two sources. *BMC Health Services Research, 10*, 111.

Gershon, A. S., Guan, J., Wang, C., & To, T. (2010). Trends in Asthma prevalence and incidence in Ontario, Canada, 1996–2005: A population study. *American Journal of Epidemiology, 172*, 728–736.

Gershon, A. S., Wang, C., Vasilevska-Ristovska, J., Guan, J., Cicutto, L., & To, T. (2009). Identifying patients with physician-diagnosed asthma in health administrative databases. *Canadian Respiratory Journal, 16*, 183–188.

Glazier, R. H., Creatore, M. I., Agha, M. M., & Steele, L. S. (2003). Socioeconomic misclassification in Ontario's health care registry. *Canadian Journal of Public Health, 94*,140–143.

Guttman, A., Nakhla, M., Henderson, M., To, T., Daneman, D., Cauch-Dudek, K., Hux, J. (2010). Validation of a health administrative data algorithm for assessing the epidemiology of diabetes in Canadian children. *Pediatric Diabetes, 11*, 122–128.

Health Council of Canada. (2007). *Population patterns of chronic health conditions in Canada. A data supplement to Why health care renewal matters: Learning from Canadians with chronic health conditions*. Toronto: Health Council of Canada.

Hux, J., Ivis, F., Flintoft, V., & Bica, A. (2002). Diabetes in Ontario: Determination of prevalence and incidence using a validated administrative data algorithm. *Diabetes Care, 25*, 512–516.

Institute for Clinical Evaluative Sciences. (2005). *Improving health care data in Ontario.* ICES investigative report. Toronto: ICES

Iron, K., & Manuel, D. (2007). *Quality Assessment of Administrative Data (QuAAD): An opportunity for enhancing Ontario's health data.* ICES investigative report. Toronto: ICES.

Iron, K., Gerson, A., Lu, H., & Manuel, D. (2011). Using linked administrative data to assess the clinical and system impact of chronic disease in Ontario. *Healthcare Quarterly, 14*(3), 23–27.

Iron, K., Zagorski, B. M., Sykora, K., & Manuel, D. G. (2008). Living and dying in Ontario: An opportunity for improved health information. ICES Investigative Report. Toronto: ICES.

Jaakkimainen, L., Barnsley, J., Klein-Geltink, J., Kopp, A., & Glazier, R. H. (2011). Did changing primary care delivery models change performance? A population-based study using health administrative data. *BMC Family Practice, 12*(44), 1–15.

Kralj, B. (2005). *Measuring "rurality" for purposes of health-care planning: An empirical measure for Ontario.* Toronto: Ontario Medical Association.

Manuel, D., Maaten, S., Rosella, L., Wilson, S., & Ho, T. (2008). *Modeling potential impact of interventions from diabetes prevention, early detection and management: Final Report.* ICES Investigative Report. Toronto: ICES.

Manuel, D., Rosella, L. C., & Stunkel, T. A. (2010). Importance of accurately identifying disease in studies using electronic health records. *BMJ, 7,* 341.

O'Halloran, J., Miller, G. C., & Britt, H. (2004). Defining chronic conditions for primary care with ICPC-2. *Family Practice, 21,* 381–386.

Public Health Agency of Canada. (2007). *Canadian Chronic Disease Surveillance System (CCDSS).* Ottawa: PHAC.

Public Health Agency of Canada. (2009). *Tracking heart disease and stroke in Canada.* Retrieved from http://www.phac-aspc.gc.ca/publicat/2009/cvd-avc/index-eng.php

Schultz, S. E., Rothwell, D. M., Chen, Z., & Tu, K. (2013). Identifying cases of congestive heart failure from administrative data: A validation study using primary care patient records. *Chronic Diseases and Injuries in Canada, 33,* 160–166.

Statistics Canada. (2007). *Leading causes of death in Canada.* Ottawa: Government of Canada.

Statistics Canada. (2010). *Canadian community health survey - Annual component (CCHS).* Ottawa: Government of Canada.

Tu, J. V., Austin, P., Naylor, D. C., Iron, K., & Zhang, H. (1999). *Acute myocardial infarction outcomes in Ontario.* Toronto: ICES.

Tu, K., Zhongliang, C., & Lipscombe, L. L. (2008). Prevalence and incidence of hypertension from 1995 to 2005: A population-based study. *Canadian Medical Association Journal, 178,* 1429–1435.

Tu, K., Campbell, N. R., Chen, Z., Cauch-Dudek, K., & McAlister, F. A. (2007). Accuracy of administrative databases in identifying patients with hypertension. *Open Medicine, 1,* 18–26.

Uijen, A. A., & van de Lisdonk, E. H. (2008). Multimorbidity in primary care: Prevalence and trend over the last 20 years. *European Journal of General Practice, 14*(Suppl. 1), 28–32.

World Health Organization (WHO). (2005). *Facing the facts: The impact of chronic disease in Canada.* Retrieved from http://www.who.int/chp/chronic_disease_report/media/CANADA.pdf

APPENDIX 6.1: CASE ASCERTAINMENT CHARACTERISTICS FOR MULTIPLE CHRONIC DISEASE DATABASE (MCDD), ICES

Disease	Age Groups	Sensitivity	Specificity	NPV	PPV	OHIP	DAD	SDS/NACRS	Diagnostic Codes	Intervention or Procedure	OHIP Fee codes	Wash out	Coverage
Asthma[1]	0-17	89.0%	72.0%			x	x	x	x			5 years	July 1991–present
	18+	84.0%	76.0%										
Congestive Heart Failure[2]		84.8%	97.0%			x	x	x	x			3 years	July 1991–present
Acute Myocardial Infarction[3]	20–105	n/a*	n/a* ('94% self-audited accuracy rates (or higher) at contributing hospitals)	n/a	n/a		x	x	x			1 year	July 1991–present
Diabetes[4,5]	<19					x			x		x	None	July 1991–present
	19					x		x	x		x		
	19+	86.0%	97.0%			x	x	x	x		x		
Hypertension[6]		72.0%	95.0%			x	x	x	x			5 years	April 1988–present
Chronic Obstructive Pulmonary Disease[1]		85.0%	78.4%			x	x	x	x			3 years	April 1988–present
Cerebral Vascular Disease[7]		n/a	n/a	n/a	n/a		x	x	x			none	April 1988–present
Peripheral Vascular Disease[7]		n/a	n/a	n/a	n/a		x	x	x (for exclusions only)	x		none	April 1988–present
End Stage Renal Disease[7]		n/a	n/a	n/a	n/a	x	x	x	x		x	none	April 1988 – present

[1] Gershon et al. 2009
[2] Schultz, Rothwell, Chen, & Tu, 2011
[3] Tu, Austin, Naylor, Iron, & Zhang, 1999
[4] Hux, Ivis, Flintoft, & Bica. 2002
[5] Guttman et al. 2010
[6] Tu et al. 2007
[7] Institute for Clinical Evaluative Sciences, 2005

APPENDIX 6.2: TECHNICAL CASE ASCERTAINMENT DEFINITIONS USED IN MULTIPLE CHRONIC DISEASE DATABASE (MCDD), ICES

Standard Exclusions Applied to All Diseases
• Valid IKN
• Must be present in RPDB
• Dead prior to April 1, 1991
• Dead before diagnosis date
• Born after diagnosis date
• Must live in Ontario
• Valid sex (M, F) in RPDB

Asthma (ICES-Derived Asthma Cohort) (29)	
Time Period	July 1991–present
Case Ascertainment	• 1 hospital admission with an asthma diagnosis code **AND/OR** • 2 OHIP claims with an asthma diagnosis code in 2 years
Washout Period	5 years
Sensitivity/ Specificity	• For 0–17 year olds: 89%/72% • For 18+: 84%/76%
Data Sources	• OHIP (July 1991 forward) • DAD/SDS (April 1991 forward) • NACRS (SDS only) (F2003-04 forward)
Codes Used	• ICD-9: 493 (any type) • ICD-10-CA: J45, J46 (any type) • OHIP dxcode: 493
Notes	• Prevalence starts in 1993 (b/c need 2 years to ascertain a case) • Incidence starts in 1996 • Must live in Ontario at prevalent start date

Congestive Heart Failure (CHF) (ICES-Derived Cohort) (30)	
Time Period	July 1991–present
Case Ascertainment	• 1 hospital admission with a CHF diagnosis code **OR** • 1 OHIP/NACRS record with a CHF diagnosis code, followed within 2 years by another OHIP/NACRS record or a hospital admission with a CHF diagnosis code
Washout Period	3 years
Sensitivity/ Specificity	84.8%/97.0%
Data Sources	• OHIP (July 1991 forward) • DAD/SDS (April 1991 forward) • NACRS (SDS only) (F2003-04 forward) • NACRS (ED only) (F2002-03 forward) • OHMRS (October 2005 forward)
Codes Used	• ICD-9: 428 (any type) • ICD-10-CA: I50.0, I50.1, I50.9 (any type) • OHIP dxcode: 428 (only 1 rec per person per service date)

Ontario Myocardial Infarction Database (OMID) (ICES Derived Cohort) (31)	
Time Period	April 1991–present
Case Ascertainment	· 1 hospital admission with an AMI diagnosis code (MRDx only) **AND** · **NO** other AMI diagnosis code with a type 2 on same record **AND** · None of the exclusion criteria listed below are applicable.
Washout Period	1 year
Sensitivity/ Specificity	N/A
Data Sources	DAD (April 1991 forward)
Codes Used	· ICD-9: 410 · ICD-10-CA: I21
Notes	Exclusion criteria applied to cohort: · Non-first visit within an episode of care · Missing Year · Invalid gender, i.e., SEX ≠ M or F · Non-acute care hospital admission · Non-Ontario resident by looking at the 1st two digits of RESCODE · Age < 20 or Age > 105 · Transfer from another acute care hospital · Patient signed out or Discharge with a LOS < 3 days **and** patient was **NOT** transferred **to** another acute care hospital · Non-valid Health Card number, i.e. invalid IKN · The **main** doctor service code was one of these:

ICD-9:

o 30 General Surgery
o 32 Neurosurgery
o 33 Oral Surgery
o 34 Orthopaedic Surgery
o 35 Plastic Surgery
o 36 Thoracic Surgery
o 37 Transplant Surgery
o 38 Unknown and reference can't be located
o 39 Urology
o 50 Obstetrics & Gynaecology
o 60 Otolaryngology
o 62 Ophthalmology
o 64 Psychiatry
o 87 Dentistry
o 95 Unknown and reference can't be located

ICD-10-CA:

o 00030 General Surgery
o 00032 Neurosurgery
o 01003 Oral Surgery
o 00034 Orthopaedic Surgery
o 00035 Plastic Surgery
o 00036 Thoracic Surgery
o 00037 Transplant Surgery
o 00039 Urology
o 00050 Obstetrics & Gynaecology
o 00060 Otolaryngology
o 00062 Ophthalmology
o 00064 Psychiatry
o 00073 General Surgical Oncology
o 01000 Dentistry Group
o 01001 Dentist
o 01002 Dental Surgeon
o 01004 Orthodontist
o 01005 Paedodontist
o 01006 Periodontist
o 01007 Oral Pathologist
o 01008 Endodontist
o 01009 Oral Pathologist
o 01010 Dental Hygienist/Assistant
o 01011 Dental Mechanic

Ontario Diabetes Database (ODD) (ICES-Derived Cohort) (32;33)	
Time Period	July 1991–present
Case Ascertainment (Pediatric < 19 yrs. old)	• 4 OHIP dxcode claims **OR** • 1 OHIP feecode in 2 years and at least 1 OHIP claim prior to 19th birth date
Case Ascertainment (Bridge)	• 1 or 2 OHIP dxcode claims prior to 19th birth date **AND** • 1 OHIP claim after 19th birth date within 2 years *(19th birth date is used as incident date)*
Case Ascertainment (Adult)	• 2 OHIP dxcodes **OR** • 1 OHIP feecode **OR** • 1 CIHI admission after 19th birth date
Washout Period	None
Sensitivity/ Specificity	86%/97% for the original algorithm
Data Sources	• OHIP (July 1991 forward) • DAD/SDS (April 1988 forward) • NACRS (SDS only) (F2003-04 forward)
Codes Used	• ICD-9: 250 (any type) • ICD-10-CA: E10, E11, E13, E14 (any type) • OHIP dxcode: 250 • OHIP feecode: Q040, K029, K030
Notes	• Gestational Diabetes records excluded • Incidence not reported for first 3 years

Hypertension (ICES-Derived Cohort) (34)	
Time Period	July 1988–present
Case Ascertainment	• 1 hospital admission with a hypertension diagnosis code **OR** • 1 OHIP record with a hypertension diagnosis code, followed within 2 years by another OHIP record or a hospital admission with a hypertension diagnosis code
Washout Period	5 years
Sensitivity/ Specificity	• 72%/95% • PPV-87%; NPV-88%
Data Sources	• OHIP (July 1991 forward) • DAD/SDS (April 1988 forward) • NACRS (SDS only) (F2003-04 forward)
Codes Used	• ICD-9: 401x, 402x, 403x, 404x, 405x (any type) • ICD-10-CA: I10, I11, I12, I13, I15 (any type) • OHIP dxcode: 401, 402, 403, 404, 405 (any type)
Notes	• Gestational hypertension records excluded • Generic exclusions do not apply to this cohort

Chronic Obstructive Pulmonary Disease (COPD)(ICES-Derived Cohort) (29)

Time Period	April 1988–present
Case Ascertainment	• 1 hospital admission with a COPD diagnosis code **OR** • 1 OHIP record with a COPD diagnosis code
Washout Period	6 years
Sensitivity/ Specificity	85.0%/78.4%
Data Sources	• OHIP (July 1991 forward) • DAD/SDS (April 1988 forward) • NACRS (SDS only) (F2003-04 forward)
Codes Used	• ICD-9: 491, 492, 496 (any type) • ICD-10-CA: J41, J42, J43, J44 (any type) • OHIP dxcode: 491, 492, 496
Notes	• Sensitive definition used • Includes only people age 35–99 years • Incidence 1994 forward

Cerebral Vascular Disease (CVD) (12)

Time Period	April 1988–present
Case Ascertainment	1 hospital admission with a CVD diagnosis code
Washout Period	None
Sensitivity/ Specificity	N/A
Data Sources	• DAD/SDS (April 1988 forward) • NACRS (SDS only) (F2003-04 forward)
Codes Used	• ICD-9: 430, 431, 432, 434, 436 (any type) • ICD-10-CA: I60, I61, I62, I63, I64, G46 (any type)
Notes	• Definition from the undiagnosed diabetes study

Peripheral Vascular Disease (PVD) (12)

Time Period	April 1988–present
Case Ascertainment	• 1 hospital admission with a PVD intervention code **AND** • Without specified diagnosis codes on the same abstract
Washout Period	None
Sensitivity/ Specificity	N/A
Data Sources	• DAD/SDS (April 1988 forward) • NACRS (SDS only) (F2003-04 forward)

Codes Used	*Major:*
	• CCP: 96.14, 96.15
	• CCI: 1VQ93, 1VC93, 1VG93
	Minor:
	• CCP: 96.11, 96.12, 96.13 WITHOUT
	  o ICD-9: 170, 171, 213, 730, 740-759, 800-900, 901-904, 940-950 **on the abstract**
	• CCI: 1WL93, 1WA93, 1WE93, 1WJ93, 1WM93 **WITHOUT**
	  o ICD-10-CA: C40, C41, C46.1, C47, C49, D16.0, M46.2, M86, M87, M89.6, M90.0-M90.5, Q00, Q38-Q40, S02.0, S09.0, S15, S25, T26 **on the abstract**

	Bypass:
	• CCP: 51.25, 51.29, 50.18 **WITHOUT**
	   o ICD-9: 4141, 441, 442 **on the abstract**
	• CCI: 1KG50, 1KG57, 1KG76, 1KG35HAC1, 1KG35HHC1 **WITHOUT**
	   o ICD-10-CA: I67.1, I71, I72, I60, I77.0, I79.0, Q codes **on the abstract**

Notes	Definition from the undiagnosed diabetes study

End Stage Renal Disease (ESRD) (12)

Time Period	April 1988–present
Case Ascertainment	• 1 hospital admission with a ESRD diagnosis code or a kidney transplant code **OR** • 1 OHIP dxcode or feecode for blindness, hypertensive retinopathy, retinal photocoagulation or eye vitreous vitrectomy
Washout Period	None
Sensitivity/ Specificity	N/A
Data Sources	• OHIP (July 1991 forward) • DAD/SDS (April 1988 forward) • NACRS (SDS only) (F2003-04 forward)
Codes Used	• ICD-9: 584, 585, 586, 4039, 4049, 7885 (any type) • ICD-10-CA: N17, N18, N19, I12, I13, R34 (any type) • OHIP dxcode: 369, 362 • OHIP feecode: E154, E148
Notes	Definition from the undiagnosed diabetes study

CHAPTER 7

Exploring the Social Determinants of Mental Health Service Use Using Intersectionality Theory and CART Analysis*

John Cairney, Scott Veldhuizen, Simone Vigod, David L. Streiner, Terrance J. Wade, and Paul Kurdyak

TAKE-HOME MESSAGE

- Most research examining how social positions are associated with health and health service use outcomes relies on statistical models of competing risks, which test the independent contribution of multiple social positions. Theoretically, this approach is problematic and may misrepresent relationships because it does not take into account the fact that people occupy multiple social positions that may interact in complex ways to predict a variety of health and health service use outcomes. This view is sometimes referred to as the *double* or *triple jeopardy* hypothesis.
- While theoretically intuitive, intersectionality is difficult to explore methodologically. Linear regression models examining intersectionality through statistical interactions require large sample sizes, produce models that are complex and difficult to interpret, are often plagued by multicollinearity and other problems, and assume linear relationships between variables.
- A possible solution is to use a Classification and Regression Tree (CART) approach that does not depend on the same assumptions of traditional linear regression. The CART approach involves recursively identifying rules that distinguish between groups, usually with certain constraints to avoid over-fitting.
- Although it does not permit the formal testing of hypotheses, CART has three important advantages: it makes no assumptions about variable distributions or relationships; it is capable of identifying complex and unsuspected interactions; and its results yield decision rules that can be used to identify at-risk individuals more instinctively than traditional linear regression coefficients.

* This chapter first appeared as an a article in 2014 in the *Journal of Epidemiology and Community Health*, Volume 68, Issue 2. It is rerpoduced with permission from BMJ Publishing Group Limited.

INTRODUCTION

Although effective treatments for mental health conditions such as depression and anxiety have been available for some time, fewer than half of individuals with a mental disorder seek formal care from a primary care physician or psychiatrist (Andrews, Henderson, & Hall, 2001; Kessler et al., 1994; Wang et al., 2005). Understanding the factors predicting mental health care–seeking behaviours is crucial for the formulation of health policy and the design of interventions to address mental health service access inequities.

In what is arguably the most influential model of health care utilization, Andersen (Andersen, 1995; Andersen, 2008; Andersen & Newman, 1973) proposed three sets of factors, which together can be used to predict use of services at the individual and population levels: predisposing, enabling, and need factors. Predisposing and enabling factors are composed mostly, though not exclusively, of social (e.g., gender, age) and economic (e.g., household income) variables, whereas need factors are indicators of objective need (e.g., presence of a health condition) and perceived need (e.g., self-rated health) for care. In an equitable system, need for care should be the most important determinant of service use. As such, the identification of non-need factors associated with service use serves a critical role in assessing systems of care. When factors such as gender, socioeconomic status, or insurance coverage are found to influence use, it raises questions about possible inequities. Examination of enabling and predisposing factors that predict mental health care service use is especially pertinent, given the long-standing concern over stigma associated with having a disorder (Leong & Zachar, 1999) and with seeking care for it (MacKenzie, Gekoski, & Knox, 2006).

A variety of predisposing and enabling factors have been identified as non-need determinants of use of mental health care services. These include age (Klap, Unroe, & Unützer, 2003; Lin et al., 1996), gender (Bland, Newman, & Orn, 1997; Kessler et al., 1994; Kessler, Chiu, et al., 2005; Parslow & Jorm, 2000), socioeconomic status (Parslow & Jorm, 2000; Steele et al., 2007; Steele, Glazier, & Lin, 2006), ethnicity (Hyman, 2001; Laroche, 2000; Wang et al., 2005; Whitley, Kirmayer, & Groleau, 2006), and marital status (Cairney et al., 2004). As several of these factors are social status positions, concerns around equity appear to be legitimate. It is not clear, however, that the influence of these factors has been thoroughly examined.

Existing research on social factors associated with mental health service use rely on statistical models of competing risks. Need and non-need factors are tested simultaneously, and those effects that are statistically significant become the focus of interpretation. With respect to social determinants, this approach is problematic, because it does not take into account the fact that the social positions occupied by each individual may interact in complex ways. The circumstances of a teenaged single mother, for example, may not be adequately described by the independent effects of marital status, parent status, age, and gender.

Intersectionality theory (e.g., Atkinson & Therneau, 2000; Cairney, Veldhuizen, & Wade, 2010) challenges us to consider social determinants not in terms of single factors (e.g., gender or SES), but in terms of multiple, interacting factors. In this framework, social disadvantage arises from a constellation of interrelated and intersecting social roles. This view, sometimes referred to as the double or triple jeopardy hypothesis, has informed considerable research on health. Applications in the mental health care utilization literature include work showing that single mothers are more likely to seek care for mental health problems than their married counterparts (Cairney, Boyle, Lipman, & Racine, 2004).

While intuitive, intersectionality is difficult to explore empirically. In linear models, interactions involving more than two variables tend to require large sample sizes, and also to produce models that are complex, difficult to interpret, and often plagued by multicollinearity or other problems. Moreover, interactions involving non-linear effects are usually difficult to detect. Something as apparently simple as an age-by-sex interaction, for example, can be complicated not only by a non-linear association between age and the outcome, but by the fact that the interaction with sex may itself vary with age in a non-linear way.

One solution to this problem is to eschew linear models entirely. Classification Trees (CART) are one alternative popular in machine learning and data mining applications (Health Canada, 2006; Lemon, Roy, & Clark, 2003; Marshall, 2000). The CART approach involves recursively identifying rules that distinguish between groups, usually with certain constraints to avoid over-fitting. Although it does not permit the testing of hypotheses in the usual sense, CART has two important advantages: (1) it makes no assumptions about variable distributions or relationships; and (2) it is capable of identifying complex and unsuspected interactions. CART results can also be useful from a clinical and health policy perspective, because they yield decision rules that can be used to identify at-risk individuals more easily than, for example, regression coefficients.

In the present study, we use CART to examine the social determinants of mental health service use in a general population sample. Specifically, we are interested in exploring complex interactions between different social determinants and their impact on mental health care use. Our focus on social determinants is related to Andersen's concern regarding equity: in a country with a "universal" health care system (Gravel & Béland, 2005), it is critical to evaluate whether factors other than need are influencing use of services.

METHODS

Data come from Cycle 1.2 of the Canadian Community Health Survey (CCHS 1.2), a population survey conducted by Statistics Canada in 2002–2003 (Wang, Nie, & Upshur, 2009). The sampling frame of CCHS 1.2 included all Canadians aged 15 or older living in private dwellings, with the exception of full-time members of the armed forces and residents of remote areas or First Nations reserves. The final sample size was 36,984. Statistics Canada linked participants from Ontario (n=13,184) to administrative health data; 10,600 (81 percent) were linked successfully. From this sample, we selected all participants (n=1,213) who met past-year criteria for one or more of five mood and anxiety disorders, with and without substance dependence. The merged dataset was accessed at the Institute for Clinical Evaluative Sciences.

MEASURES

Outpatient Mental Health Service Use

We used physician billing records in the Ontario Health Insurance Plan (OHIP) database to determine whether each respondent used physician-provided mental health services in the year following the survey. In Ontario, medically necessary care coverage is fully financed by a government-funded health insurance program. Within this universal health care coverage setting, 94 percent of physicians have a fee-for-service practice that is captured by OHIP billing submission data (Steele et al., 2004), and physicians who provide services on a salary are mandated to submit "shadow billings" for accountability purposes, resulting in a highly accurate and comprehensive physician activity data source. A visit for mental health care was defined as any outpatient encounter with a psychiatrist, or a visit with a primary care provider (e.g., family physician) or geriatrician with both a mental health and/or addictions ICD-9 diagnosis and a mental health and/or addictions service billing code. Mental health visits with a primary care provider or geriatrician are defined based on a validated algorithm developed by Steele and colleagues (Steele, Glazier, Lin, & Evans, 2004), with modifications to include contacts with specialist physicians.

Mental Disorders

CCHS 1.2 assessed all respondents for six conditions (major depressive disorder, bipolar disorder, social phobia, panic disorder, agoraphobia, and substance abuse or dependence) based on symptom reporting in the 12 months prior to the time of the survey, using the World Mental Health–Composite International Diagnostic Interview (WMH-CIDI). The WMH-CIDI was developed and validated using the Structured Clinical Interview for DSM-IV (SCID) as a reference standard, and is now widely used in epidemiological surveys (Kessler et al., 1994; McGibbon, 2009). In CCHS 1.2, the WMH-CIDI was administered by trained lay interviewers. Details of the administration and psychometric properties of the measure are provided in Gravel and Béland (2005).

Social Determinants

We selected eight variables capturing different social factors previously shown to be associated with the use of mental health care: age (in years), gender (males, females), marital status (married or cohabitating, formerly married [including separated, divorced, or widowed], never married), parental status (parent living with children, other), income adequacy (low, moderate, or high), education (less than secondary, secondary graduate, some post-secondary, post-secondary graduate), rurality (rural, urban), and visible minority status (white, visible minority). Age was entered as a continuous variable; all others were dummy-coded. Income adequacy is a derived variable, produced by Statistics

Canada, that combines household income and household size. Household incomes are "low," in 2002 Canadian dollars, if they are less than $15,000 for 1–2 residents, less than $20,000 for 3–4 residents, or less than $30,000 for 5 or more residents.

ANALYSIS

We conducted descriptive, univariate, and logistic regression analyses. For the logistic regression models, we modelled any service use and specialist care. We used Stata 9 for these analyses, and bootstrapped all statistical tests using a set of replication weights supplied by Statistics Canada.

We performed CART analyses using the rpart package and R 2.13. We used the Gini index, a measure of heterogeneity that reflects the difference across groups in the probability of the outcome, to select decision rules. We required a minimum terminal node size of 30 individuals and assigned cost weights of [(1–P) / P] to cases (where P is the prevalence, in this case of help-seeking) and 1 to non-cases. This weighting scheme yields equal sums of weights for cases and non-cases, and therefore assigns equal importance to sensitivity and specificity. This is comparable to the weighting used implicitly in, for example, receiver operating characteristic curve analysis. After fitting, trees were "pruned" by retaining the set of decision rules that minimized the cross-validated error. In the CART analysis, we modelled the "any service use" outcome only, as the sample size for specialist care (n=312) was too small to produce meaningful results.

To take into account the complex design of CCHS 1.2, we applied sampling weights in the CART analysis. We used the master survey weights provided by Statistics Canada, rescaled to have a mean of 1.

RESULTS

The prevalence of any past-year disorder was 9.2 percent (unweighted n=1213; 95% CI = 8.6% to 9.9%). Twenty-four percent (unweighted n=312) of people with a disorder had one or more mental health consultations in the year following the survey. Of those who sought care, 52 percent had seen a psychiatrist in the year preceding the survey. In the univariate analysis (not shown), service use was significantly associated with female gender, low income adequacy, and greater age.

Table 7.1 shows the results of two logistic regression models: one for any service use and one for use of specialist services. Initial analyses revealed that the association between age and any service was not linear. For this outcome, we therefore included two non-linear variables for age, obtained with Stata's fracpoly procedure. For any service use, age, gender, and marital status were significant in the main effects model. Age terms for this outcome yielded an inverted U form, with probability of service use lowest at the youngest and oldest ages and peaking at approximately age 55. Women (OR=1.64; 95% CI=1.03–2.60) and those who were never married (OR=1.88; 95% CI=1.04–3.39) were more likely

Table 7.1: Logistic Regression Models Predicting Any Service Use and Use of Specialist Care

	Any Service Use (n=1213)		Specialist Care (n=312)	
	OR (95% CI)	p	OR (95% CI)	p
Age				
Linear			1.02 (0.99–1.05)	0.20
Age^0.5	13.8 (3.4–56.0)	<0.001		
Age^3	0.99 (0.989–0.998)	0.003		
Female	1.6 (1–2.6)	0.04	0.4 (0.1–0.9)	0.02
Education				
< Secondary	1 (0.5–1.8)	0.95	1.3 (0.4–4)	0.62
Secondary	(reference)	0.77	(reference)	0.65
Some post-secondary	0.9 (0.4–1.9)	0.34	0.7 (0.1–3.3)	0.75
Post-secondary graduate	1.3 (0.8–2.1)		1.2 (0.4–3.4)	
Marital status				
Married	(reference)	0.09	(reference)	0.12
Formerly married	1.6 (0.9–2.7)	0.04	0.5 (0.2–1.2)	0.75
Never married	1.9 (1–3.4)		1.2 (0.5–3)	
Visible minority	0.8 (0.3–2)	0.60	1.4 (0.3–7.2)	0.66
Parent	1.2 (0.7–2)	0.54	0.8 (0.3–1.8)	0.57
Low income adequacy	1.5 (0.9–2.7)	0.15	1.2 (0.5–3.1)	0.66
Rural residence	0.8 (0.3–1.9)	0.55	1 (0.2–5.2)	0.98

to have sought any care for mental health than men and those who were married, respectively. Only one variable, gender, significantly predicted specialist care among those who had consulted a physician: this outcome was less common among women (OR=0.36, 95% CI=0.15–0.87). This effect, however, largely reflects the fact that women were more likely to have consulted a primary care provider, and thus to be included in this analysis. In the sample as a whole, men and women were equally likely to have consulted a specialist (men, 13.7%, 95% CI=10.5–17.0%; women, 13.1%, 95% CI=9.3–16.9%).

Classification and Regression Tree (CART) Analysis

The final Classification Tree for any service use included decision rules based on four of the eight social determinant variables included in this study: age, sex, income adequacy, and marital status. Detailed results are shown in Figure 7.1 and Table 7.2. Groups more likely to use services were formerly-married men aged 23 to 46; all participants older than 46; and low-income women aged 23 to 46. Although CART decision rules do not necessarily reflect meaningful or replicable difference, the final tree implies the possibility that income adequacy plays an important role among women, while marital status is of greater importance among men. In terms of overall fit, the effectiveness of the tree as a classifier was moderate, with overall agreement of 60 percent, sensitivity of 82 percent, and specificity of 53 percent.

Table 7.2: Detailed Classification and Regression Tree (CART) Results for Any Service Use

Nodes	People	Prediction	Proportions	
			No	Yes
Root				
Age under 23	266	No	0.92	0.08
Age 23+				
Age 47+	315	Yes	0.63	0.37
Age 23 to 46				
Male				
Not formerly married	223	No	0.86	0.14
Formerly married	47	Yes	0.60	0.40
Female				
Not low income	278	No	0.72	0.28
Low income	84	Yes	0.48	0.52

DISCUSSION

We applied two different methods to explore the social determinants of mental health service use in a population-based sample linked to health administrative data. The results of the conventional regression analysis demonstrated that physician mental health service use has a complex relationship with age, and is positively associated with being female and never having been married. This is broadly consistent with previous research (Bland, Newman, & Orn, 1997; Kessler, Chiu et al., 2005; Kessler et al., 1994; Klap, Unroe, & Unützer, 2003; Lin et al., 1996; Parslow & Jorm, 2000).

The CART analysis also supports the finding of a complex relationship between age and service use, but in addition it suggests interactions between gender and other social determinants that were not apparent in the regression analysis. Marital status, for example, appeared to be more important among young and middle-aged men (from approximately age 25 to 50), while income adequacy played a larger role among women.

To our knowledge, this is the first study that shows the complex interactions of gender, age, income, and marital status to be associated with use of mental health services in the formal health care sector. The comparison of regression and the CART models in our study confirm that the inability of linear models to identify complex interactions is a limitation. When such interactions are likely to be present, data mining techniques merit serious consideration.

Our results are broadly consistent with intersectionality theory (Cairney, Veldhuizen, & Wade, 2010; Atkinson & Therneau, 2000), which holds that health outcomes (including service use) are differentially affected by multiple, interacting facets of social advantage and disadvantage. Our results are also consistent with empirical work on the social determinants of

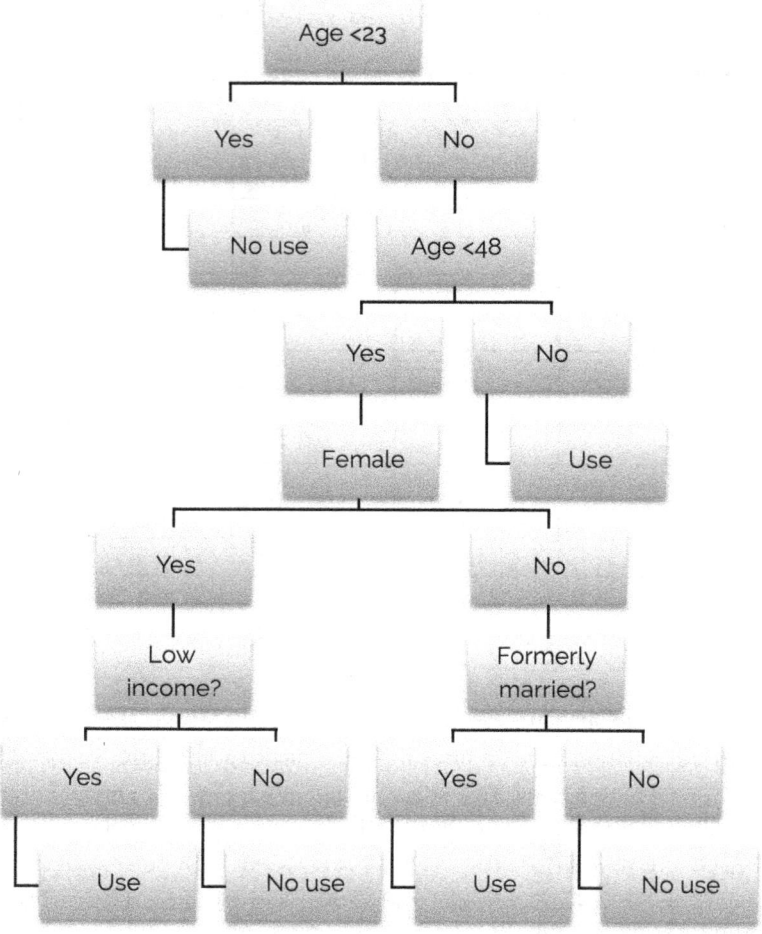

Figure 7.1: Final Classification and Regression Tree, Any Service Use 12 Months
Following Survey

health care use, showing use of services to be influenced by the joint effects of parental status, marital status, and gender. For example, single parent mothers have been shown to be much more likely to use mental health care services than married mothers (Cairney et al., 2004).

Importantly, our findings raise some important concerns about the role of non-need factors as important determinants of mental health care use in a public system. Splits involving age highlight the low levels of service use among young people. This may reflect, in part, the lower propensity of young people to use treatment services (Mackenzie, Gekoski, & Knox, 2006). For young and middle-aged men, consultations were more common among those who were separated or divorced. Although CART does not tell us whether this effect differs significantly between the sexes, one interpretation of this result is that the loss of spousal support increases the likelihood of help-seeking in the formal care sector. The role of low income among young and middle-aged women may also bear further examination. Greater contact with social services might facilitate contact with the medical sector. Conversely, higher-income women may be able to access mental health care from non-physicians (e.g., psychologists). Variables such as marital status and income may also function, in part, as indicators of illness type (e.g., substance-related) or severity. Nevertheless, results suggest the presence of intriguing differences between men and women in the importance of these social variables as determinants of mental health service use. Bearing in mind the limited sample and the nature of the methods used, we would cautiously suggest that differential use of services by men and women is itself conditioned by other social factors (notably social support and income). While women have may a greater propensity to seek care, results suggest that this is not a simple gender difference, and that interactions with other social and structural factors influence help-seeking for mental health.

There are several limitations that warrant caution when drawing conclusions based on these results. One concerns the difficulty CART methods experience in treating continuous variables: although true age effects are usually incremental, CART is obliged to select specific cut-off points. More important is the fact that CART is an exploratory technique unsuited to hypothesis testing. This makes replication of these results in a different dataset imperative. At present, no such comparable data exist in Ontario. However, a new national survey of mental health is currently underway, and if these data can be linked to health administrative data as has been done for CCHS 1.2, it will be possible to test these classifications using comparable data.

We have also limited our analysis to social determinants. There are many other factors related to need (e.g., severity, co-morbidity), the health care system (e.g., availability of psychiatrists), and cultural or individual characteristics (e.g., personality, perception of stigma) that influence help-seeking, and these are best considered together. Sample size and other data limitations circumscribed our analysis. Future work, however, may be able to explore how these other factors interact with social determinants in shaping help-seeking behavior.

Further, we included all individuals meeting diagnostic criteria for one or more of the six disorders included in CCHS 1.2. This approach has well-known drawbacks (Kurdyak & Gnam, 2005). Individuals with other disorders (e.g., generalised anxiety disorder) were not included unless they also had one of the six mentioned; and, more importantly, not everyone who meets diagnostic criteria requires formal care.

Finally, unmet need in our sample was, at almost 75 percent, somewhat higher than previous estimates. Research based on self-report has estimated this proportion at 66 percent (Kessler, Demler, et al., 2005). One explanation for this discrepancy is that we had no data on non-physician services. Some individuals without service use in our data may have been adequately treated by other providers, especially if suffering from mild to moderate illness.

Strengths should also be acknowledged. By using survey data to identify individuals in need of care and administrative data to identify service use, we address two important methodological issues: recall and other biases associated with the self-report of care, and the problem of relying solely on treatment data to define need. The combination of both data sources allows us to first measure untreated prevalence and then examine service use in this sample.

CONCLUSION

Using a data mining technique, we identified a set of complex interactions not apparent using more conventional methods. While further research (including replication) is needed, we believe the approach used in this paper warrants serious consideration as a method for understanding factors associated with help-seeking in general, and mental health care in particular.

GLOSSARY

Classification and Regression Tree (CART): A data-mining technique using machine-learning methods to build prediction models.

DSM-IV: *Diagnostic and Statistical Manual of Mental Disorders*, Fourth Edition, from the American Psychiatric Association, used to classify psychiatric disorders.

ICD-9: *International Classification of Diseases*, Ninth Edition, by the World Health Organization, used to promote international comparability of disease and treatment.

Income adequacy: A measure of income that takes into account the number of persons in the household being supported by that income.

Logistic regression: A regression model that uses a binary outcome (e.g., yes/no) as the outcome variable that yields findings based on an odds ratio, modelling the likelihood of an outcome occurring over the likelihood of it not occurring.

Sample weights: A factor that differentially gives greater or lesser influence to a sample participant based on the number of people that participant represents in the target population.

DISCUSSION QUESTIONS

1. Discuss other possible areas in health research where the double or triple jeopardy hypothesis is plausible and how you would implement a CART-based analysis to address it.
2. Identify two or three findings in the health literature examining how various social positions are connected to health and/or health service use outcomes, and assess whether they have miss-specified the results based on their choice of methodology.
3. One of the most common findings in psychiatric epidemiology is the roughly two-fold higher prevalence rate of depression and mood disorders among women compared to men. Discuss how a CART analysis may alter this by considering how additional social positions (e.g., age, race, poverty) may influence this finding.

REFERENCES

Andersen, R. M. (1995). Revisiting the behavioral model and access to medical care: Does it matter? *Journal of Health and Social Behavior, 36*, 1–10.

Andersen, R. M. (2008). National heath surveys and the behavioral model of health services use. *Medical Care, 46*, 647–653.

Andersen, R. M., & Newman, J. F. (1973). Societal and individual determinants of medical care utilization in the United States. *The Milbank Quarterly, 51*, 95–124.

Andrews, G., Henderson, S., & Hall, W. (2001). Prevalence, comorbidity, disability and service utilization. Overview of the Australian National Mental Health Survey. *British Journal of Psychiatry, 178*, 145–53.

Atkinson, E. J, & Therneau, T. M. (2000). *An introduction to recursive partitioning using the RPART routines*. Rochester, MN: Mayo Foundation.

Bland, R. C., Newman, S. C., & Orn, H. (1997). Health care utilization for emotional problems: Results from a community survey. *Canadian Journal of Psychiatry, 42*, 935–942.

Cairney, J., Boyle, M. H., Lipman, E., & Racine, Y. (2004). Single mothers and the use of professionals for mental health care reasons. *Social Science & Medicine, 59*, 2535–2546.

Cairney, J., Veldhuizen, S., & Wade, T. J. (2010). Intersecting social statuses and psychiatric disorder: New conceptual directions in the social epidemiology of mental disorder. In J. Cairney & D. L. Streiner (eds.), Mental Disorder in Canada (pp. 48–70). Toronto: University of Toronto Press.

Gravel, R., & Béland, Y. (2005). The Canadian community health survey: Mental health and well-being. *Canadian Journal of Psychiatry, 50*, 573–590.

Health Canada. (2006). *Canada Health Act: Annual report 2005–2006*. Retrieved from http://www.hc-sc.gc.ca/hcs-sss/alt_formats/hpb-dgps/pdf/pubs/chaar-ralcs-0506/chaar-ralcs-0506-eng.pdf

Hyman, I. (2001) *Immigration and health*. Health policy working paper series, working paper 01-05. Ottawa: Health Canada.

Kessler, R. C., Chiu, W. T., Demler, O., Merikangas, K. R., & Walters, E. E. (2005). Prevalence, severity, comorbidity of 12-month DSM-IV disorders in the National Comorbidity Survey Replication. *Archives of General Psychiatry, 62*, 617–627.

Kessler, R. C., Demler, O., Frank, R. G., Olfson, M., Pincus, H. A., Walters, E. E., Wang, P., Wells, K. B., & Zaslavsky, A. M. (2005). Prevalence and treatment of mental disorders, 1990 to 2003. *New England Journal of Medicine, 352*(24), 2515–2523.

Kessler, R. C., McGonagle, K. A., Zhao, S., Nelson, C. B., Hughes, M., Eshleman, S., Wittchen, H. U., & Kendler, K. S. (1994). Lifetime and 12-month prevalence of DSM-III-R psychiatric disorders in the United States. Results from the National Comorbidity Survey. *Archive of General Psychiatry, 51*, 8–19.

Kessler, R. C., & Ustün, T. B. (2004). The World Mental Health (WMH) Survey Initiative version of the World Health Organization (WHO) Composite International Diagnostic Interview (CIDI). *The International Journal of Methods in Psychiatric Research, 13*(2), 93–121.

Klap, R., Unroe, K. T., & Unützer, J. (2003). Caring for mental illness in the United States: A focus on older adults. *American Journal of Geriatric Psychiatry, 11*, 517–524.

Kurdyak, P. A., & Gnam, W. H. (2005). Small signal, big noise: Performance of the CIDI depression module. *Canadian Journal of Psychiatry, 50*(13), 851–856.

Laroche, M. (2000). Health status and health services utilization of Canada's immigrant and non-immigrant populations. *Canadian Public Policy, 26*, 51–73.

Lemon, S. C., Roy J., & Clark, M. A. (2003). Classification and regression tree analysis in public health: Methodological review and comparison with logistic regression. *Annals of Behavioral Medicine, 26*(3), 172–181.

Leong, F. T. L., & Zachar, P. (1999). Gender and opinions about mental illness as predictors of attitudes toward seeking professional psychological help. *British Journal of Guidance & Counselling, 27*(1), 123–132.

Lin, E., Goering, P., Offord, D. R., Campbell, D., & Boyle, M. H. (1996). The use of mental health services in Ontario: Epidemiologic findings. *Canadian Journal of Psychiatry, 41*, 572–577.

Mackenzie, C. S., Gekoski, W. L., & Knox, V. J. (2006). Age, gender, and the underutilization of mental health services: The influence of help-seeking attitudes. *Aging & Mental Health, 10*(6), 574–582.

Marshall, R. J. (2000). The use of classification and regression trees in clinical epidemiology. *Journal of Clinical Epidemiology, 54*, 603–609.

McGibbon, E. (2009). Health and health care: A human rights perspective. In D. Raphael (ed.), *The social determinants of health* (2nd ed., pp. 319–339). Toronto: Canadian Scholar's Press.

Parslow, R. A., & Jorm, A. F. (2000). Who uses mental health services in Australia? An analysis of data from the National Survey of Mental Health and Wellbeing. *Australian and New Zealand Journal of Psychiatry, 34*, 997–1008.

Steele, L. S., Glazier, E., & Lin, E. (2006). Inequity in mental health care under Canadian universal health coverage. *Psychiatric Services, 57*, 317–324.

Steele, L. S., Dewa, C. S., Lin E., & Lee, K. L. (2007). Education level, income level and mental health services use in Canada: Associations and policy implications. *Healthcare Policy, 3*, 96–106.

Steele, L. S., Glazier, R. H., Lin, E., & Evans, M. (2004). Using administrative data to measure ambulatory mental health service provision in primary care. *Medical Care, 42*, 960–965.

Wang, L., Nie, J. X., & Upshur, R. E. G. (2009). Determining use of preventive health care in Ontario: Comparison of 3 maneuvers in administrative and survey data. *Canadian Family Physician, 55*, 178–179.e15.

Wang, P. S., Lane, M., Olfson, M., Pincus, H. A., Wells, K. B., & Kessler, R. C. (2005). Twelve-month use of mental health services in the United States: Results from the National Comorbidity Survey Replication. *Archive of General Psychiatry, 62*, 629–640.

Whitley, R., Kirmayer, L. J., & Groleau, D. (2006). Understanding immigrants' reluctance to use mental health services: A qualitative study from Montreal. *Canadian Journal of Psychiatry, 51*, 205–209.

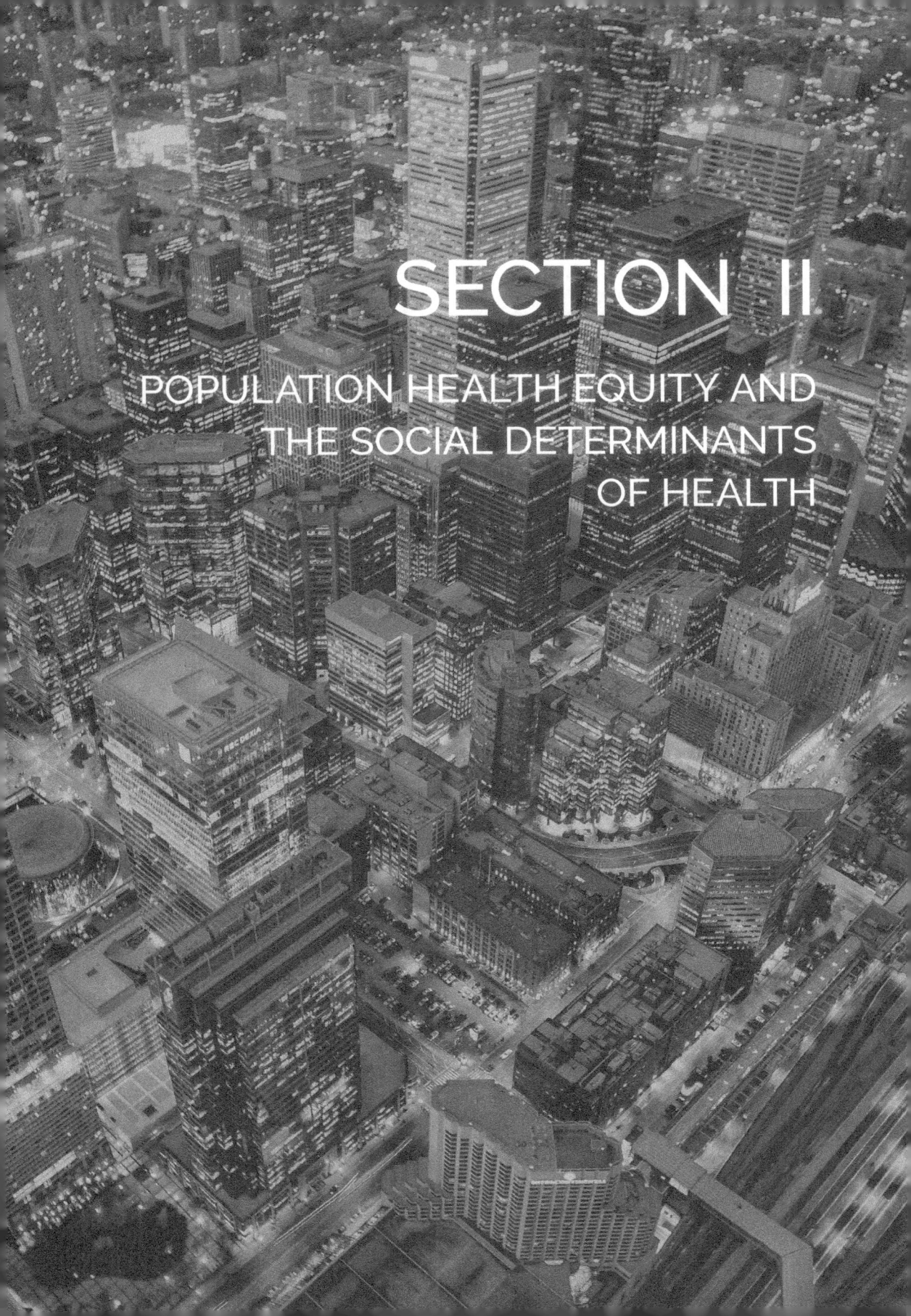

SECTION II

POPULATION HEALTH EQUITY AND THE SOCIAL DETERMINANTS OF HEALTH

CHAPTER 8

The State of Health Equity in Ontario

Dennis Raphael

TAKE-HOME MESSAGE

- Health inequities in Ontario are widespread and significant.
- To date, government policy in Ontario appears unwilling to address health inequities.
- It will take an aroused public literally forcing governments to take action to address health inequities.

INTRODUCTION

Working towards health equity is about creating the circumstances in which avoidable differences or inequalities in health among groups—that is, *health inequities*—are reduced and eventually eliminated (Braveman & Gruskin, 2003). There is increasing consensus that the key path towards health equity is creating public policy that strengthens and makes more equitable the distribution of the social determinants of health—the living and working conditions that are the primary factors that shape health outcomes (World Health Organization, 2008).

Social determinants of health refer to the economic and social conditions that shape health and create health inequities (Raphael, 2009). They include amount of income, quality of employment, working conditions, and features of housing. When these factors are inadequate, they contribute to material deprivation, stress, a higher likelihood of adopting health-threatening coping behaviours, and lower levels of access to quality health care, among other things (see Table 8.1). Canada's distribution of the social determinants of health is among the most unequal of wealthy developed nations (Bryant, Raphael, Schrecker, & Labonté, 2011). In this chapter, I detail the current state of health equity in Ontario and recommend ways to address health inequity through public policy action.

Table 8.1: The Social Determinants of Health

Aboriginal Status	Health Services
Disability Status	Housing
Early Life	Income and Income Distribution
Education	Race
Employment and Working Conditions	Social Exclusion
Food Security	Social Safety Net
Gender	Unemployment and Employment Security

Source: Mikkonen & Raphael, 2010

THE HEALTH GAP IN ONTARIO

There is an extensive literature on health inequities in Ontario (Gardner, 2010; Project for an Ontario Women's Health Evidence-Based Report, 2012). Health inequities exist for life expectancy, infant mortality, and mortality rates from a number of diseases among those differing in incomes and living in urban versus rural settings. There are also income-related inequities in the incidence and prevalence of various diseases and injuries. Two illustrative examples of such inequities are provided here: (1) premature mortality prior to age 75 as a function of income, and (2) differences in incidence of injuries among Ontarians of differing ages and income.

Differences in Mortality Prior to Age 75

One study provides data on premature mortality (percentage of the population who died before age 75) by gender and neighbourhood income quintile in Ontario for the year 2001 (Project for an Ontario Women's Health Evidence-Based Report, 2012; see Figure 8.1). Premature mortality is distinctively higher among residents of the poorest 20 percent of Ontario neighbourhoods. The lowest-income men have a 41 percent chance of dying before age 75, while the best-off men have a 28 percent chance. This 13 percent absolute difference translates into a relative greater risk of dying prior to age 75 for the lowest income men of 45 percent using the best-off group as a baseline. For women, the absolute difference of 7 percent between the lowest income women (26 percent) and best-off women (19 percent) converts into a 35 percent greater risk of dying prior to age 75 for the lowest income women.

Differences in Injuries as a Function of Age and Income

Profound differences in injuries are seen in Ontario between those of differing incomes. Figure 8.2 provides rates of injury-related hospitalizations per 100,000 population, by age group and income quintile in Ontario for the period 2002–2003 (Macpherson et al., 2005). Amongst the

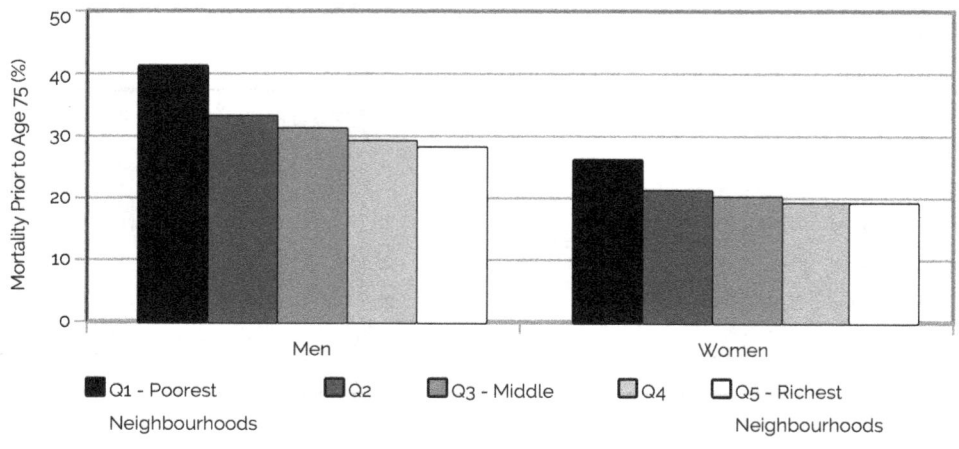

Figure 8.1: Premature Mortality of Men and Women in Ontario by Neighbourhood Quintille, 2001 (Percentage)

Source: Wilkins, 2007

youngest age group, the rate for hospitalizations for the lowest income group (287/100,000) is 35 percent higher than for the most well-off group (213/100,000). Among the oldest group, the hospitalization rate for the lowest income group (566/100,000) is 42 percent higher than for the most well-off group (1269/100,000). These inequities in health status as a function of income are seen for just about every disease or affliction. Further examples of health inequities in Ontario, including inequities in access to health care, are available (Raphael, 2012).

FACTORS DRIVING THESE HEALTH INEQUITIES IN ONTARIO

Consistent with the social and health inequalities literature, the World Health Organization argues that health inequities result from the inequitable distribution of power, money, and resources. A good indicator of these inequities is the poverty rate, which reflects the inequitable distribution of monetary resources. Figure 8.3 provides evidence of the extent of poverty among Ontarians across the life span using the after-tax low-income measure (LIM), a measure that demonstrates that people with less than half the average income are denied access to the resources necessary for health.

Poverty rates for Ontario children are above 14 percent and rates across all age groups have increased since the mid-1990s. The trend for those over 65 years is particularly striking, with their rates growing to close to 10 percent after the lows of 4 percent seen during the mid-1990s. Canada—including Ontario—is one of the very few wealthy developed nations whose poverty rates for children are higher than for the general population, a finding noted by UNICEF in its most recent report on child poverty (Innocenti Research Centre, 2012).

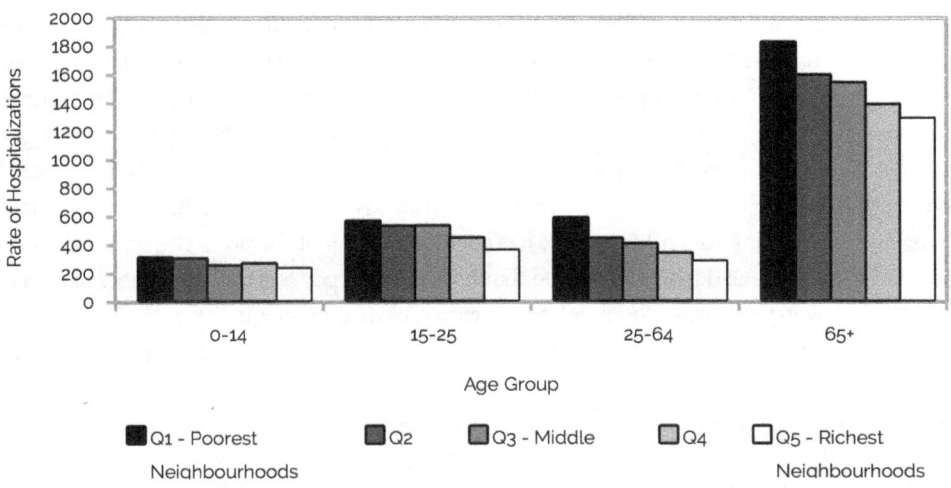

Figure 8.2: Rates of Injury-Related Hospitalization per 100,000 Population, by Age Group and Income Quintile, Ontario, 2001

Source: Macpherson et al., 2005.

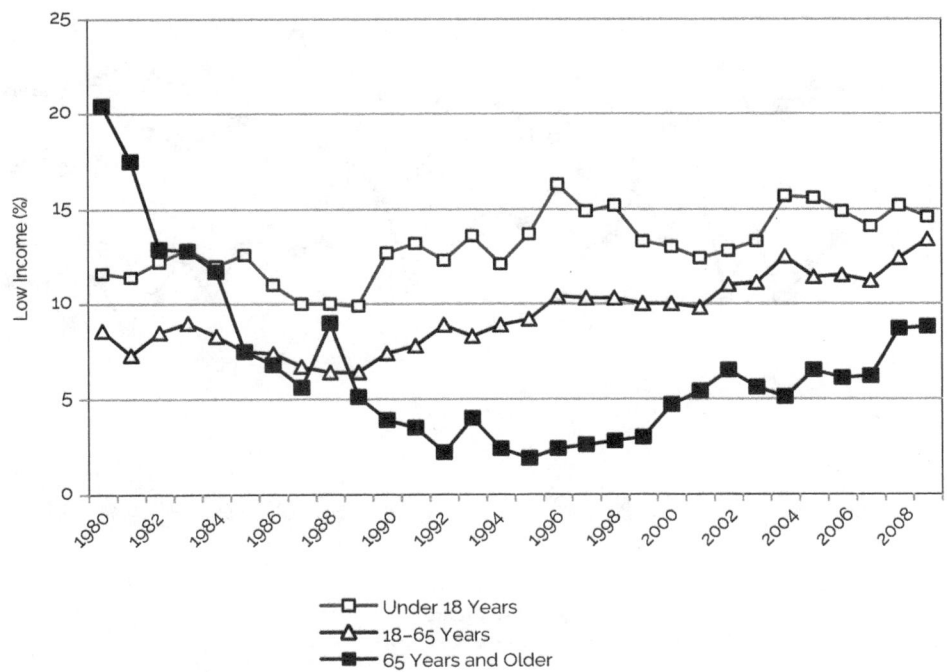

Figure 8.3: Percentage Living in Poverty, Using Low-Income Measures, after Tax, by Age Group, Ontario, 1980–2010

Source: Statistics Canada, 2016

An important question is how much, on average, those identified as living in poverty are below the poverty line. Are poor people in Ontario just below the poverty line or are they very much below? Figure 8.4 provides a measure of how far below the poverty line people in Ontario living in poverty are as a percentage of the poverty line. The gap is rather large. For poor children the gap is currently is 24 percent, for adults aged 18–65 it is 33 percent, and for those older than 65 it is 17 percent. For adults aged 18–65 these figures show little change since 1980, but for children there has been a lessening of the poverty gap. For seniors there is a slight decline during this period, but note that the poverty rate for seniors has been increasing. Poverty rates are closely related to extent of income inequality within a jurisdiction, and evidence shows that income inequality is on the rise in Ontario (Raphael, 2012).

PROMOTING HEALTH EQUITY IN ONTARIO

The World Health Organization suggests that health equity can be promoted by improving living conditions and considering health equity in all policies, systems, and programmes. This includes promoting fair financing and market responsibility so that no

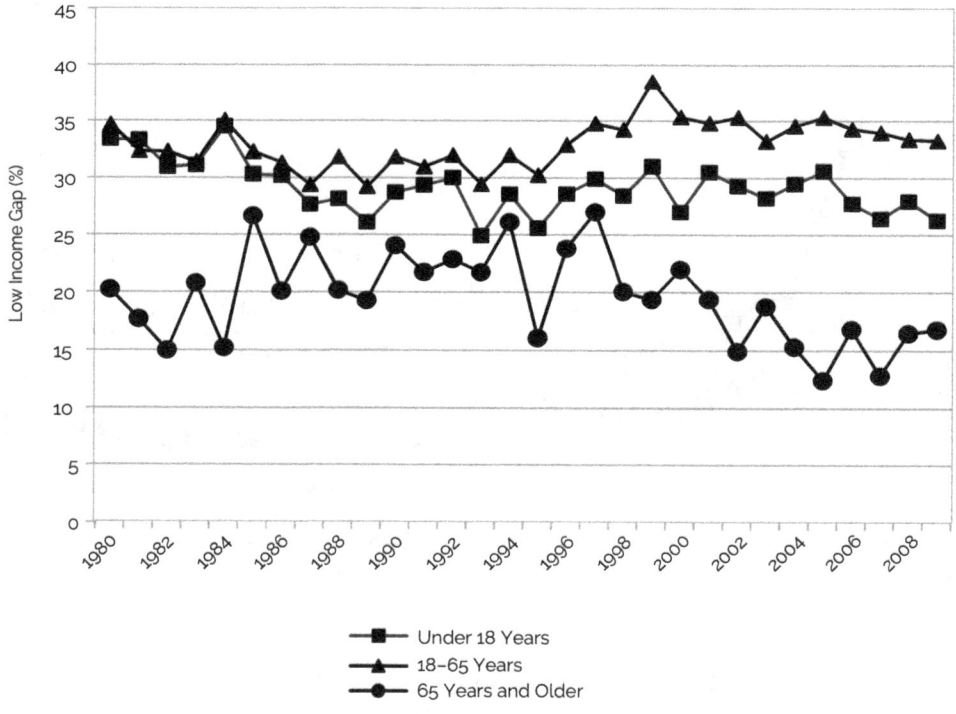

Figure 8.4: Low Income Gap, Using Low-Income Measures, after Tax, by Age Group, Ontario, 1980–2010

Source: Statistics Canada, 2016

one is denied the economic and social resources necessary for health. Raphael (2012) suggests that the following steps, if immediately taken, would help create living conditions that would reduce health inequities in Ontario:

- raising minimum wage, social assistance, and child benefit levels to a level that would assure health;
- improving working conditions and employment standards and making it easier for workplaces to unionize;
- creating a fairer tax system;
- providing an affordable, regulated childcare system;
- ensuring affordable healthy foods and adequate housing;
- including a consideration of health impacts when developing economic and other policies; and
- ensuring public support through raising awareness for a health equity agenda.

Building Long-Term Commitments

Currently, the political context in Ontario is not one that easily aligns with the promotion of health equity through public policy action. The Health Council of Canada (2010) provides an analysis of what is needed to have governments address health inequities through a whole-of-government approach. Their checklist specifies what values, information, and government infrastructure would be needed to tackle health inequities in Ontario (see Box 8.1). Without such commitments, we can expect little government action to address health inequities through public policy action.

Box 8.1: The Health Council of Canada's Checklist for a Whole-of-Government or Intersectoral Approach to Promoting Health Equity

The checklist on this page synthesizes key pieces of information from Canadian and international reports and documents about implementing intersectoral and whole-of-government approaches; our consultants' experience working with Canadian governments, agencies, and organizations; and the information gathered from interviews with officials from across Canada.

Values and Commitment
- ☐ An overriding philosophy that health initiatives will be viewed through a population health lens.
- ☐ Leadership at the top from the prime minister, premiers, ministers, cabinet secretaries, and others.
- ☐ Recognition and awareness among elected representatives of the importance of the determinants of health for promoting population health and reducing health inequities.

☐   Recognition that it may take years, even decades, for benefits to materialize.

☐   Willingness to name the difficult problems and barriers that exist, and to provide the resources necessary to transcend them.

☐   Commitment of civil servants to undertake a broader approach to addressing population health and reducing health inequities.

☐   Willingness and commitment to ensure a structural approach to placing health projects on the public policy agenda.

☐   Allocation of significant funding that allows for governmental commissioning of research, analysis, and policy implementation.

Information and Data

☐   Decisions should be made and actions taken based on available evidence without necessarily waiting for conclusive evidence.

☐   Information and evidence on the state of population health and the presence of health inequities is presented in a government-instigated integrative report or statement.

☐   Development of clear, identifiable, and measurable goals and targets.

☐   Focusing on explicit concrete objectives and visible results. Ensuring transparency in governmental efforts and activities.

☐   Messaging to the public, including media support, about the importance of dealing with population health and reducing health inequities through action on the determinants of health.

☐   Development of practical models, tools, and mechanisms, such as health impact assessment, to support the implementation.

☐   Setting of realistic timelines.

☐   Support for academic and agency researchers who provide data and evaluation.

☐   Provision of ongoing public reports that document successes and challenges.

Governmental Infrastructure

☐   Governments must establish the means for society's participation in the initiatives.

☐   Establishment of an independent authority within government that will be responsible for coordinating activity across ministries and departments.

☐   Cross-ministry structures and processes that provide a basis for these kinds of whole-of-government or intersectoral approaches.

☐   Contacting and drawing support from various external organizations that would be responsive to governmental action on the determinants of health.

☐   Government civil servants' capacity to carry out the task.

☐   Ensuring that leadership, accountability, and rewards are shared among partners.

☐   Provision of adequate resources to sustain activities beyond the tenure of the present governing authority.

☐ Establishment of a balance between central direction and discretion of local authorities to implement goals and objectives.

☐ Establishment of accountability and evaluation frameworks.

☐ Building of stable teams of people who work well together, with appropriate support systems.

Source: Health Council of Canada, 2010, p. 25

Unfortunately, there is little evidence that governing authorities—or opposition parties, for that matter—are concerned with addressing health inequities and the conditions that create them. There is, however, grassroots activity on the part of the public health community to draw public attention to these issues. Local public health units across Canada are engaging in public education activities (Raphael, Brassolotto, & Baldeo, 2014). One public health unit in Ontario created the video animation "Let's Start a Conversation about Health and Not Talk about Health Care at All" (Sudbury and District Health Unit, 2011), which has been adapted for use by no fewer than 18 other public health units in Ontario (out of a total of 36).

Mikkonen and Raphael created the public primer *Social Determinants of Health: The Canadian Facts*, which has been downloaded over 300,000 times since April 2010. Eighty-five percent of these downloads are by Canadians (Mikkonen & Raphael, 2010). Also, a new Canadian organization, Upstream Action, aims to start a movement to create a healthy society through disseminating to the public—as well as policy-makers—evidence-based, people-centred ideas (Upstream Action, 2013). Hopefully, these activities will create a groundswell of public interest and concern that will force Ontario to take seriously the issue of addressing health inequities.

GLOSSARY

Health equity: "Equity in health can be defined as the absence of systematic disparities in health (or in the major social determinants of health) between social groups that have different levels of underlying social advantage/disadvantage—that is, different positions in a social hierarchy" (Braveman & Gruskin, 2003).

Public policy: "A course of action or inaction chosen by public authorities to address a given problem or interrelated set of problems" (Pal, 2006).

Social determinants of health: "The social determinants of health are composed of the conditions in which people are born, grow up, live, work, and age, together with the systems that are put in place to deal with illness" (World Health Organization, 2008).

DISCUSSION QUESTIONS

1. Prior to reading this, what did you think were the primary factors affecting health?
2. What are the reasons that a wealthy province like Ontario seems unable to create public policy that will reduce health inequities?
3. Who benefits from the presence of the social conditions that spawn health inequities?

REFERENCES

Braveman, P., & Gruskin, S. (2003). Defining equity in health. *Journal of Epidemiology and Community Health, 57,* 254–258.

Bryant, T., Raphael, D., Schrecker, T., & Labonté R. (2011). Canada: A land of missed opportunity for addressing the social determinants of health. *Health Policy, 101*(1), 44–58.

Gardner, B. (2010). Health equity into action: Planning and other resources for LHINs. Retrieved from http://www.wellesleyinstitute.com/publication/health-equity-into-action-planning-and-other-resources-for-lhins

Health Council of Canada. (2010). *Stepping it up: Moving the focus from health care in Canada to a healthier Canada.* Toronto: Health Council of Canada.

Innocenti Research Centre. (2012). *Measuring Child Poverty: New league tables of child poverty in the world's rich countries.* Florence: Innocenti Research Centre.

Macpherson, A. K., Schull, M., Manuel, D., Cernat, G., Redelmeier, D. A., & Laupacis, A. (2005). *Injuries in Ontario.* ICES Atlas. Toronto: Institute for Clinical Evaluative Sciences.

Mikkonen, J., & Raphael, D. (2010). *Social determinants of health: The Canadian facts.* Retrieved from http://www.thecanadianfacts.org

Pal, L. (2006). *Beyond policy analysis: Public issue management in turbulent times.* Toronto: Nelson.

Project for an Ontario Women's Health Evidence-Based Report. (2012). *POWER: Project for an Ontario women's health evidence-based report.* Retrieved from http://www.powerstudy.ca

Raphael, D. (2012). *Working towards health equity-related policymaking in Ontario.* Retrieved from http://www.rrasp-phirn.ca/images/stories/Download_937_KBl.pdf

Raphael, D. (Ed.). (2009). *Social determinants of health: Canadian perspectives* (2nd ed.). Toronto: Canadian Scholars' Press.

Raphael, D., Brassolotto, J., & Baldeo, N. (2014). Ideological and organizational components of differing public health strategies for addressing the social determinants of health. *Health Promotion International, 30*(4), 855–867.

Statistics Canada (2016). *CANSIM tables: Income, pensions, spending and wealth.* Retrieved from http://www5.statcan.gc.ca/cansim/a33?lang=eng&spMode=master&themeID=3868&RT=TABLE

Sudbury and District Health Unit. (2011). *Let's start a conversation about health . . . and not talk about health care at all.* Retrieved from http://tinyurl.com/7t8476f

Upstream Action. (2013). *Upstream Action is a movement to create a healthy society through evidence-based, people-centred ideas.* Retrieved from http://www.thinkupstream.net/

World Health Organization. (2008). *Closing the gap in a generation: Health equity through action on the social determinants of health*. Geneva: World Health Organization.

Wilkins, R. (2007). *Mortality by neighbourhood income in urban Canada from 1971 to 2001*. Statistics Canada, Health Analysis and Measurement Group (HAMG). HAMG Seminar, and Special Compilations.

CHAPTER 9

How to Think about Social Determinants of Health: Revitalizing the Agenda in Canada

Ted Schrecker and Vanessa Taler

TAKE-HOME MESSAGE

- Approaches to health equity that emphasize individual lifestyles are pernicious.
- Decisions about how much evidence is "enough" are complex, political, and a matter of public health ethics.
- Public finance is a public health issue.

INTRODUCTION

> "Realism is to put our ambition at the level of our challenges."
> —José Manuel Barroso (2012),
> then President of the European Commission

In August 2008, the World Health Organization's Commission on Social Determinants of Health released its final report. The report, a product of three years' work by 19 commission members (with Sir Michael Marmot as chair) and a large multinational supporting cast of researchers, was organized around the concepts of health equity and socioeconomic gradients in health. Health equity was defined with reference to the absence of systematic differences in health that are avoidable by reasonable action, and the commission emphasized that it considered most such differences to be avoidable and therefore inequitable (Commission, 2007, p. 2). The commission further emphasized that the "unequal distribution of health-damaging experiences is not in any sense a 'natural' phenomenon but is the result of a toxic combination of poor social policies and programmes, unfair economic arrangements, and bad politics" (Commission, 2008, p. 1) .

Canada has a long history of highlighting the importance of social determinants of health (SDH) well before the term was in widespread use (Evans & Stoddart, 1990).

More recently, the Code Red study of Hamilton, Ontario—a novel collaboration be-tween university researchers and an investigative journalist in a metropolitan area whose economy had been devastated by the loss of manufacturing jobs—found a difference of 21 years in average age of death between one of the wealthiest neighbourhoods and one of the poorest (Buist, 2010). Yet in 2011, leading researchers described Canada as "a land of missed opportunity" for action on SDH (Bryant, Raphael, Schrecker, & Labonté, 2011). In this chapter, we first outline three ways of rethinking public policy to incorporate concern for health inequalities and SDH. We conclude with observations about breaking down the "silos" that impede governmental action on SDH, and about the need to build public support for such action more effectively than has been the case to date.

THINKING DIFFERENTLY: CHALLENGING "LIFESTYLE DRIFT"

Popay, Whitehead, and Hunter describe lifestyle drift as "the tendency for policy to start off recognizing the need for action on upstream social determinants of health inequalities only to drift downstream to focus largely on individual lifestyle factors" (2010, p. 148). Lifestyle drift is endemic in Canadian health promotion and public health (Dupéré et al., 2007, p. 373; Frohlich & Poland, 2007, p. 47; Low & Thériault, 2008).

For example, a survey of initiatives related to healthy eating and physical activity in Ontario and British Columbia (Gore & Kothari, 2012) found a preponderance of life-style- or environment-based rather than structure-based initiatives, even using a broad and inclusive definition of the latter category, despite abundant demonstrations of the unaffordability of a healthy diet for low-income Canadians (Dietitians of Canada, 2012; Ottawa Public Health, 2011; Toronto Medical Officer of Health, 2010; Williams et al., 2012). A study of how to make the province of Ontario a leader in population health argues for a focus on improved health behaviours such as healthy eating, physical activ-ity, maintaining healthy body weight, avoiding tobacco, and reducing stress (Manuel, Creatore, Rosella, & Henry, 2009). The authors acknowledge that "it is fundamentally unfair to try and change social attitudes or to tell poor people they should take more re-sponsibility for their health if governments do not remove societal barriers which might prevent them from doing so" (Manuel, Creatore, Rosella, & Henry, 2009, p. 6). However, in the text of the document as a whole there is one reference to poverty, one to unemploy-ment, no reference to food insecurity (despite a substantial body of research on its extent in Canada), but 65 mentions of health behaviours, health behaviour strategies, health be-haviour targets, and the like. It is hard to reconcile this emphasis with the realities of life in a neighbourhood like one in downtown Halifax, where a wheelchair-bound resident spends $20 on taxis every time he goes to the nearest supermarket; the taxis are a necessity because purchases in his wheelchair basket may otherwise be stolen (Beaumont, 2012).

As this example suggests, the complexities of diet, overweight, and obesity illustrate the importance of challenging lifestyle drift. "The causes of the obesity epidemic are multifacto-rial, having much more to do with the absence of sidewalks and the limited availability of healthy and affordable foods than a lack of personal responsibility" (Institute of Medicine, 2012, summarizing Glickman et al., 2012). Deprived parts of many North American metropolitan areas lack full service grocery stores but abound in convenience stores and fast food outlets—the "food deserts" phenomenon (Beaulac, Kristjansson, & Cummins, 2009; Treuhaft & Karpyn, 2010); and when healthy food is accessible, it may be unaffordable for many—the "food mirage" problem (Breyer & Voss-Andreae, 2013). In addition, low-income neighbourhoods may not be activity-friendly, for reasons including heavy traffic and the associated air pollution, lack of recreational amenities, and the risk of violence.

In their work on social conditions as fundamental causes of disease, Link and Phelan warn that such causes "can defy efforts to eliminate their effects when attempts to do so focus solely on the mechanisms that happen to link them to disease in a particular situation" (1995, p. 81). Nowhere is this insight more applicable than in the case of stress and health. Many Canadian health promotion efforts, not just in the report cited above, treat stress as something under an individual's control, rather than as primarily a function of social position and structural economic influences (Schrecker, 2013a). Abundant evidence supports the latter view, and shows how stress can wear people out over time in biologically measurable ways (Geronimus, Hicken, Keene, & Bound, 2006; Marmot, 2004, p. 107–141; Seeman et al., 2010). Indeed, the treatment of stress in public health policy as a whole needs to be fundamentally rethought, with reference to external influences like the widespread job losses associated with deindustrialization.

THINKING DIFFERENTLY: HOW MUCH EVIDENCE IS ENOUGH? WHAT KIND OF EVIDENCE? WHO DECIDES?

Given the popularity of evidence-based medicine and health policy, critical perspectives on these questions are especially important. Health researchers and those making use of their findings often operate on the basis of a hierarchy of evidence with randomized controlled trials (RCTs), ideally repeated to test transferability, and large-scale prospective epidemiological studies at the top.

This is an inappropriate approach to understanding SDH and interventions to address them, running the risk of reaching the (inaccurate) conclusion that almost nothing works. Insistence on RCTs builds into intervention research a bias against larger-scale, contextual interventions that are difficult if not impossible to evaluate in this manner (National Research Council & Institute of Medicine, 2013, pp. 164, 262–263; Schrecker, Acosta, Somerville, & Bursztajn, 2001, pp. 1679–1682). This bias may contribute to lifestyle drift, since interventions that focus on changes in individual behaviour are more amenable to RCT study designs, and easier to manage and less demanding in terms of their resource requirements. Marmot (2000, p. 308) has noted that "the further upstream we go in our search for causes, the less applicable is the randomized controlled trial.... We must therefore rely on observational evidence and judgment in formulating policies to reduce inequalities in health."

Waiting for epidemiological evidence raises similar problems. Even in high-income jurisdictions with extensive health data, mortality measures may be insufficiently sensitive to capture deteriorations in health status, except in the case of catastrophic disruptions like the collapse of the former Soviet economy. For how long is it justifiable to defer action while waiting for health outcome data that may, given the accumulation of effects of disadvantage over the life course, be decades in materializing (Frank & Haw, 2011)? Instead, should evidence of causal relations with such risk factors as overweight or allostatic load—a key concept in the physiology of stress—be sufficient to justify policy change? Even this strategy may not cast the net widely enough. As noted in a recent literature review,

> many strategies aimed at obesity prevention may not be expected to have a direct impact on BMI [body mass index], but rather on pathways that will alter the context in which eating, physical activity and weight control occur. Any restriction on the concept of a successful outcome, to either weight-maintenance or BMI measures alone, is therefore likely to overlook many possible intervention measures that could contribute to obesity prevention. (Mooney, Haw, & Frank, 2011, p. 22)

No simple algorithm will answer these and similar questions, which should be addressed directly as matters of public health ethics (Schrecker, 2013b), but it is worth noting Marmot's (2000) view that "the best should not be the enemy of the good. While we should not formulate policies in the absence of evidence to support them, we must not be paralyzed into inaction while we wait for the evidence to be absolutely unimpeachable" (p. 308). This observation applies with special force to the health consequences of the expenditure restraint (austerity) programs that have been adopted in many jurisdictions following the financial crisis. Stuckler and Basu correctly observe that "in countries where austerity is ascendant, we're undergoing a massive and untested experiment on human health, and left to count the dead" (2013, p. xxi). In 10 or 20 years, that experiment may provide answers to some of the questions epidemiologists would like to ask about SDH, although there will always be uncertainty because in the real world many things go on in people's lives at the same time.

That is too long to wait. A preferable approach addresses complex population health problems by way of what has been called a "portfolio of evidence" (Kim, 2003) that includes both qualitative and quantitative findings, and a "portfolio of interventions" (Swinburn, Gill, & Kumanyika, 2005) supported by distinctive evidence bases. Obviously, ongoing evaluation of interventions and policy changes is important—and of course, unless undertaken on a meaningful scale, they cannot be evaluated! But how much more evidence is needed to demonstrate, for example, the public health imperative of increasing the incomes of people for whom eating a healthy diet while keeping a roof over their heads is arithmetically impossible?

THINKING DIFFERENTLY: PUBLIC FINANCE AS A PUBLIC HEALTH ISSUE

In June 2011, with Ontario's government facing a $14 billion budget deficit, it neverthe-less found more than $200 million to widen a short stretch of freeway on the eastern edge of Ottawa. This announcement was made the day after the Ontario Non-Profit Housing Association released an annual survey showing that more than 150,000 households were on waiting lists for affordable housing; by 2016 the waiting list had grown to 171,000 (Ontario Non-Profit Housing Association, 2016). The $200 million could have been used, instead, as seed money for an expanded program of building affordable housing, or in a variety of other ways that could have made a direct contribution to reducing health disparities by way of acting on SDH (cf. Labonté, 1990). It's a matter of priorities: if the SDH agenda is to be revitalized, then advocates, including public health professionals, must be willing to trespass on the sacred terrain of public budgets to argue for different priorities. Although the connection between economic inequality (rather than specific manifestations or corollaries of inequality) and health outcomes is contested, the case for trespassing is strengthened by evidence that the distribution and objectives of govern-ment expenditure have a more powerful role than the structure of taxation in reducing economic inequality and its manifestations, such as poverty (Campbell, 2012).

Public finance, in other words, is a public health issue. This includes the revenue as well as the expenditure side of the equation, as pointed out in *Tax Is Not a Four Letter Word*, a book co-edited by Alex Himelfarb, who retired as Canada's most senior public servant (Himelfarb & Himelfarb, 2013). The importance of the revenue side was illus-trated, perhaps unintentionally, by a report on Ontario's financial future that envisioned no new spending on increasing social assistance rates or affordable housing until after the anticipated balancing of the provincial budget in 2017–2018 (Commission, 2012). The Commission on the Reform of Ontario's Public Services had been directed not to con-sider any form of new taxation, resulting in a set of fiscal projections in which government revenues as a percentage of the province's economic product actually decline slightly. The report did, however, provide the basis for an alternative revenue assumption in which the provincial treasury's "own source" revenues—that is, revenues from provincial taxes and fees rather than federal transfers—rise to their 1999–2000 level of 15.9 percent of the province's economic product. Under this scenario, using the report's expenditure assump-tions, the province would be running a $22.6 billion budget surplus in 2017–2018, or, looking at the issue another way, $22.6 billion would be available for program spending while balancing the budget in that fiscal year.

What steps could be taken to reduce health inequities if even some of those re-sources were directed towards SDH? This should not be treated as a rhetorical question. Encouragingly, the government of Ontario that was re-elected in 2014 signalled an incre-mental shift from an anti-tax position and a willingness to tax high earners more heavily, a position that has abundant support outside the narrow confines of Canadian policy debates (Saez & Piketty, 2013). Budgetary priorities matter in health research as well, and so long as adequate support is not available for research that specifically addresses SDH, "biomedical individualism" (Baum, Bégin, Houweling, & Taylor, 2009, pp. 1968–1969) will dominate discussions of how to reduce health inequity. It is fair to say that, at least in Canada, the budget for research on SDH is minuscule relative to what is available for research on curative interventions. The point is not that less should be spent on research to improve patient care, but that research budgets that continue to devote the lion's share of funding to biomedical and clinical research mean that the body of evidence that many knowledge users will demand before acting on SDH simply will not be generated.

NEXT STEPS: BREAKING DOWN SILOS, REFRAMING HEALTH DISPARITIES

As an oversimplification, two distinctive perspectives, which are not mutually exclusive, emerge from discussions on how the SDH agenda can be moved forward.

The first perspective emphasizes reorganizing public sector institutions and processes around concepts like intersectoral action, health in all policies—the focus adopted by Finland during its rotating presidency of the European Union in 2006 (Ståhl et al., 2006)—or a whole-of-government approach. These concepts respond to the "silo problem" that is widely recognized as a defining characteristic of contemporary government organization. Less often acknowledged is the fact that many of the largest silos, with the strongest walls, are defined and defended by relations with powerful client groups outside government—think of ministries of agriculture, transportation, industry, or for that matter, health (care). Social policy ministries and agencies, by contrast, seldom if ever have a comparably cohesive or influential clientele. The economic management role of ministries of finance and their lead role in public budgeting automatically confers special importance in an "unequal structure of representation" within government (Mahon, 1977).

A review of the health divide in WHO's European Region was emphatic about the need to integrate "the views of ministers of health and social affairs" into economic and fiscal policy, specifically in the current context of austerity (Marmot et al., 2012, p. 1013). This proposal is laudable for its understanding of the influence of economic policy on health, which is a central theme of the review; disturbingly, it has been noted that "public health voices have been largely absent from the debate" about responses to the financial crisis in Europe (Karanikolos et al., 2013, p. 1329). At the same time, it is not clear that being at the table will necessarily make a difference, given the unequal structure of representation (and the shift of power from elected governments to financial markets that is a defining characteristic of contemporary globalization). It is also unclear whether health ministries have either the capacity or the commitment to advance health equity in a way that goes beyond the narrowly behavioural.

The second perspective looks outside government and emphasizes the need to build widespread support for action on SDH. Policy change and new initiatives to address the underlying causes of health disparities will rarely, if ever, be achieved simply by assembling evidence, however compelling, that social conditions contribute to health disparities. Sir Michael Marmot has said that "a social movement to advance the cause of health equity through action on the social determinants of health" was one of the objectives of the commission he chaired (Marmot, Allen, & Goldblatt, 2010, p. 1254). However, social movements concerned with health equity and SDH may lack natural constituencies, complicating the task of building the necessary coalitions and mobilizing their support (see chapter 28, this volume).

Here, the concept of *framing* is central. Framing refers to the way in which an issue is presented (see Lakoff, 1996). For example, presenting a taxation issue in terms of "tax burden" will encourage a different view on the issue than referring to "taxes for education." In the context of policies that address SDH, frames that involve attributions of responsibility may be especially important (Niederdeppe et al., 2008). To the extent that health and illness are seen as consequences of individual choices, rather than as consequences of a social and economic environment in which the opportunities to lead a healthy life are distributed unequally, health disparities are less likely to be viewed as an important issue that merits policy attention, and lifestyle drift is likely to be pervasive. In the British context in which one of the authors (TS) now lives and works, Owen Jones (2011) has noted the emergence since the 1980s of a political culture that embraced "aspiration" and presumed that, if not wealth, then at least a comfortable middle-class existence was available to anyone willing to work hard. He argues that this presumption was assiduously cultivated by the media, yet is increasingly at odds with the realities of deindustrialization; the spread of low-wage, precarious employment; growing inequality in access to education; and the erosion of various forms of social protection—ironically, on the watch of the same Labour government that was targeting health inequalities.

Thus, "a short-term goal of population health researchers and advocates should be to convey to both key stakeholders (policymakers, opinion leaders) and the broader public that health is produced not only by access to health care and individual health behaviors but also by other social and economic factors such as poverty, education, and racial discrimination" (Niederdeppe et al., 2008, p. 483). But making that case is not enough. It is also essential to question the presumption that people's social and economic position is a consequence of their own efforts and initiative—or, conversely, of their lack of responsibility—rather than of a background set of conditions in which "the inequality machine is reshaping the whole planet" (Halimi, 2013). Deindustrialization and, more recently, the financial crisis of 2008 and its aftermath, should have underscored the reality that people's social and economic position and life chances are often the result of choices made and processes operating entirely outside their control. Challenging what Jones calls a pernicious "doctrine of personal responsibility" (2011, p. 183) may take many health practitioners and researchers far outside their comfort zone, but revitalizing the SDH agenda is likely to depend on the forceful articulation of that challenge.

GLOSSARY

Neoliberalism: A political perspective that considers markets the normal and natural way of organizing most forms of human interaction (not just economic transactions); public policy that produces outcomes different from those that would result from markets working as they do in economics textbooks to require justification; and the primary objective of government to ensure the efficient functioning of markets. The term *neoliberalism* was coined by the Walter Lippmann Colloquium, a meeting of academics, in 1938. (See Dardot & Laval, 2013; Schrecker & Bambra, 2015; Ward & England, 2007.)

Progressive and regressive taxation: Essential concepts for understanding public finance as a public health issue. A progressive tax is one that is paid at a proportionately higher rate by people or households with higher incomes or more wealth. Many income taxes are progressive in theory because the marginal rate of taxation—the proportion of income paid as tax on each additional dollar of income—increases above a certain threshold. (These thresholds are often referred to as tax brackets.) The real-world progressivity of income taxes depends not only on these thresholds, but also on whether exemptions exist, such as a lower rates of tax on capital gains—income from the sale of shares or commercial property, forms of income that are mainly the province of the wealthy. Consumption taxes like sales or value-added taxes (the GST/HST in Canada) are generally regressive; as a proportion of income, they fall more heavily on people and households with low incomes that spend most if not all of their incomes on daily necessities. Taxes on luxury goods are an exception to this general rule. Fixed user charges for public health care and other services are an especially significant example of a regressive tax.

DISCUSSION QUESTIONS

1. What examples of lifestyle drift can you identify from your own experience?
2. What are the most important pieces of evidence about social determinants of health that are still not available? (See the discussion in Östlin et al., 2011, if in need of ideas.)
3. What would a social movement to advance health equity look like?
4. How can public health researchers and practitioners most effectively use the material in this chapter to reframe discussions of health disparities?

REFERENCES

Barroso, J. M. (2012). *State of the union 2012 address*. European Commission. Retrieved from http://europa.eu/rapid/pressReleasesAction.do?reference=SPEECH/12/596

Basu, S., Carney, M.A., & Kenworthy, N.J. (2017). Ten years after the financial crisis: The long reach of austerity and its global impacts on health. *Social Science & Medicine, 187*, 203–207.

Baum, F. E., Bégin, M., Houweling, T. A. J., & Taylor, S. (2009). Changes not for the fainthearted: Reorienting health care systems toward health equity through action on the social determinants of health. *American Journal of Public Health, 99*, 1967–1974.

Beaulac, J., Kristjansson, E., & Cummins, S. (2009). A systematic review of food deserts, 1966–2007. *Preventing Chronic Disease, 6*. Retrieved from http://www.cdc.gov/pcd/issues/2009/jul/08_0163.htm?s_cid=pcd63a105_e

Beaumont, H. (2012, November 4). Everyday life's a challenge in a 'food desert.' *Chronicle-Herald*. Retrieved from http://thechronicleherald.ca/thenovascotian/161761-everyday-life-s-a-challenge-in-a-food-desert

Breyer, B., & Voss-Andreae, A. (2013). Food Mirages: Geographic and economic barriers to healthful food access in Portland, Oregon. *Health & Place, 24*, 131–139.

Bryant, T., Raphael, D., Schrecker, T., & Labonté, R. (2011). Canada: A land of missed opportunity for addressing the social determinants of health. *Health Policy, 101*, 44–58.

Buist, S. (2010, August 25). Worlds apart. *Hamilton Spectator*. Retrieved from http://www.thespec.com/news-story/2168237-worlds-apart

Campbell, A. L. (2012). America the undertaxed: U.S. fiscal policy in perspective. *Foreign Affairs, 91*(5), 99–112.

Commission on Social Determinants of Health (2007). *Achieving health equity: From root causes to fair outcomes.* Interim Statement. Geneva: World Health Organization. Retrieved from http://www.who.int/social_determinants/resources/csdh_media/csdh_interim_statement_07.pdf

Commission on Social Determinants of Health (2008). *Closing the gap in a generation: Health equity through action on the social determinants of health.* Final report. Geneva: World Health Organization. Retrieved from http://whqlibdoc.who.int/publications/2008/9789241563703_eng.pdf

Commission on the Reform of Ontario's Public Services. (2012). *Public services for Ontarians: A path to sustainability and excellence.* Toronto: Ontario Ministry of Finance. Retrieved from http://www.fin.gov.on.ca/en/reformcommission/chapters/report.pdf

Dardot, P., & Laval, C. (2013). *The new way of the world: On neoliberal society.* English translation; original French edition 2009. London: Verso.

Dietitians of Canada (2012). *Cost of eating in British Columbia 2011.* Vancouver: Dietitians of Canada, BC Region. Retrieved from http://www.dietitians.ca/DownloadableContent/Public/CostofEatingBC2011_FINAL.aspx

Dupéré, S., Ridde, V., Carroll, S., O'Neill, M., Rootman, I., & Pederson, A. (2007). Conclusion: The rhizome and the tree. In M. O'Neill, A. Pederson, S. Dupéré, & I. Rootman (eds.), *Health promotion in Canada: Critical perspectives* (pp. 371–388). Toronto: Canadian Scholars' Press.

Evans, R. G., & Stoddart, G. L. (1990). Producing health, consuming health care. *Social Science & Medicine, 31*, 1347–1363.

Frank, J., & Haw, S. (2011). Best practice guidelines for monitoring socioeconomic inequalities in health status: Lessons from Scotland. *Milbank Quarterly, 89*, 658–693.

Frohlich, K. L., & Poland, B. (2007). Points of intervention in health promotion practice. In M. O'Neill, A. Pederson, S. Dupéré, & I. Rootman (eds.), *Health promotion in Canada: Critical perspectives* (pp. 46–60). Toronto: Canadian Scholars' Press.

Geronimus, A. T., Hicken, M., Keene, D., & Bound, J. (2006). "Weathering" and age patterns of allostatic load scores among blacks and whites in the United States. *American Journal of Public Health, 96*, 826–833.

Glickman, D., Parker, L., Sim, L. J., Cook, H. D. V., & Miller, E. A. (eds.) (2012). *Accelerating progress in obesity prevention: Solving the weight of the nation.* Washington, DC: National Academies Press for the Institute of Medicine. Retrieved from http://www.nap.edu/catalog.php?record_id=13275

Gore, D., & Kothari, A. (2012). Social determinants of health in Canada: Are healthy living initiatives there yet? A policy analysis. *International Journal for Equity in Health, 11*, 41. Retrieved from http://www.equityhealthj.com/content/11/1/41

Halimi, S. (2013, May). Tyranny of the one per cent. *Le Monde diplomatique* (English edition).

Himelfarb, A., & Himelfarb, J. (eds.) (2013). *Tax is not a four letter word: A different take on taxes in Canada.* Waterloo, ON: Wilfrid Laurier University Press.

Institute of Medicine. (2012). *Accelerating progress in obesity prevention: Solving the weight of the nation.* Washington, DC: National Academies Press. Retrieved from http://www.nap.edu/catalog.php?record_id=13275

Jones, O. (2011). *Chavs: The demonization of the working class.* London: Verso.

Karanikolos, M., Mladovsky, P., Cylus, J., Thomson, S., Basu, S., Stuckler, D., McKee, M. (2013). Financial crisis, austerity, and health in Europe. *The Lancet, 381*, 1323–1331.

Kim, Y. I. (2003). Role of folate in colon cancer development and progression. *The Journal of Nutrition, 133*, 3731S–3739S.

Labonté, R. (1990). Health-care spending as a risk to health. *Canadian Journal of Public Health, 81*, 251–253.

Lakoff, G. (1996) *Moral politics: What conservatives know that liberals don't.* Chicago: University of Chicago Press.

Link, B. G., & Phelan, J. (1995). Social conditions as fundamental causes of disease. *Journal of Health and Social Behavior, 35*, 80–94.

Low, J., & Thériault, L. (2008). Health promotion policy in Canada: Lessons forgotten, lessons still to learn. *Health Promotion International, 23*, 200–206.

Mahon, R. (1977). Canadian public policy: The unequal structure of representation. In L. Panitch (ed.), *The Canadian state: Political economy and political power* (pp. 165–198). Toronto: University of Toronto Press.

Manuel, D., Creatore, M. I., Rosella, L. C. A., & Henry, D. A. (2009). *What does it take to make a healthy province? A benchmark study of jurisdictions in Canada and around the world with the highest levels of health and the best health behaviours.* Toronto: Institute for Clinical Evaluative Sciences. Retrieved from http://www.ices.on.ca/file/Healthy%20province%20November%20release.pdf

Marmot, M. (2004). *Status syndrome: How your social standing directly affects your health and life expectancy.* London: Bloomsbury.

Marmot, M. (2000). Inequalities in health: causes and policy implications. In A. Tarlov & R. St. Peter (eds.), *The society and population health reader, vol. 2: A state and community perspective* (pp. 293–309). New York: New Press.

Marmot, M., Allen, J., & Goldblatt, P. (2010). A social movement, based on evidence, to reduce inequalities in health. *Social Science & Medicine, 71*, 1254–1258.

Marmot, M., Allen, J., Bell, R., Bloomer, E., & Goldblatt, P. (2012). WHO European review of social determinants of health and the health divide. *The Lancet, 380*, 1011–1029.

Mooney, J., Haw, S., & Frank, J. (2011). *Policy interventions to tackle the obesogenic environment: Focusing on adults of working age in Scotland.* Edinburgh: Scottish Collaboration for Public Health Research and Policy. Retrieved from https://www.scphrp.ac.uk/system/files/publications/policy_interventions_to_tackle_the_besogenic_environment_0.pdf

National Research Council & Institute of Medicine. (2013). *U.S. health in international perspective: Shorter lives, poorer health.* Washington, DC: National Academies Press. Retrieved from http://www.nap.edu/catalog.php?record_id=13497

Niederdeppe, J., Bu, Q. L., Borah, P., Kindig, D. A., & Robert, S. A. (2008). Message design strategies to raise public awareness of social determinants of health and population health disparities. *Milbank Quarterly, 86*, 481–513.

Ontario Non-Profit Housing Association. (2016). *Waiting lists survey 2016.* Toronto: ONPHA. Retrieved from http://www.onpha.on.ca/CMDownload.aspx?ContentKey=85812d7f-2d88-4b28-bbb2-9a76990de22d&ContentItemKey=bdeeb1f1-c466-4ffe-a10e-a2b35370e7fe

Östlin, P., Schrecker, T., Sadana, R., Bonnefoy, J., Gilson, L., Hertzman, C., Vaghri, Z. (2011). Priorities for research on equity and health: Towards an equity-focused health research agenda. *PLoS Medicine, 8*(11), e1001115. Retrieved from http://dx.doi.org/10.1371%2Fjournal.pmed.1001115

Ottawa Public Health. (2011). *The price of eating well in Ottawa 2011.* Ottawa: City of Ottawa. Retrieved from http://ottawa.ca/cs/groups/content/@webottawa/documents/pdf/mdaw/mdqw/~edisp/dev020395.pdf

Popay, J., Whitehead, M., & Hunter, D. J. (2010). Injustice is killing people on a large scale—but what is to be done about it? *Journal of Public Health, 32*, 148–149.

Saez, E., & Piketty, T. (2013, October 24). Why the 1% should pay tax at 80%. *The Guardian.*

Schrecker, T. (2013a). Beyond 'run, knit and relax': Can health promotion in Canada advance the social determinants of health agenda? *Healthcare Policy, 9*, 48–58.

Schrecker, T. (2013b). Can health equity survive epidemiology? Standards of proof and social determinants of health. *Preventive Medicine, 57*, 741–744.

Schrecker, T., & Bambra, C. (2015). *How politics makes us sick: Neoliberal epidemics.* Houndmills, UK: Palgrave Macmillan.

Schrecker, T., Acosta, L., Somerville, M. A., & Bursztajn, H. (2001). The Ethics of social risk reduction in the era of the biological brain. *Social Science & Medicine, 52*, 1677–1687.

Seeman, T., Epel, E., Gruenewald, T., Karlamangla, A., & McEwen, B. S. (2010). Socio-economic differentials in peripheral biology: Cumulative allostatic load. *Annals of the New York Academy of Sciences, 1186*, 223–239.

Ståhl, T., Wismar, M., Ollila, E., Lahtinen, E., & Leppo, K. (eds.) (2006). *Health in all policies: Prospects and potentials.* Helsinki: Ministry of Social Affairs and Health. Retrieved from http://ec.europa.eu/health/ph_information/documents/health_in_all_policies.pdf

Stuckler, D., & Basu, S. (2013). *The body economic: Why austerity kills.* London: Allèn Lane.

Swinburn, B., Gill, T., & Kumanyika, S. (2005). Obesity prevention: a proposed framework for translating evidence into action. *Obesity Reviews, 6*, 23–33.

Toronto Medical Officer of Health. (2010). *Cost of the nutritious food basket – Toronto 2010.* Staff Report. Toronto: Department of Public Health. Retrieved from http://www.toronto.ca/legdocs/mmis/2010/hl/bgrd/backgroundfile-33845.pdf

Treuhaft, S., & Karpyn, A. (2010). *The grocery gap: Who has access to healthy food and why it matters.* Oakland, CA: PolicyLink. Retrieved from http://www.policylink.org/atf/cf/%7B97C6D565-BB43-406D-A6D5-ECA3BBF35AF0%7D/FINALGroceryGap.pdf

Ward, K., & England, K. (2007). Introduction: Reading neoliberalization. In K. England & K. Ward (eds.), *Neoliberalization: States, networks, people* (pp. 1–22). Oxford: Blackwell.

Williams, P. L., Watt, C. G., Amero, M., Anderson, B. J., Blum, I., Green-LaPierre, R., … Reimer, D. E. (2012). Affordability of a nutritious diet for income assistance recipients in Nova Scotia (2002–2010). *Canadian Journal of Public Health, 103,* 183–188.

CHAPTER 10

Synthesizing Review Evidence on Community-Based Diet and Nutrition, Built Environment, and the Social Determinants of Health in Canada

Maureen Dobbins, Daiva Tirilis, and Kara Decorby

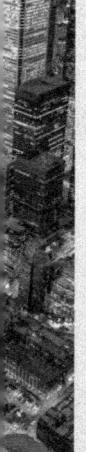

TAKE-HOME MESSAGE

- Community-based diet and nutrition interventions appear most promising for those with pre-existing conditions in relation to weight loss, but less so as a preventive strategy to maintain a healthy weight.
- Built environment interventions focused on improving street lighting, safety, ease of street crossing, sidewalk continuity, and traffic calming was associated with increased physical activity.
- While many public health interventions may result in improved health outcomes at the population level, evidence suggests intervention effects are not equally distributed across the population with those at a lower socioeconomic status experiencing fewer health improvements..

INTRODUCTION

A growing incidence of chronic diseases has contributed to increased political and societal pressure to ensure public funds are allocated to services with known effectiveness. This call to action is intended to result in improved health outcomes for Canadians. Evidence suggests that current practices related to the promotion of healthy dietary behaviours, the built environment, and social determinants of health may not adequately address health inequities and may even increase disparities. This paper identifies and summarizes research findings on the effectiveness of population-based interventions identified as priority areas in the Ontario Chief Medical Officer of Health's annual report to the legislative assembly: (1) community-based diet and nutrition; (2) built environment; and (3) social determinants of health.

Community-Based Diet and Nutrition

Proper nutrition is essential to the growth and development of children and youth, as well as maintaining health in adulthood. While the Canadian Food Guide suggests a minimum of 5 daily servings of vegetables and fruit, 7 out of 10 children aged 4 to 8 and half of all adults are not meeting this recommended minimum (Garriguet, 2004; Health Canada, 2011). Over 25 percent of Canadians aged 31 to 50 get more than 35 percent of their total calories from fat, increasing their health risks, such as elevating their BMI (Garriguet, 2004). Additionally, children and adults in low- and lower-income households are more likely than those in higher-income households to get more than 35 percent of their daily calories from fat (Garriguet, 2004).

Built Environment

As defined by the Public Agency of Canada (n.d), *built environment* "is part of our physical surroundings and includes the buildings, parks, schools, road systems, and other infrastructure that we encounter in our daily lives." These environments can influence physical and mental health through factors such as community design, safe water, safe neighbourhoods, and access to education, public transit, and recreation services. Built environment also includes adequate housing, since it is a critical component to each individual's environment. As such, housing outcomes can directly and indirectly impact health. For example, respiratory illnesses and allergies can be related to mould, dampness, or poorly ventilated houses (World Health Organization, 2009). Subsequently, the built environment also has an impact on and contributes to the social determinants of health (Frohlich, Ross, & Richmond, 2006).

Social Determinants of Health

Social determinants of health include a wide range of factors, such as social class, income, education and literacy, race and ethnicity, and housing quality (Halfon, Larson, & Russ, 2010). Social relationships are also factors considered part of the social determinants of health, and can have an influence, such as chronic illness in later life, being the product of adverse early social exposures (Halfon, Larson, & Russ, 2010). As the boundaries of social determinants expand, it is important to synthesize what is known and how the health of individuals can be improved.

Evidence-Informed Decision Making

Evidence-informed decision making (EIDM) is accepted in Canada as necessary for the provision of effective health care services. The goal of the public health sector in Canada is to promote health and reduce the amount of disease, premature death, and pain and suffering in the population through health promotion, disease and injury prevention, and health protection (Naylor et al., 2003). The effectiveness of public health services has direct implications for health system outcomes and expenditures, as the following example illustrates. In 2005, chronic diseases such as cardiovascular disease (CVD), cancer, emphysema, and diabetes accounted for 35 million deaths worldwide (Catford, 2007); had been increasing steadily over the past two decades; and in 2002, the economic burden of CVD and cancer alone in Canada was $32.7 billion (Health Canada, 2002). Overweight and physical inactivity, recognized risk factors for chronic diseases (Centers for Disease Control, 2000; Lobstein, Baur, & Uauy, 2004), have also risen steadily in the past two decades. Canadian data suggests a 10 percent decrease in sedentary behaviour would result in health savings of $150 million per year (Katzmarzyk, Gledhill, & Shephard, 2000).

METHODS

Healthevidence.org was searched in May 2011 for evidence reviews evaluating interventions targeted at diet and nutrition, built environment, and SDH. A standardized quality assessment tool used by two independent reviewers appraised relevant reviews. Only reviews deemed to be of strong methodological quality were retained for this synthesis. Data extracted included participant age, research design, quality rating, intervention details, outcomes evaluated and how they were measured, and actual outcome data.

RESULTS

Community-Based Diet and Nutrition

Thirty-three high-quality reviews were identified, with 17 reporting relevant outcomes: improved diet (N=10), weight change (N=5), and reduced body mass index (BMI) (N=5). Participants ranged from healthy adults to obese adults and adults diagnosed with pre-diabetes, as well as children, adolescents, and ethnic and low-income populations. Interventions varied significantly across included reviews but can be classified as follows: improving diet, weight management, fruit and vegetable consumption, nutrition education, sodium reduction, cognitive/behavioural change strategies, lifestyle interventions, self-help interventions, and incentives.

Cognitive/behavioural change strategies result in significantly large effects on eating behaviours among adults. Evidence supports the provision of behaviour change interventions—self-monitoring plus one other self-regulating intervention (intention formation, feedback, goal setting, review of behavioural goals)—to improve healthy eating. While behavioural- and education-based nutrition strategies are associated with healthier diets, some evidence suggests nutrition interventions may be associated with increased health disparities. This finding is discussed in the full report (Dobbins & Tirilis, 2011).

Community-based interventions significantly increase fruit and vegetable consumption among preschoolers, school-aged children, and adults (when implemented in workplaces). However, the magnitude of effect may not produce clinically significant health benefits. Much of the evidence suggests that community-based diet and nutrition interventions do not impact BMI among children, adolescents, or adults, although some evidence suggests these interventions may be effective among those diagnosed with pre-diabetes.

Overall, evidence suggests weight loss interventions are effective, particularly in obese and high-risk (pre-diabetes) groups. Significant effects at 2 to 3 years post-intervention are not maintained long-term (5 years). Incentives are effective in reducing weight, but long-term impact is unknown. The impact of incentives on subgroups (low SES, different ethnicities) has not yet been studied.

Built Environment

Thirty-seven high-quality reviews were identified, with 27 reporting relevant outcomes: injuries and safety (N=11), mental health (N=8), physical activity behaviour (N=7), and household air quality (N=5). Participants ranged from the general population to children, adults, older adults, and ethnic and low-income populations. Settings included roadways, worksites, and homes. Interventions included traffic safety, occupational health, supportive housing, physical environment, falls prevention, home safety, child safety, and physical activity.

Injury Prevention: Home safety education and/or provision of low-cost or free equipment did not result in fewer injuries among children in homes, or fewer visits to the emergency department.

Mental Health: There is evidence of a positive effect of housing on mental health outcomes among adults and male children, but not female children. Positive effects lasted as long as 2 to 3 years post-intervention in some studies. A number of less rigorous studies show that access to green spaces, rehousing, refurbishment, and relocation interventions are associated with better mental health. Where the impact of witnessing crime or being a victim of crime was explored, evidence illustrates poorer mental health outcomes for both adults and children, with similar results for neighbourhood disorder. Evidence on the relationship between population density and psychological outcomes is mixed, with some reporting worse psychological outcomes for adults in high density areas, and others reporting no association.

Household Air Quality: Education about allergen exposure and provision of allergen-reduction equipment shows significant reductions in physician-diagnosed asthma and sick days in children, but not symptoms (wheezing and lung function). Evidence on dust mite control is not rigorous but illustrates that mite-impermeable bedding significantly reduced dust mite load but not dust levels. A growing body of evidence suggests interventions targeting children's exposure to environmental tobacco smoke, particularly at home, achieves some reduction in exposure.

Physical Activity: Evidence on travel behaviour change is mixed and is not high quality. Limited evidence shows people are using cars less and walking more, with an equal amount of evidence reporting no impact on behaviour. Limited evidence shows that subsidy of employees who choose not to drive positively impacts travel behaviour. Interventions targeting promoting walking and cycling during leisure time appear to have beneficial effects on behaviour. (Examples of effective interventions and important components and elements of their delivery are explored in greater detail in the full report; see Dobbins & Tirilis, 2011.) Interventions focused on promoting active and educational activities and improving cycle route networks increase the proportion of people cycling, frequency of cycling, and distance travelled. However, the overall effect size remains relatively small. Bike path use increases with media and social marketing campaigns and is sustained long-term, but did not translate into increased cycling prevalence in the population. Lastly, improved street lighting or infrastructure that increases ease and safety of street crossing, ensures sidewalk continuity, introduces or enhances traffic calming, or enhances the aesthetics of the street (e.g., landscaping) were found to have positive effects on physical activity behaviour.

Social Determinants of Health

Thirty-one high-quality reviews were identified, with 17 reporting relevant outcomes: health care utilization (N=10), mental health (N=9), physical health (N=6), and behavioural problems (N=6). Participants ranged from the general population with low literacy to adults with mental disorders and homeless persons, as well as children, adults, and health professionals. Interventions can be classified as improving health, supportive housing, home visiting/social support programs, improving literacy, after-school programs, gang/violence prevention, monetary incentives, reducing disparities, and prevention of sexually transmitted infections.

Nursing home visits in the prenatal period were associated with increased awareness of available community services, greater attendance at childbirth education classes, and speaking more frequently with service providers. Furthermore, social support interventions for at-risk pregnant women resulted in significantly fewer hospital admissions during pregnancy.

In contrast, health interventions among those with low literacy had no impact on health-related outcomes or mammography screening rates in the long term, though positive effects for screening rates were observed at six months. Assertive community treatment (ACT) reduced homelessness and hospitalization outcomes. A single study illustrated that combining case management and subsidized housing reduced inpatient and outpatient health care utilization. However, no impact was observed for substance use, psychiatric symptoms, or outpatient mental health care use. Finally, strategies to prevent HIV and other sexually transmitted infections among female sex workers in resource-poor settings effectively increased use of preventive services.

Evidence on the impact of social determinants of health interventions on mental health is mixed. Some suggest that for homeless persons with severe mental illness, ACT significantly reduced homelessness and improved psychiatric symptom severity. Additional evidence indicates that intensive case management with access to drop-in services, temporary housing, and rehabilitation improves symptoms and perceived quality of life compared to usual care. Among those with a substance use disorder, case management vs. standard care did not significantly affect psychiatric symptoms. However, among those with intellectual disability and concurrent physical, mental, or behavioural problems, and in homeless populations with concurrent mental illness and substance use disorders, ACT did not improve psychological and psychiatric function or reduce substance use. Those receiving housing support spent less time hospitalized and reported more days housed, but did not experience fewer symptoms or reduced substance use.

The evidence indicates that health care services for populations with intellectual disabilities were not effective in improving behavioural issues such as adaptive behaviours. Similarly, the provision of financial resources to families with low SES did not lead to significant improvements in problem behaviour among children nor delinquent behaviour in adolescents. Evidence illustrates that a universal school-based program to prevent violent and aggressive behaviour resulted in a 15 percent reduction school-wide, with the greatest impact observed in pre-kindergarten, kindergarten, and high school students. Equal impact was demonstrated in schools located in low SES and high-crime environments. A description of interventions, topics, and elements of effective interventions are discussed in the full report (Dobbins & Tirilis, 2011).

Postnatal home visiting for teenaged mothers with low SES resulted in significant weight and height gain in infants and better Denver Developmental Screening Test scores at four months, compared to infants of mothers in standard care. Among very low-weight infants, telephone support and home visiting together resulted in significantly fewer re-hospitalizations and acute care visits, as well as less failure to thrive, child abuse, and foster placement. High-risk mothers with low SES receiving prenatal and postnatal visits reported fewer bladder infections and cigarettes smoked daily, and improved nutrition. Provision of financial resources to low SES families did not reduce child maltreatment, physical/emotional/sexual abuse, emergency department visits, or injuries.

CONCLUSION

This review represents many systematic reviews, meta-analyses, primary studies, and thousands of participants. Results illustrate that many population health and public health programs are associated with benefits to particular populations, especially related to outcomes such as healthy eating, physical activity, mental health symptoms, more stable housing, and, in some populations, substance use. There is cause for concern given that evidence suggests some interventions may in fact widen health disparities. As a result, higher SES and white populations benefit from certain interventions more than others. More research is needed to fully explore whether and how interventions impact heath in different subpopulations. However, review evidence provides direction, draws attention to areas requiring ongoing evaluation, and identifies practices that may not produce the expected impact, which should be examined critically in terms of future investment. While a great deal has been accomplished in population and public health programs, there is still much work to be done!

GLOSSARY

Built environment: The human-made space in which people live, work, and play on a day-to-day basis.

Evidence-informed decision making: The process of distilling and disseminating the best available evidence from research, practice, and experience and using that evidence to inform and improve public health policy and practice.

Health disparities: The variation in rates of disease occurrence and disabilities between socioeconomic and/or geographically defined population groups.

Health equity: The study and causes of differences in the quality of health and health care across different populations.

Health inequities: Differences in health status or in the distribution of health determinants between different population groups.

Social determinants of health (SDH): Economic and social conditions and their distribution among the population that influence individual and group differences in health status.

Socioeconomic status: An economic and sociological measure of a person's work experience and of an individual's or a family's economic and social position in relation to others, based on income, education, and occupation.

DISCUSSION QUESTIONS

1.   Are population-based strategies effective in promoting healthier eating across populations? If, yes, which strategies appear to be most promising?
2.   Which built environment interventions are most likely to result in significant improvements in mental health outcomes?
3.   Which strategies are effective in improving future health outcomes of babies born to adolescent mothers with low socioeconomic status?

REFERENCES

Catford, J. (2007). Chronic disease: preventing the world's next tidal wave—The challenge for Canada 2007? *Health Promotion International, 22,* 1–4.

Centers for Disease Control. (2000). *Nutrition and physical activity.* Atlanta: Centers for Disease Control.

Dobbins, M., & Tirilis, D. (2011). *A synthesis of review evidence: An overview of systematic review evidence on the effectiveness of community-based interventions to promote healthy diet and nutrition, built environment, and social determinants of health.* Hamilton, ON: McMaster University.

Frohlich, K., Ross, N., & Richmond, C. (2006). Health disparities in Canada today: Some evidence and a theoretical framework. *Health Policy, 79*(2–3), 132–143.

Garriguet, D. (2004). *Overview of Canadians' eating habits.* Ottawa: Statistics Canada.

Halfon, N., Larson, K., & Russ, S. (2010). Why social determinants? *Healthcare Quarterly, 14*(Special Issue 1), 8–20.

Health Canada. (2002). *Economic burden of illness in Canada, 1998.* Ottawa: Health Canada.

Health Canada. (2011). *Canada's food guide.* Ottawa: Health Canada.

Katzmarzyk P. T, Gledhill, N., & Shephard, R. J. (2000). The economic burden of physical inactivity in Canada. *Canadian Medical Association Journal, 163*(11), 1435–1440.

Lobstein, T., Baur, L., & Uauy, R. (2004). Obesity in children and young people: A crisis in public health. *Obesity Reviews, 5*(Suppl. 1), 4–85.

Naylor, D., Basrur, S., Bergeron, M. G., Brunham, R.C., Butler-Jones, D., Dafoe, G., Plummer, F. (2003). *Learning from SARS: Renewal of public health in Canada.* Ottawa: Health Canada.

Public Health Agency of Canada. (n.d.). *Supportive environments for physical activity: How the built environment affects our health.* Ottawa: Public Health Agency of Canada. Retrieved from http://www.phac-aspc.gc.ca/hp-ps/hl-mvs/be-eb-eng.php#1

World Health Organization. (2009). *Damp and Mould: Health risks, prevention and remedial actions.* Copenhagen: WHO Regional Office for Europe.

CHAPTER 11

Inequities in Housing and the Health of Recent Immigrants to Canada: Summary of a Literature Review

Ronald Labonté, Abdullahel Hadi, Corinne Packer, Vivien Runnels, and Arne Ruckert

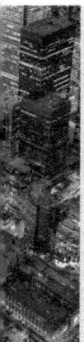

TAKE-HOME MESSAGE

- The lack of adequate and affordable housing continues to have detrimental effects on the health of recent immigrants to Canada, with the medium- and long-term health costs of inadequate housing greater than the costs of ensuring affordable housing in the short-term.
- New policy directions are required if inadequate housing conditions are to be prevented.

INTRODUCTION

The important role of housing as a determinant of health has been well documented in population health literature (Bryant, 2003; Dunn & Dyck, 2000; Miles & Jacobs, 2008; National Center for Healthy Housing, 2009; Stewart & Rhoden, 2006). Housing has an impact on health through a number of direct and indirect pathways, including the presence of lead and mould, poor heating and drafts, inadequate ventilation, the presence of vermin, and other determinants of adverse health effects (Mikkonen & Raphael, 2010). Overcrowding enables the speedy transmission of respiratory and other illnesses, while high housing costs can diminish the resources available to support other social determinants of health. The effects of housing conditions on health have been extensively reviewed among most major population sub-groups in Canada. However, although there is growing interest in immigrant access to affordable housing, very few studies attempted to assess the effects of housing on immigrant health.

The purpose of this narrative review is to fill this gap and assess the evidence base for the effects of housing on the health and well-being of recent immigrants to Canada. Specific objectives were to review the profiles of recent immigrants to Canada and examine the accessibility of recent immigrants to adequate and affordable housing compared to other Canadians. The review also assessed the effects of housing on health, in particular with regards to recent immigrant communities. We further considered the changes to housing policies that might have created inequities in housing affordability among Canadian populations. Finally, we identified policy options that can promote adequate and affordable housing for recent immigrants, thereby reducing housing-related health inequities in Canada.

METHODS

We adopted a systematic approach composed of the following sequence of activities: determine the synthesis questions; conduct a mapping exercise; refine the search strategy; appraise and classify evidence; synthesize selected evidence; adapt international findings to the Canadian context; and summarize potential policy implications of the findings. Literature was sought through a variety of sources, including electronic databases, reference lists, and hand-searching of key journals. The primary database was Medline, Embase and Web of Science (SSCI). Other databases such as Google Scholar, GreyNet International, ISI Web of Knowledge, and Scopus were also searched. We also reviewed reference lists of the relevant studies on housing and health that met the inclusion/exclusion criteria. Keywords used were *housing, shelter, housing policy, immigrant, newcomer, settlement, health, equity,* and *well-being.*

The inclusion and exclusion criteria used to select studies were articles/reports that were: about the housing and health of immigrants; published in English; published from January 1991 to August 2010; and relevant to the Canadian context. The final search provided 318 citation titles, 77 of which met the inclusion criteria, although not all of these are referenced in this article.

RESULTS

The Changing Profiles of Immigrants to Canada

While Europe has long been the primary source of immigration to Canada, most recent immigrants (those who have entered the country within the past 10 years) have come from East and South Asia, followed by the Middle East and Africa. This is changing the traditional mosaic of ethnic groups, particularly in large metropolitan centres (Wayland, 2007). Although recent immigrants are better educated and skilled than their earlier counterparts, they experience extreme difficulties in the job market (Statistics Canada, 2005), largely because of the lack of Canadian experience and skills (Wayland, 2007). Evidence indicates that people with non-Canadian education earned 30 percent less than those with a Canadian education after arriving in Canada (Alboim, Finnie, & Meng, 2005). Also, overseas labour market experience is associated with reduced earnings of 25 to 50 percent relative to comparable Canadian experience (Alboim, Finnie, & Meng, 2005; Aydemir

& Skuterud, 2004). The overall slower growth of the Canadian economy in recent decades is also considered an employment-related barrier for newcomers (Wayland, 2007). Recent immigrants, therefore, have tended to rent rather than own their homes. Housing "pathways" also differ by ethnicity of recent immigrants. Immigrants from southern Europe in the past and China in recent years have been the most successful in becoming homeowners, while Caribbean and South Asian immigrants have experienced difficulties in affording homes (Wayland, 2007). Regardless of their country of origin, most recent immigrants settle in one of three large metropolitan areas: Toronto, Vancouver, and Montreal (Wayland, 2007).

Poverty and Affordability of Housing for Recent Immigrants

Recent immigrants are generally poorer compared to earlier immigrants and native-born Canadians, and the income gap between recent immigrants and other Canadians has been increasing (Picot, 2004). Poverty and poor economic standing, in turn, are associated with limited access to housing and other needed services (Reid, Vittinghoff, & Kushel, 2008). In a study on changes in housing affordability and Toronto's rental market, Murdie (2003) found that recent immigrants with low income had very limited access to affordable housing, paid a large share of their income on housing, and were unlikely to have enough money to spend on food, clothing, transportation, and educational supplies. This resulted in a weakened ability to improve their quality of life. Opportunities in the labour and housing markets, the study notes, have worsened substantially for recent immigrants compared to earlier immigrants to the area.

Other studies have found that most recent immigrants spend more than 30 percent of household earnings on accommodation (Carter, Polevychok, Friesen, & Osborne, 2008) while a small proportion spend 50 percent of their incomes on rent (CMHC [Canada Mortgage and Housing Corporation], 2004). On average, recent immigrants have to spend 6.3 percent more of their income for housing than other Canadians, while their average income was 18.9 percent less (CHMC, 2004; Wachsmuth, 2008). Unsurprisingly, a study of early settlement experiences found that 31 percent of recent immigrants identified high housing cost as the greatest problem they encountered (Statistics Canada, 2005). Compared to the Canadian average, only a small proportion of recent immigrants have been successful in owning homes in recent years (CMHC, 2004).

Barriers, discrimination, and challenges in the housing market in Canada by ethnicity are well known (Murdie, Preston, Ghosh, & Chevalier, 2006; Teixeira, 2008; Wachsmuth, 2008). Immigrants with minority identities have greater difficulties finding appropriate housing (Wachsmuth, 2008) than whites, and racialized immigrants (notably Black African immigrants) are generally treated differently in housing markets (Danso & Grant, 2001; Hulchanski, 1997). Using the housing experience of Black African immigrant communities in Calgary, Danso and Grant (2001) identified various difficulties in the employment market and ethnicity-based discrimination in the housing market. These findings suggest the existence of racial inequity that reinforces residential inequalities by ethnicity (Dion, 2001).

Of particular concern in the Canadian context is the fact that Canada's housing market in recent decades has become increasingly inaccessible to low-income individuals and households, resulting in inequities in housing accessibility, affordability, and adequacy (Hulchanski, 2007).

Housing and Health

The correlations between housing and health outcomes have been extensively studied (Bryant, 2003; Dunn & Dyck, 2000; Miles & Jacobs, 2008; National Center for Healthy Housing, 2009; Stewart & Rhoden, 2006). Poor housing conditions affect various dimensions of health. Krieger and Higgins (2002) synthesized evidence that shows how overcrowding with poor ventilation increases interior moisture; exposure to organic compounds such as lead can cause asthma; exposure to deteriorating insulation can cause lung cancer; dirty carpeting contains dust and allergens; and toxic substances can result in allergic, respiratory, neurological, and haematological illnesses and chronic health problems. The WHO (2004), in a review of housing and health, found poor housing (with potential exposure to toxins, lead, asbestos, or carbon monoxide) to be associated with higher incidence of asthma, respiratory and skin allergies, and lung diseases. Several studies conducted in the UK found that poor environmental conditions, such as dampness and exposure to asbestos and radon, led to higher prevalence of asthma, meningitis, hypothermia, skin and eye irritation, and coronary heart disease (Care Services Improvement Partnership, 2010; Harker, 2006). In a literature review of over 100 research studies undertaken in the UK, bad housing, defined by homelessness, overcrowding, and poor physical conditions, was found to be associated with a higher incidence of childhood accidents and poor health status in children (Harker, 2006). Overcrowding, generally associated with poverty, can aggravate existing health problems and increase the risk of skin infections, meningitis, respiratory infections, childhood tuberculosis, and poor mental health (Australian Indigenous Health, 2008; Goux & Maurin, 2005; Harker, 2006; Murphy, 2006).

Housing and Immigrant Health

For recent immigrants, access to adequate and suitable housing with security of tenure is an important facilitator of integration into a new society (Ley, Murphy, Olds, & Randolph, 2001, pp. 141–152; Murdie, Preston, Ghosh, & Chevalier, 2006). Good housing not only reduces the length of resettlement for immigrants, but also reduces long-term costs to society in other areas such as health, education, social assistance, and employment insurance (Ambrose, 2001; Carter & Polevychok, 2004; Dunn & Dyck, 2000; Jacobs et al., 2009; Thompson, Petticrew, & Morrison, 2001). Immigrants, compared to native-born

Canadians, have better health status when they arrive in Canada (Chiu et al., 2009; Dean & Wilson, 2010; Perez, 2002), partly because persons with serious health problems are screened in the immigration process (Ali, McDermott, & Gravel, 2004). Over time, the health status of immigrants declines compared to that of the average native-born population (Dean & Wilson, 2010). How much of this decline might be attributed to poor housing has not been systematically reviewed, and only a few Canadian studies have attempted to assess specifically the effects of housing on migrant health (Mattu, 2002; Murdie, Preston, Ghosh, & Chevalier, 2006). However, in Canada, recent immigrants with low incomes have experienced substantial housing deprivation (such as poor environmental conditions, overcrowding, and homelessness), which can have serious health implications (Marsh, 1999).

Hyman (2004) found resettlement stress among Canadian immigrants to be associated with diabetes, the re-activation of tuberculosis (from their previous infections in countries of origin), and a decline in mental health. The decline of the "healthy immigrant effect" noted earlier has been explained in a US study by, in part, the low income of recent immigrants and associated poor physical facilities, overcrowding, and inappropriate housing environments (Early et al., 2006).

Public Housing and Health

There has been some academic and research interest in understanding the social and economic returns of housing investment. A decade-old systematic review found that public investment in housing can significantly reduce heating and cooling costs and improve physical and mental health (Thompson, Petticrew, & Morrison, 2001). A British intervention study—conducted in an overcrowded, poor, and inner urban area of West London with a matched control community—showed a seven-fold improvement in health, measured in self-rated illness days (Ambrose, 2001). A recent Canadian review argues that the cost needed to provide affordable housing is much less than the costs required to provide health care, education, and other social services for those who would benefit from better housing (Wellesley Institute, 2010). Overall, evidence suggests that investing in housing reduces health care and welfare costs. Spending on housing programs for marginalized communities can also generate desired social returns in the long run. Housing support for low-income households has already been adopted as a policy tool to de-concentrate poverty (Suttor, 2007). Such programs (for example, shelter allowance in Canada and rental voucher programs in the UK) have been effective in improving household safety and security (Strange, 2003; Taske, Taylor, Mulcihill, & Doyle, 2005).

Public Housing Policy in Canada

Government shifts in ideology have led to an emphasis on private markets—markets that create the conditions that reduce the affordability of housing (Bryant, 2003). Canada now has the largest market-based private housing sector of the developed countries after the US. This strategy has not only been discriminatory in the way it treats owners and renters (Hulchanski, 2007); it has also shifted from providing affordable housing to low-income households to relying on market mechanisms to do so. Property investment decisions are left primarily to private markets, which in turn are shaped largely by corporate strategic interests where investing for affordable housing is not a priority (Hulchanski, 2007).

Another key concern in Ontario is the downloading of responsibilities for housing and homelessness policies to the municipal level, implemented as part of Ontario's Long-Term Affordable Housing Strategy, without providing the financial and programmatic tools for municipalities to properly administer affordable housing and homelessness programs. Programmed cutbacks and devolution of authority come at a time when the affordable housing wait list in Toronto has reached an all-time high at 90,000 households, representing a 25 percent increase since 2009. In Ontario, a record 167,000 households are currently on the wait list for affordable housing (Shapcott, 2014).

CONCLUSION

The lack of adequate and affordable housing has and will continue to have detrimental effects on the health of recent immigrants to Canada. It also compounds other stresses (such as higher rates of poverty, and the stresses of settlement) that affect recent immigrants' health. Some studies suggest that the medium- and long-term health costs of inadequate housing could be greater than the costs of ensuring affordable housing in the short-term.

If inadequate housing conditions are to be prevented, several policy directions are suggested by the available evidence, including: (i) the provision of rental subsidies, including a targeted subsidy for recent immigrants in need; (ii) consideration of the reinstatement of rent control by provincial governments affecting all population groups experiencing difficulty in accessing affordable housing; and (iii) a needs-based share of the current stock of affordable housing dedicated to recent immigrants.

GLOSSARY

Housing "pathways": Housing impacts health through a number of direct and indirect pathways, including the presence of lead and mould, poor heating and drafts, inadequate ventilation, the presence of vermin, and other determinants of adverse health effects (Mikkonen & Raphael, 2010).

DISCUSSION QUESTIONS

1. What are some of the factors that could explain why immigrants from southern Europe and China have been more successful in becoming homeowners than Caribbean or South Asian immigrants?

2. To what extent is the decline of the health status of immigrants over time attributable to poor housing?

3. What are some of the solutions that would allow Ontario municipalities to effectively implement the Long-Term Affordable Housing Strategy given the prohibitively high rate of households on the wait list for affordable housing?

REFERENCES

Alboim, N., Finnie, R., & Meng, R. (2005). The discounting of immigrants' skills in Canada: Evidence and policy recommendations. *IRPP Choices, 11*, 1–26.

Ali, J. S., McDermott, S., & Gravel, R. G. (2004). Recent research on immigrant health from Statistics Canada's population surveys. *Canadian Journal of Public Health, 95*(3), 1–9.

Ambrose, P. J. (2001). Living conditions and health promotion strategies. Journal of the Royal *Society for the Promotion of Health, 121*(1), 9–15.

Australian Indigenous HealthInfoNet. (2008). *Review of the impact of housing and health-related infrastructure on indigenous health.* Retrieved from http://www.healthinfonet.ecu.edu.au/determinants/physical-environment/reviews/our-review

Aydemir, A., & Skuterud, M. (2004). *Explaining the deteriorating entry earnings of Canada's immigrant cohorts: 1966–2000.* Economics Working Paper, Labour and Demography Series. Ottawa: Statistics Canada.

Bryant, T. (2003). The current state of housing in Canada as a social determinant of health. *Policy Options, 24*, 52–56.

Carter, T., & Polevychok, C. (2004). *Housing is good social policy.* Ottawa: Canadian Policy Research Networks Inc.

Carter, T., Polevychok, C., Friesen, A., & Osborne, J. (2008). *The housing circumstances of recently arrived refugees: The Winnipeg experience.* Edmonton: Prairie Metropolis Centre.

Chiu, S., Redelmeier, D. A., Tolomiczenko, G., Kiss, A., & Hwang, S. W. (2009). The health of homeless immigrants. *Journal of Epidemiology and Community Health, 63*(11), 943–948.

Canada Mortgage and Housing Corporation. (2004). *2001 census housing series issue 7 revised: Immigrant households.* Socio economic Series 04-042. Ottawa: CMHC.

Care Services Improvement Partnership. (2010). *Good housing and good health? A review and recommendations for housing and health practitioners.* Sector Study, Care Services Improvement Partnership, UK. Retrieved from http://www.healthimpactproject.org/resources/document/Good_housing_and_good_health.pdf

Danso, R., & Grant, M. (2001). Access to housing as an adaptive strategy for immigrant groups: Africans in Calgary. *Canadian Ethnic Studies, 32*, 19–43.

Dean, J.A., & Wilson, K. (2010). "My health has improved because I always have everything I need here.": A qualitative exploration of health improvement and decline among immigrants. *Social Science & Medicine, 70*, 1219–1228.

Dion, K.L. (2001). Immigrants' perceptions of housing discrimination in Toronto: The housing new Canadians project. *Journal of Social Issues, 57*, 523–539.

Dunn, J.R., & Dyck, I. (2000). Social determinants of health in Canada's immigrant population: Results from the National Population Health Survey. *Social Science & Medicine, 51*, 1573–1593.

Early, J., Davis, S. W., Quandt, S. A., Rao, P., Snively, B. M., & Arcury, T. A. (2006). Housing characteristics of farmworker families in North Carolina. *Journal of Immigrant and Minority Health, 8*, 173–184.

Goux, D., & Maurin, E. (2005). The effect of overcrowded housing on children's performance at school. *Journal of Public Economics, 89*, 797–819.

Harker, L. (2006). Chance of a lifetime: The impact of bad housing on children's lives. Edinburgh: Shelter.

Hulchanski, J. D. (1997). *Immigrants and access to housing: How welcome are newcomers to Canada?* Metropolis year II Conference, The Development of a Comparative Research Agenda, Montreal, November 23–26, 1997.

Hulchanski, J. D. (2007). *Canada's dual housing policy: Assisting owners, neglecting renters: Research bulletin no. 38.* Toronto: Centre for Urban and Community Studies, University of Toronto.

Hyman, I. (2004). Setting the stage: Reviewing current knowledge on the health of Canadian immigrants. *Canadian Journal of Public Health, 95*(3), 1–8.

Jacobs, D. E., Wilson, J., Dixon, S. L., Smith, J., & Evens, A. (2009). The relationship of housing and population health: A 30-year retrospective analysis. *Environmental Health Perspectives, 117*(4), 597–604.

Krieger, J., & Higgins, D. (2002). Housing and health: Time again for public health action. *American Journal of Public Health, 92*(5), 758–768.

Ley, D., Murphy, P., Olds, K., & Randolph, B. (2001). Immigration in gateway cities: Sydney and Vancouver in comparative perspective. *Progress in Planning, 55*, 119–194.

Marsh, A. (1999). Housing and health: The nature of the connection. *Radical Statistics, 72*.

Mattu, P. (2002). *A survey on the extent of substandard housing problems faced by immigrants and refugees in the lower mainland of British Columbia.* Vancouver, BC: MOSAIC. Retrieved from https://www.mosaicbc.org/wp-content/uploads/2017/01/SCPI-Summary-Report_0.pdf

Mikkonen, J., & Raphael, D. (2010). *Social determinants of health: The Canadian facts.* Toronto: York University School of Health Policy and Management.

Miles, R., & Jacobs, D.E. (2008). Future directions in housing and public health: Findings from Europe with broader implications for planners. *Journal of the American Planning Association, 74*(1), 77–89.

Murdie, R.A. (2003). Housing affordability and Toronto's rental market: Perspectives from the housing careers of Jamaican, Polish and Somali newcomers. *Housing, Theory and Society, 20*, 183–196.

Murdie, R., Preston, V., Ghosh, S., & Chevalier, M. (2006). *Immigrants and housing: A review of Canadian literature from 1990 to 2005.* Ottawa: Canada Mortgage and Housing Corporation.

Murphy, D. (2006). *Exploring the complex relationship between housing and health through consideration of the health needs of people who are homeless.* Prepared for the 2006 ENHR Conference Workshop 5, "The Residential Context of Health," Brussels, June 2006.

National Center for Healthy Housing. (2009). *Housing interventions and health: A review of the evidence.* Columbia, MD: NCHH.

Perez, C.E. (2002). Health status and health behaviour among immigrants. *Supplement to Health Reports, 13.* Ottawa: Statistics Canada.

Picot, G. (2004). The deteriorating economic welfare of Canadian immigrants. *Canadian Journal of Urban Research, 13,* 25–45.

Reid, K. W., Vittinghoff, E., & Kushel, M. B. (2008). Association between the level of housing instability, economic standing and health care access: A meta-regression. *Journal of Health Care for the Poor and Underserved, 19,* 1212–1228.

Shapcott, M. (2014). *Federal budget 2014 fails to deliver housing investments to meet national needs.* Retrieved from http://www.wellesleyinstitute.com/housing/federal-budget-2014-fails-to-deliver-housing-investments-to-meet-national-needs

Statistics Canada. (2005). *Longitudinal survey of immigrants to Canada: A portrait of early settlement experiences.* Catalogue No. 89-614-XIE. Ottawa: Statistics Canada.

Stewart, J., & Rhoden, M. (2006). Children, housing and health. *International Journal of Sociology and Social Policy, 26,* 326–341.

Strange, W. C. (2003). *The unintended consequences of housing policy.* Toronto: C.D. Howe Institute.

Suttor, G. (2007). Growth management and affordable housing in greater Toronto: A macro view of Toronto social mix and polarization. Ottawa: Canada Mortgage and Housing Corporation.

Taske, N., Taylor, L., Mulvihill, C., & Doyle, N. (2005). *Housing and public health: A review of reviews of interventions for improving health.* London: National Institute for Health and Clinical Excellence.

Teixeira, C. (2008). Barriers and outcomes in the housing searches of new immigrants and refugees: A case study of "Black" Africans in Toronto's rental market. *Journal of Housing and the Built Environment, 23,* 253–276.

Thompson, H., Petticrew, M., & Morrison, D. (2001). Health effects of housing improvement: Systematic review of intervention studies. *BMJ, 323*(7306), 187–190.

Wachsmuth, D. (2008). *Housing for immigrants in Ontario's medium-sized cities.* Ottawa & Toronto: Canadian Policy Research Networks Inc. & Social Housing Services Corporation.

Wayland, S.V. (2007). *The housing needs of immigrants and refugees in Canada.* Ottawa: Canadian Housing and Renewal Association.

Wellesley Institute. (2010). *Precarious housing in Canada.* Toronto: Wellesley Institute.

World Health Organization. (2004). *Review of evidence on housing and health: Background document.* Fourth Ministerial Conference on Environment and Health. Budapest, Hungary, 23–25 June, 2004.

CHAPTER 12

Wildfires and Population Health in Northeastern Ontario

K. S. Mohindra

TAKE-HOME MESSAGE

- Wildfires are an important and growing threat to population health, particularly in remote areas and among First Nation communities.
- Wildfires can affect both physical and psychological dimensions of population health.
- Addressing public health implications of wildfires will require multi-disciplinary approaches, involving multiple stakeholders.

INTRODUCTION

According to ancient Greek medicine, fire was one of the four elements of the human body, and its metabolic agent was yellow bile. Together fire and bile digest, consume, metabolize, and transform; they provoke, excite, and inflame, causing anger and irritability. This description could easily be given to the effects of wildfires, potentially sweeping and destructive forces on populations living in parts of rural and northern Canada.

Wildfires are not new, but rather have been a longstanding part of Canada's natural ecology. Experiences with wildfires, however, are a growing reality for Canadians, due to a combination of climate change, altered forest conditions, and an increasing number of houses being built in fire-prone areas. There has been a rise in the frequency of wildfires in Canada over the past 10 years. Many of these fires have been large, leading to widespread effects on the land and on the well-being of the population. In severe cases, evacuations are mandated for health concerns due to nearby fires or direct fire threats. Evacuation orders occur either because an area is under direct fire threat or community members are exposed to indirect threats from the fires, including biomass smoke, power outages, food shortages, and a lack of food storage capacity (some communities are only accessible by air).

In this chapter, we aim to draw greater attention to the population health issues related to wildfires for research and practice. First, we review the evidence linking wildfires and population health. Second, we discuss the specific impact of wildfires on population health in a fire-prone area in Canada: northeastern Ontario. Third, we highlight some of the roles that public health practitioners can assume prior to and after a wildfire.

WHAT DO WILDFIRES HAVE TO DO WITH POPULATION HEALTH?

The public safety implications of wildfires are evident and have been well established, but the population health issues have received relatively little attention. Moreover, there are important methodological difficulties in studying the health impacts of wildfires. Recent attention to this topic, with researchers applying innovative methods, has begun to yield some findings. The evidence base, however, remains small. In this chapter, we focus on the health effects supported by solid scientific evidence.

Wildfires can affect both the physical and psychological health of communities. Close proximity to fires can result in burns and heat-related illnesses; however, these are predominantly a concern for those engaged in firefighting and are beyond the scope of this chapter. We focus on three main pathways in which wildfires can affect the health of the general population.

The first pathway is through air pollution, which is produced by the combustion of biomass, yielding a range of pollutants—although elevated levels of fine particulate matter present the greatest risk to human health (Johnston et al., 2012). Studies have found that populations exposed to a deterioration of air quality during a wildfire have an increased risk of respiratory illnesses, including chronic obstructive pulmonary disease, bronchitis, asthma, and chest pain (Caamano-Isorna et al., 2011; Moore et al., 2006; Mott et al., 2002). Adverse effects of biomass smoke on respiratory health tend to be short term, although the effects may be more severe and long term for populations vulnerable to biomass smoke, notably young children, the elderly, those with pre-existing conditions, and smokers (Fowler, 2003; Sim, 2002). Other potential health consequences that arise from biomass smoke include eye irritations and traffic accidents due to reduced visibility (Finlay et al., 2012; Fowler, 2003).

The second pathway is via the economic and psychosocial determinants of health. Wildfires can lead to destruction of household or community property and loss of employment. These may be felt not only as economic losses, but as emotional losses as well. This grief, compounded by the stress of disruptions to family or social life, particularly during an evacuation, can be a major source of stress (Fowler, 2003). Wildfires are uncertain events; their strength and direction can change unexpectedly, leading to a sudden need to evacuate, which can compound the levels of stress experienced in a population (American Psychological Association, 2011). How individuals react and cope with a wildfire can vary tremendously. The psychological effects tend to be delayed, felt most deeply after the initial shock, and range from symptoms such as changes in mood and behaviour (e.g., heightened irritability, difficulty sleeping) to more severe illness, such as post-traumatic stress disorder (PTSD) or depression (American Psychological Association, 2011; Caamano-Isorna et al., 2011; Fowler, 2003; Marshall et al., 2007). There can also be positive psychosocial influences on health through resiliency, driven by community solidarity or the spirit of voluntarism.

The third pathway is through environmental contamination. Chemicals may be leached into ecosystems, which can occur through direct diffusion of chemicals from biomass smoke or increased erosion, which can lead to contamination of the soil or water supply (Fowler, 2003). There can also be widespread public exposure to chemicals from ash and debris (Wittig, Williams, & DuTeaux, 2008). The effects of these health risks from these sources of contamination are long term but have yet to be well established.

THE CASE OF NORTHEASTERN ONTARIO

In 1916, the great Matheson fire burned through northeastern Ontario, killing 224 people; it was the world's seventh-largest fire in terms of loss of life (Buse & Mount, 2011). More recently, the number of wildfires and the size of areas burned have been increasing across northern Ontario, with large-ranging effects (Box 12.1).

Box 12.1: Notable Wildfires in Northern Ontario

Northern Ontario: Over 120 wildfires between July 6 and July 25, 2011. Evacuations were required in a number of areas, leading to a total of 3,292 people evacuated. More than 85 hydro poles and over 13 km of hydro wire were damaged, which caused power outages across the north.

Mishkeegogamang Ojibway First Nation (New Osnaburgh): June 22 to 27, 2011. A state of emergency was declared as the First Nation community was overcome by smoke from more than 17 wildfires burning within 10 km of the community's housing area. A total of 423 residents were evacuated.

Chapleau: May 27, 2010. A wildfire burned through approximately 22 hydro poles and caused a power outage affecting approximately 2,000 local residents.

Northwest Ontario: May 13, 2007. A large fire 75 km west of Thunder Bay led to the evacuation of 300 residents.

Keewaywin First Nation, Townships of Terrace Bay and Schreiber, Village of Rossport, Pays Plat First Nation, and Deer Lake First Nation: July 1, 2002. Members of several communities were concerned by nearby fires and smoke. More than 1,000 people were evacuated to Thunder Bay, Geraldton, and Sioux Lookout. Municipal emergency declarations occurred in six communities.

Source: Public Safety Canada, n.d.

Vulnerability to wildfires (and other similar disasters) is a complex phenomenon, involving two components: (1) the degree of exposure to a wildfire, or *susceptibility*; and (2) the capacity to recover and cope with the consequences of a wildfire (Keim, 2008). Northeastern communities in Ontario are susceptible to wildfires since the forest coverage in this region is both vast (about 13.5 million hectares of production forests, approximately half of Ontario's managed forest area) and diverse, including stunted spruce, tamarack, and willow in the Hudson Bay Lowlands; boreal forests dominated by spruce, jack pine, poplar, and birch; and the transition forests, filled with hardwoods, of the Great Lakes St. Lawrence region (Buse & Mount, 2011). In addition, people who live and work in northeastern Ontario face threats to their capacity to cope with the consequences of wildfires; these encompass both geographical and health vulnerabilities.

Geographical Vulnerability

Ontario's northeast is characterized by vast land with a low population density. While there are four main urban centres, the northeast is largely rural and remote. There are over 100 single-tier municipalities as well as smaller towns and hamlets, which are settlements with a population below 500 that do not have a municipal authority. Many residents living in remote areas are at a great distance from other households and public services. This has implications for accessing health care (described below) and affects communication, which is critical during crisis situations. In the rural and remote areas of the northeast, there are some areas that lack road access. In addition, the large distances, low population density, weather, and technological challenges can hamper communication strategies. A recent survey of communication tools in the northeast found that conventional communication tools (e.g., high-speed internet, cellular phones) were not reliable tools to use during a crisis situation since not all areas could access them (Morris, 2009). Local media communication has become difficult; in 2009 the Canadian Broadcasting Corporation (CBC) reduced radio, television, and internet programs on their English and French networks due to financial cutbacks, and disproportionate cuts were made in northern Ontario, affecting local programming despite a wide audience (Grenier, 2009).

Health Vulnerability

According to the 2011 census, the population for Ontario's northeast was 508,982, which is about 4 percent of the population of the province. The percentage of senior residents (over 65 years of age) is about 18 percent and is expected to almost double by 2036 (to 30 percent). The northeast includes a diversity of linguistic and cultural groups. The largest proportion of French-speaking communities in Ontario resides in the northeast (23 percent) (North East LHIN, 2012); the francophone population is older and has lower levels of education compared to the northeast overall (North East LHIN, 2006). Ten percent of the population is Aboriginal, which includes 56 First Nations (51 percent of whom live off reserve) and Métis communities (North East LHIN, 2011). As in other parts of Canada, our colonial history and discriminatory policies have contributed to the marginalization of First Nations groups, which has resulted in lack of land, economic deprivation, and loss of cultural traditions and practices.

Mortality rates and the burden of ill health are higher in the northeast compared to the provincial averages, especially in the more remote areas. Infant mortality rate is 6.2 and 5.1 per 1000 people for the northeast and Ontario, respectively (MOHLTC, 2010). Life expectancy in the northeast is 76.5 years for men and 81.4 years for women, while in Ontario, male and female life expectancy is respectively 79.2 years 83.6 years (MOHLTC, 2010). The prevalence of several chronic diseases is higher in the northeast compared to Ontario, including asthma, diabetes, arthritis, chronic obstructive pulmonary disease (COPD), ischaemic heart disease, and some cancers. Of particular interest are the higher rates of respiratory illnesses, since people living with pre-existing respiratory conditions are more vulnerable if exposed to biomass smoke from wildfires. The elevated rates of chronic disease in the northeast are attributed partly to higher rates of disease key risk factors, such as high blood pressure, obesity and overweight, smoking, and heavy drinking. Again, the higher smoking rates are of particular concern for communities exposed to biomass smoke—in the northeast almost a quarter of men smoke, and about 15 percent of women. Smoking rates are elevated among francophone and First Nation populations (North East LHIN, 2006, 2011). The higher rates of chronic disease are also attributed to fundamental social causes of disease, notably poverty.

There is also a heavier burden of poor mental health in northeastern Ontario, which is particularly important given that experiencing a wildfire is associated with poorer mental health. The prevalence of major depressive disorders and other mood disorders, as well as suicides, is higher in the northeast than for the province (CMHA, 2009). Rates of depression and suicide are especially elevated among First Nation populations (North East LHIN, 2012). Self-reported mental health is also poorer, and there are higher rates of medication use and hospitalization for mental health disorders (CMHA, 2009).

Access to quality health care, including primary health care, mental health services, and tertiary care, is poorer in the northern and remote communities of Ontario compared to the rest of the province (CMHA, 2009; North East LHIN, 2012). The barriers to care include a short supply of health care providers, as well as geographical remoteness, long distances, low population density, and frequent poor weather conditions. Francophone and Aboriginal populations face further cultural and linguistic barriers to quality health care services (North East LHIN, 2006, 2011). These barriers preclude optimal access to those health services that would contribute to relieving health conditions in general, and those caused or exacerbated by a wildfire in particular.

IMPLICATIONS OF WILDFIRES FOR PUBLIC HEALTH PRACTICE IN NORTHEASTERN ONTARIO

The main public health issues of concern are: (1) the effects of air pollution on respiratory health, eye irritations, and traffic accidents due to reduced visibility (including signs and symptoms, how to reduce the severity of symptoms, and when and where to seek treatment); (2) the effects that wildfires have on social and economic determinants of health; and (3) potential mental health consequences (including signs and symptoms, how to reduce stress during a wildfire, and when and where to seek care). There is also less robust evidence linking wildfires, environmental contamination, and population health, which could potentially require explicit interventions in the future.

The geographic and health vulnerabilities in the northeast can be countered by building resilience among communities through strengthening public health preparedness and responses. There are a number of important roles for public health practioners, including promoting public understanding, monitoring and reporting the health effects of wildfires, and working with communities to protect their health during and following a wildfire (Box 12.2).

In addition, there is a need to work closely with local communities. Despite the diversity of people, there continues to be a strong connection between the people and the land

---

Box 12.2: Roles of Public Health Practitioners

Prior to a wildfire:

- Provide public education (e.g., population health and public safety resources for communities to consult when dealing with a wildfire and potential evacuation)
- Set up preventive programmes (e.g., public health considerations during evacuations; road safety during disasters)
- Survey diseases (e.g., COPD) and key risk factors (e.g., smoking) exacerbated by wildfires
- Forecast future health risks from projected wildfires

After a wildfire:

- Assess affected communities to identify health and medical needs and priorities
- Provide health care, food supplies, shelter, and adequate water and sanitation among displaced communities
- Provide health care (especially mental health) for communities affected by a wildfire
- Set up cleanup campaigns after a wildfire (notably in communities where high levels of toxins have been identified)
- Conduct environmental health assessments

that is unique and is claimed by the residents of northeastern Ontario as their own (Abel, 2006). This has helped to create a social identity that includes shared beliefs, values, and norms, which contributes to similar needs and a commitment to address them.

CONCLUSION

Given the growing influence of climate change, the threat of wildfires is expected to continue to increase (Keim, 2008). Moreover, some communities, such as those in northeastern Ontario, are already facing greater susceptibility and vulnerability to wildfires and their negative consequences on health, thereby perpetuating existing health inequities between the northeast and other regions of Ontario. Public health practicioners have an important role to play in developing a greater understanding of the health implications of wildfires and implementing appropriate responses, which will ultimately contribute to health equity in the province.

GLOSSARY

Biomass smoke: Smoke from biomass burning (e.g., burning of wood, leaves, trees, grass) resulting in increased levels of fine particulate matter (Curtis, 2002).
Wildfire: A large, destructive fire that spreads quickly over woodland or brush (Oxford Living Dictionaries, n.d.).

DISCUSSION QUESTIONS

1. What are the health equity implications of wildfires?
2. What potential population health interventions (local, regional, global) could help address health issues related to wildfires?

REFERENCES

Abel, K. (2006). *Changing places: History, community, and identity in Northeastern Ontario.* Montreal & Kingston: McGill-Queen's University Press.

American Psychological Association. (2011). *Recovering from the wildfires.* Retrieved from http://www.apa.org/helpcenter/wildfire.aspx

Buse, D., & Mount, G. (2011). *Come on Over! Northeastern Ontario A to Z.* Sudbury: Scrivener Press.

Caamano-Isorna, F., Figueiras, A., Sastre, I., Montes-Martínez, A., Taracido, M., & Piñeiro-Lamas, M. (2011). Respiratory and mental health effects of wildfires: an ecological study in Galician municipalities (north-west Spain). *Environmental Health, 10,* 48.

Curtis, L. (2002, November 11). Biomass burning. *Burning Issues, Special Issue.*

CMHA. (2009). *Rural and northern community issues in mental health.* Toronto: Canadian Mental Health Association.

Finlay, S., Moffat, A., Gazzard, R., Baker, D., & Murray, V. (2012). Health impacts of wildfires. *PLoS Current Disasters, 1*. Retrieved from http://dx.doi.org/10.1371/4f959951cce2c

Fowler, C. (2003). Human health impacts of forest fires in the southern United States: A literature review. *Journal of Ecological Anthropology, 7*, 39–63. Retrieved from http://dx.doi.org/10.5038/2162-4593.7.1.3

Grenier, R. (2009, March 31). Northern Ontario losing out in wake of CBC media cuts. Editorial. *The Northern Life*, 8.

Johnston, F., Henderson, S., Chen, Y., Randerson, J., Marlier, M., DeFries, R., Brauer, M. (2012). Estimated global mortality attributable to smoke from landscape fires. *Environmental Health Perspectives, 120*(5), 695–701.

Keim, M. (2008). Building human resilience: the role of public health preparedness and response as an adaptation to climate change. *American Journal of Preventive Medicine, 35*, 508–516.

Marshall, G., Schell, T., Elliott, M., Rayburn, N., & Jaycox, L. (2007). Psychiatric disorders among adults seeking emergency disaster assistance after a wildland-urban interface fire. *Psychiatric Services, 58*, 509–514.

Ministry of Health and Long Term Care (MOHLTC). (2010). *Rural and northern health care framework/plan*. Retrieved from http://www.health.gov.on.ca/en/public/programs/ruralnorthern/report.aspx

Moore, D., Copes, R., Fisk, R., Joy, R., Chan, K., & Brauer, M. (2006). Population health effects of air quality changes due to forest fires in British Columbia in 2003. *Canadian Journal of Public Health, 97*(2), 105–108.

Morris, K. (2009). Crisis communications: Challenges faced by remote and rural communities in north eastern Ontario. *McMaster Journal of Communications, 6*, 82–100. Retrieved from https://journals.mcmaster.ca/mjc/article/view/248

Mott, J., Meyer, P., Mannino, D., Redd, S., Smith, E., Gotway-Crawford, C., & Chase, E. (2002). Wildland forest fire smoke: Health effects and intervention evaluation, Hoopa, California, 1999. *Western Journal of Medicine, 176*(3), 157–162.

North East LHIN. (2012). *Population health profile*. Retrieved from http://www.nelhin.on.ca/WorkArea/showcontent.aspx?id=13182

North East LHIN. (2011). *NE LHIN Aboriginal/First Nation and Métis mental health and addictions framework*. Retrieved from http://www.nelhin.on.ca/aboriginalhealthservices.aspx

North East LHIN. (2006). *Integrated health service plan*. Retrieved from http://www.nelhin.on.ca/newsandevents/internalpublications.aspx

Oxford University Press. (n.d.). *Wildfire*. Retrieved from https://en.oxforddictionaries.com/definition/wildfire

Public Safety Canada. (n.d.). *Canadian disaster database*. Retrieved from http://cdd.publicsafety.gc.ca/srchpg-eng.aspx

Sim, M. (2002). Bushfires: Are we doing enough to reduce the human impact? *Occupational and Environmental Medicine, 59*, 215–216.

Wittig, V., Williams, S., & DuTeaux, S. (2008). Public health impacts of residential wildfires: Analysis of ash and debris from the 2007 southern California fires. *Epidemiology, 19*, S207.

CHAPTER 13

Global Finance's Impacts on Social Determinants of Health and Health Equity

Ronald Labonté

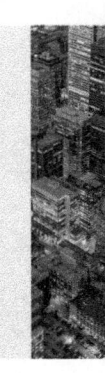

TAKE-HOME MESSAGE

- Many of the improvements needed in the social determinants of health involve structural conflicts of interest between public and private sectors, and elite and non-elite groups.
- Improving health equity requires strong governmental policy action focused on the redistribution of social policies, regulation of international trade through use of health equity impact assessments, and strengthening of human rights.

INTRODUCTION

In considering what actions must be undertaken to achieve greater health equity, there are three global finance phenomena that we simply cannot ignore because of their knock-on effects on the social determinants of health. The first is the crisis in global capitalism and financial markets, brought on by some 35 years of inadequate or indifferent regulation. The second is that, even if we manage to re-regulate banking, capital, and corporate behaviours, "there is as yet no credible, socially just, ecologically sustainable scenario of continually growing incomes for a world of nine billion people" (Sustainable Development Commission, 2009, p. 8). The third phenomenon is that a political and economic orthodoxy emerged in the 1970s and 1980s that unleashed an unprecedented and extreme maldistribution of wealth, which is bad for societies and their economies. Not all countries have followed the same trend. For instance, economic growth and redistributive social policies have begun to reduce inequalities in some countries, such as in Brazil, Argentina, and other Latin American nations (Birdsall, Lustig, & McLeaod, 2011), although they have been plagued with economic downturns following the 2008 global financial crisis. For other countries where inequalities are worsening, they are doing so slowly and from a base that was far more equal to begin with, such as the case in many northern European nations. But these are the exceptions. Elsewhere inequalities have worsened, sometimes dramatically: in the US, South Africa, China, India, even Canada. The rise in economic inequalities in these countries reflects a larger global trend.

GLOBAL ECONOMIC CRISES AND THE SOCIAL DETERMINANTS OF HEALTH

Most attention on the health impacts of recent global economic crises focuses on the ongoing fallout of the 2008 global near-collapse of the international banking system. We know from three decades of previous financial crises that the impacts ripple across global production chains, with recessionary consequences. When debt-financed consumption by people in wealthier countries contracts, so does employment for the poor in poorer nations. The International Labour Organization (ILO) estimates that at least 20 million jobs disappeared between 2008 and 2011 alone (2011), with the total reaching closer to 70 million by late 2013 (2014).

Such health-harming contractions grate against multilaterally agreed best practices. The United Nations has been actively promoting its Social Protection Floor Initiative to encourage countries to systematically build up their social protection systems. The argument for such an initiative is simple and compelling: social protection equitably redistributes wealth, opportunity, and health, and it is rooted in globally shared principles of social justice and human rights. It is supported by a large number of UN agencies, development banks, and government development agencies. There are glimmers of its implementation in different parts of the world: extended health coverage, social cash transfers, and public sector and rural employment guarantee schemes. Consistent with the Globalization Knowledge Network's findings for the Commission on Social Determinants of Health (CSDH), the initiative highlights the important role that a strong and tax-supported social protection system can play in times of economic crises. But while the Social Protection Floor Initiative offers countries good technical advice, it does not and cannot address the political will needed to implement such schemes. Nor does it examine the global economic practices that give rise to economic crises.

CAPITAL MOBILITY, GLOBAL TAXATION, AND BANKING REFORM

Notwithstanding the post-2008 "credit crunch," there remains the problem of global capital mobility. In 2008, the total annual amount of foreign direct investment going into production and services was USD $1.7 trillion—a substantial sum. But in 2007 the daily amount of currency exchange, most of it speculative and highly leveraged, was USD $3.2 trillion (Labonté, Mohindra, & Schrecker, 2011). It is time to re-valorize the use of border controls over capital (Wade, 2009), something Brazil is doing now, much to the irritation of the International Monetary Fund (although by 2015 it was changing its tune somewhat on this issue). Such controls can stem from destructively speculative inflows and outflows, but more importantly from capital flight and tax avoidance, clamping down on the estimated USD $32 trillion in personal wealth untaxed in offshore financial centres operating under British, European, and American protection, which government treasuries as much as USD $250 billion a year in foregone tax revenues on growth on the principal alone (Henry, 2012; Oxfam International, 2013).

A globalized economy also calls out for global systems of taxation. There is now some willingness for such taxation, particularly the French and German push to implement an EU-wide financial transaction tax. Although such a tax may not have quite the speculative dampening outcome that its first proponent, the Nobel economist James Tobin, envisioned, it is a simple means of generating considerable revenue for the public good. At a low rate of 0.05 percent (5 cents/100 dollars) on foreign currency, it would raise USD $250 billion annually. Applied to all currency transactions, including bonds and over-the-counter trades, the tax could raise USD $8.63 trillion annually (McCulloch & Pacillo, 2011), a sum that would go a long way towards stabilizing global finances, covering sovereign debts, and financing climate change mitigation. There are other hopeful precedents. The formation of the Leading Group on Innovative Financing for Development in 2006 provided impetus for the Unitaid airline tax, the International Financial Facility for Immunization, and the Advanced Market Commitment agreement on pneumococcal vaccines—all small steps towards a more global health equitable future. Now numbering 63 nations (neither Canada nor the United States has opted in), it supports financial transaction taxes as a globally just system for financing development and dealing with climate change.

However, banking reform remains. Many reformers have argued for the necessity of clearly separating commercial banking from investment banking. There is some willingness in the high-income countries from which the banking collapse emanated to ensure that a minority portion of bank assets are "ring-fenced" for commercial lending (rather than casino betting), as well as a willingness to increase the amount capital banks must have based on their risk-weighted assets (Bank for International Settlements, 2011; Independent Commission on Banking, 2011). The 2008 crisis was partly precipitated by the US decision to allow the loan-to-reserve ratio of banks to increase from 17:1 to 40:1. But there are concerns that these are limited interventions with implementation still many years away, leaving more time for more financial chicanery.

STRENGTHENING LABOUR MARKETS?

As many countries around the world brace for a potential double-dip recession (including Canada in 2015), the political moment has become dominated by one word: jobs. Another CSDH recommendation urged international institutions and national policy to support full and fair employment, extending core labour standards for formal and informal workers to reduce the health-damaging insecurities of precarious work. The ILO had already taken up this task, promoting its Decent Work Agenda, which includes active labour market policies to create more jobs; guaranteed workers' rights of representation, participation, and security; and extended social protection through safe workplaces and adequate income. Again, reasonable sentiments clash with a globalized economy that so far has failed to provide much movement in these directions. Instead, we are witnessing a steady erosion in labour rights, with evidence suggesting ongoing and marked increases in precisely the insecure and unhealthy work the ILO's Decent Work Agenda has been attempting to remedy (Inter-American Development Bank, 2011; Schrecker & Labonté, 2010; Standing, 2011).

TRADE, HEALTH, AND THE NEW PANDEMIC OF NON-COMMUNICABLE DISEASES

Trade liberalization plays an important role in increasing labour market insecurities, an outcome only offset through generous active labour programs and social protection safety nets (Labonté et al. 2008). But there are other and more direct ways in which international trade treaties can compromise both health and its social determinants, apart from the long-festering and much-publicized issue of intellectual property rights and access to essential medicines. Consider these examples below.

First, reductions in revenue from tariffs or border taxes may reduce a country's public policy capacity. The theoretical claim that liberalization-related growth should allow countries to develop new forms of taxation to replace lost revenue has rarely been realized, largely due to weak infrastructure and capacity (Labonté et al. 2008). Many countries have failed to recover these losses, reducing what they have available for social protection or spending on social determinants of health. The health equity implication is straightforward: trade negotiation pressure for such countries to reduce tariffs should not be made until there is evidence that they have developed equitable, effective, and transparent tax systems.

Second, trade treaties play a role in creating the communicable vectors of the new pandemic of non-communicable diseases. As smoking rates decline in developed countries, tobacco transnational corporations target developing nations. Trade treaties have been used successfully to block developing country efforts to limit the introduction of new foreign brands through tariffs, with WTO's dispute panel ruling border tax policies discriminatory, even if they are invoked under the WTO's health defense. This argument, while technically correct, ignores the fact that as tobacco products exposure increases in any given market, price competition leads to increased consumption. Liberalized investment is an even more important means by which tobacco consumption rises, with transnational tobacco corporations buying out domestic manufacturers or creating new manufacturing facilities within developing countries: as foreign direct investment in tobacco rises so does tobacco consumption, sometimes quite dramatically (Labonté, Mohindra, & Lencucha, 2011).

The Framework Convention on Tobacco Control (FCTC), although a groundbreaking global health agreement, failed to deal with the one global dimension of its control: the role trade and investment policies play in allowing tobacco use to continue to rise by 2 percent each year. Tobacco companies, or the governments they persuade to act on their behalf, are now using trade and bilateral investment treaties to challenge the very control measures advocated by the FCTC. In several instances one finds governments simultaneously adopting a control measure (such as restrictions on flavoured cigarettes) while challenging other governments' identical efforts: a clear case of the lack of policy coherence between trade and public health. A similar situation exists with trade, food, and the obesity pandemic. We can welcome the UN's 2011 High-level Meeting on Prevention and Control of Non-communicable Diseases, and applaud that its Political Declaration made several references to the social determinants of health. But like the FCTC, it is almost completely silent on trade and wholly silent on the role played by global investment. When a US representative was asked why his country was not promoting its own obesity control program at the summit, he reportedly responded that it would hurt US trade export interests. The lack of targets in the Political Declaration on tobacco control and salt reduction was similarly attributed to corporate pressure and trade export interests (Boseley, 2011).

Third, rather than tackle the economic interests underlying the pandemic of chronic disease, the UN Summit's Political Declaration (United Nations, 2011) talks of private sector partnerships, urging companies to "consider producing and promoting more food products consistent with a healthy diet" (para.44 (b)) and to "take measures … to reduce the impact of the marketing of unhealthy foods and non-alcoholic beverages [i.e., soft drinks] to children" (para. 44 (a)). Ironically, around the same time, PepsiCo, which had let its soft-drink advertising budget lag in order to promote its healthier products, lost ground to rival Coca-Cola, resulting in an about-face and a plan to massively increase its soft-drink promotion budget (iStockAnalyst, 2011). The US-based Campbell's, seen as a leader in voluntarily reducing salt in some of its products, announced just prior to the Summit an almost 50 percent increase in the salt of one its previously low-sodium soup brands due to flagging market sales, a move welcomed by the Salt Institute as a cautionary tale for companies wanting to cut sodium in their products (Weeks, 2011). Voluntary codes do not produce the level playing field that profit-driven companies need in order to act in socially responsible ways—enforceable regulations do.

Bearing these examples in mind, how can we ensure that social determinants of health are not undermined? Optimistically, this past decade has seen a global diffusion of human rights, gender empowerment, and increased aid for both health and (at least some) of its social determinants. An ambitious set of Sustainable Development Goals, to replace 2000's Millennium Development Goals, was finalized by the UN General Assembly in September 2015. A new "health and foreign policy" discourse also emerged, emanating from the 2007 Ministerial Declaration led by the Norwegian foreign minister, which proposes to align health and foreign policy goals more closely (Foreign Ministers of Brazil, France, Indonesia, Norway, Senegal, South Africa & Thailand, 2007).

But are these initiatives happening? Perhaps—but they are not taking the great strides we so desperately need. A recent study found that global health was pursued by nations more for their own security and economic means than for the purposes of strengthening human rights, building global public goods, or even ensuring meaningful development assistance (Labonté & Gagnon, 2010). This suggests that our failure to act on social determinants of health is not due to our lack of technical knowledge or capacity, nor is it simply a matter of identifying the right tools. It is a matter of choosing sides. Many of the improvements needed in social determinants of health are not win/win—they are win/lose, in the sense that there are structural conflicts of interest between public and private sectors, and elite and non-elite groups. Governments must make a choice.

What is to be done? First, it is important to recognize that a good diagnosis of a problem infers a solution. The CSDH report (WHO, 2011) offered many good diagnoses from which defining the next steps—however challenging or controversial—is not difficult.

WHAT CAN BE DONE TO IMPROVE HEALTH EQUITY?

The report, emanating from the 2011 World Conference on Social Determinants of Health (WHO, 2011), identified a number of small policy actions that could become much larger policy strides. For example, governments can formalize the use of health equity impact assessments of international agreements before those agreements are ratified (and also afterwards, to see what may need re-negotiation). These assessments could consider trade, the environment, finance, or even international or bilateral codes attempting to manage more equitably the global flow of health workers. Whether they are rigorous sketches or detailed analyses, they could help to build a much-needed social determinants approach across the UN system. Given the emergent consensus on social protection floors, this should not be hard to achieve.

In all of this work, there is the unavoidable policy imperative with which this commentary began—that of redistribution, regulation, and rights. In restating this imperative the bar is set very high for the policy actions that should arise from the knowledge base generated by the CSDH, in addition to the subsequent findings and reports on how to achieve a fairer, healthier, and ecologically sustainable world. But there really is no alternative.

Many thought that the 2008 crisis would mark a turning point towards a fairer world, but this has not yet happened. Moreover, the crises are continuing, and deepening, across multiple global fronts. We should heed the wise words spoken by President Obama's chief of staff when America first started to teeter in 2008: "You never want a serious crisis to go to waste" (cited in Wade, 2009).

We must commit to the policy choices that evidence and morality tell us we must make.

GLOSSARY

Social protection (systems): Social protection equitably redistributes wealth, opportunity, and health. It is rooted in globally shared principles of social justice and human rights.

DISCUSSION QUESTIONS

1. How realistic is the potential for implementation of social protection systems in countries such as China, India, South Africa, and Canada?
2. What are some of the policy actions that could prevent social determinants of health from being undermined?

REFERENCES

Bank for International Settlements (2011). *Basel III Agreement*. Basel Committee on Banking Supervision. Retrieved from http://www.bis.org/bcbs/basel3.htm

Birdsall, N., Lustig, N., & McLeod, D. (2011). *Declining inequality in Latin America: Some economics, some politics*. Working Paper 251. Washington: Center for Global Development.

Boseley, S. (2011, September 16). UN calls summit on spread of 'lifestyle' diseases. *The Guardian*. Retrieved from http://www.guardian.co.uk/society/2011/sep/16/un-summit-spread-lifestyle-diseases

Foreign Ministers of Brazil, France, Indonesia, Norway, Senegal, South Africa and Thailand (2007). Oslo Ministerial Declaration – global health: A pressing foreign policy issue of our time. *The Lancet, 369*(9570), 1373–1378.

Henry, J. (2012). *The price of offshore revisited*. Chesham: Tax Justice Network.

Independent Commission on Banking. (2011). *Final report: Recommendations*. London: Independent Commission on Banking. Retrieved from https://www.reedsmith.com/en/perspectives/2011/09/independent-commission-on-bankings-final-report--s

Inter-American Development Bank. (2011). *Urban sustainability in Latin America and the Caribbean*. Retrieved from http://idbdocs.iadb.org/wsdocs/getdocument.aspx?docnum=35786014

International Labour Office. (2011). *Global employment trends 2011: The challenge of a jobs recovery*. Geneva: ILO. Retrieved from http://www.ilo.org/wcmsp5/groups/public/@dgreports/@dcomm/@publ/documents/publication/wcms_150440.pdf

International Labour Office. (2014). *Global employment trends 2014: Risk of a jobless recovery?* Geneva: ILO.

iStockAnalyst (2011, June 28). *Pepsi goes back to its roots with Pepsi-Cola marketing*. Retrieved from http://www.istockanalyst.com/finance/story/5258994/pepsi-goes-back-to-its-roots-with-pepsi-cola-marketing

Kentikelenis, A., Karanikolos, M., Papanicolas, I., Basu, S., McKee, M., & Stuckler, D. (2011). Health effects of financial crisis: Omens of a Greek tragedy. *The Lancet, 378*, 1457–1458.

Labonté, R., Blouin, C., Chopra, M., Lee, K., Packer, C., Rowson, M., Woodward, D., et al. (2008). *Towards health-equitable globalisation: Rights, regulation and redistribution: Final report to the Commission on Social Determinants of Health*. Retrieved from http://www.globalhealthequity.ca/projects/proj_WHO/pres_pub.shtml

Labonté, R., & Gagnon, M. (2010). Framing health and foreign policy: Lessons for global health diplomacy. *Globalization and Health, 6*(14), 1–22.

Labonté, R., Mohindra, K., & Schrecker, T. (2011). The growing impact of globalization for health and public health practice. *Annual Review of Public Health, 32*, 263–283.

Labonté, R., Mohindra, K., & Lencucha, R. (2011). Framing international trade and chronic disease. *Globalization and Health, 21*(3), 273–287.

McCulloch, N., & Pacillo, G. (2011, May). *The Tobin tax: A review of the evidence.* IDS Research Report 68. Brighton, UK: Institute of Development Studies. Retrieved from http://www.ids.ac.uk/files/dmfile/rr68.pdf

Oxfam International. (2013). *Tax on the "private" billions now stashed away in havens enough to end extreme world poverty twice over.* Oxford: Oxfam International.

Schrecker, T., & Labonté, R. (2010). Globalization and urban health. In J. Bouffard & D. Vlahov (eds.), *Urban health: Global perspectives* (pp. 13–26). New York: Jossey-Bass/John Wiley & Sons.

Standing, G. (2011). *The precariat: The new dangerous class.* London: Bloomsbury.

Sustainable Development Commission. (2009). *Prosperity without growth: The transition to a sustainable economy?* London: UK Sustainable Development Commission.

United Nations Conference on Trade and Development. (2011). *Trade and development report 2011: Post-crisis policy challenges in the world economy.* Geneva: United Nations.

United Nations. (2011). *Political declaration of the High-level Meeting of the General Assembly on the Prevention and Control of Non-communicable Diseases.* Retrieved from http://www.who.int/nmh/events/un_ncd_summit2011/political_declaration_en.pdf

Wade, R. (2009). From global imbalances to global reorganisations. *Cambridge Journal of Economics, 33*(4), 539–562.

Weeks, C. (2011, July 17). Campbell's adding salt back to its soup. *The Globe and Mail.* Retrieved from http://www.theglobeandmail.com/life/health/new-health/health-news/campbells-adding-salt-back-to-its-soups/article2097659

World Health Organization. (2011). *Closing the gap: Policy into practice on social determinants of health.* Discussion Paper. Geneva: World Health Organization.

CHAPTER 14

Complementarities or Contradictions? Scoping the Health Dimensions of "Flexicurity" Labour Market Policies*

Zabia Afzal, Carles Muntaner, Haejoo Chung, Qamar Mahmood, Edwin Ng, and Ted Schrecker

TAKE-HOME MESSAGE

- Flexicurity appears to be an institutional arrangement of labour market liberalization and social protection rather than a conscious social democratic policy.
- Flexicurity appears to be politically unstable and historically specific, in particular since 2000 and even more so during the recession.
- The effects of flexicurity on population health should be beneficial only with strong and institutionalized forms of social protection. but not if the emphasis is on flexibility.

INTRODUCTION

According to the World Health Organization Commission on Social Determinants of Health, the political configurations of labour markets are powerful factors in determining material and psychosocial working environments, which, in turn, affect patterns of health and disease in the wider society (Commission on Social Determinants of Health, 2008). Associations between health and labour market conditions suggest that non-standard employment conditions and, in particular, precarious employment practices, are major risk factors in the development of adverse health outcomes (Benach et al., 2010a, 2010b; Muntaner et al., 2010).

The current trend in labour markets to increase the flexibility of employment conditions has directly contributed to higher levels of job insecurity among workers in Canada (Vosko, 2006). In Ontario, as elsewhere, the consequences of flexible employment arrangements are disproportionately borne by vulnerable and marginalized segments of the

* This chapter first appeared as a article in 2013 in the *International Journal of Health Services*, Volume 43, Issue 3. It is reproduced with permission from Sage Publications.

labour force, including women, immigrants, and those with low credentials or disabilities (Fuller & Vosko, 2008; Lewchuk, Clarke, & De Wolff, 2011). Indeed, it has been suggested that the credential-driven character of Ontario's employment system necessitates a rethinking of its governing paradigm and calls for an alternative labour market strategy that produces equitable outcomes on measures of health and well-being (Lewchuk, Clarke, & De Wolff, 2011). Rethinking and identifying alternative labour market strategies have become particularly salient and urgent given that the current economic downturn has accelerated the pressure on governments to further deregulate labour markets and practice fiscal austerity (Ontario Progressive Conservative Caucus, 2012).

Against this background, the idea of flexicurity has been proposed as a viable alternative in Europe since the mid-1990s. *Flexicurity* refers to the simultaneous integration of labour market flexibility with social security and active labour market policies. It challenges the idea that labour and capital are intrinsically antagonistic, presenting itself as a viable third strategy. At its core, flexicurity involves substituting labour's demand for job security with employment security. Whereas job security refers to protection for the job held by workers with a particular employer, employment security ensures workers are able to find employment in the labour market. Flexicurity also involves a search for non-precarious forms of flexibility and a commitment to compensate for increases in flexibility with provisions of security. Thus, the overarching goal of flexicurity is to promote and facilitate the adaptability of both employers and workers within a global economy characterized by fluctuation and uncertainty (Wilthagen, Tros, & Van Lieshout, 2003).

Following the lead of the European Commission, a number of European nations have experimented with various flexicurity initiatives (European Expert Group on Flexicurity, 2007). Denmark and the Netherlands are, however, the only two countries that have actively restructured their social and economic institutions and labour market arrangements toward the pursuit and implementation of flexicurity. Because health outcomes have been rarely conceptualized as a deliverable of flexicurity policies, past research on the effects of flexicurity has operationalized health or health equity issues as peripheral outcomes. This brief review underscores the need to (a) systematically review the empirical literature on flexicurity policies in Europe, and (b) assess the potential of flexicurity as a strategic intervention to promote health equity within Ontario and Canada.

METHODS

Realist review methods were originally proposed for this study; however, the extant literature on labour market policies and health inequalities revealed sufficient information on social mechanisms that linked interventions and outcomes (Greenhalgh et al., 2009). Instead, we used the scoping review framework developed by Arksey and O'Malley (2005) to critically appraise the literature in three steps.

First, we searched for potentially relevant studies in digital libraries (i.e., Scopus, JSTOR, Web of Science, and Google Scholar) and gray literature sources (e.g., Organisation for Economic Co-operation and Development [OECD], International

Labour Organization, and Canadian research organizations) using the following key-words: flexicurity, health, health equit*, health promotion, active labour market policies, labour market flexibility, welfare state, corporatism, social determinants of health, social security, Denmark, Netherlands, Europe, Ontario, and Canada. Preliminary keyword searches yielded 1,246 abstracts.

Second, we evaluated these records in two stages against our exclusion criteria: dupli-cates, no references to empirical data, simulation or model-based, non-OECD countries, dated literature, addressed only the consequences of the Personal Responsibility and Work Opportunity Reconciliation Act (PROWRA), redundant articles, or full text not available online. We then retrieved the full text of 29 studies on flexicurity and activation policies.

Third, the bibliographies of these 29 studies were screened, and a targeted search on "flexicurity AND health" was conducted using Google Scholar. This third step identified an additional 10 articles that met our inclusion criteria for a final total of 39 core publications.

Our scoping review methods are outlined in a flow chart (see Figure 14.1). In our analysis of core publications, we focused on the experience of flexicurity policies in Denmark, given its expansive documentation in the extant literature, and applied a social determinants of health framework to evaluate the relevance and feasibility of flexicurity policies for Ontario and Canada.

RESULTS

Although flexicurity in Denmark does not represent a deliberately designed configura-tion, it does embody the culmination of a long developmental process (Bredgaard, Larsen, & Madsen, 2006) that involved a pragmatic process of trial-and-error reforms (Andersen & Svarer, 2007). The Danish labour market largely derives its flexible character from non-restrictive employment protection legislation (EPL) dating back to the 19th century. By design, EPL lowers the costs associated with hiring and firing workers and enables companies to adapt easily to economic periods of increased fluctuations and intense com-petition. This particular attribute of the labour market links Denmark with the liberal economies of the United States and the United Kingdom and represents a clear departure from Scandinavian welfare regimes (Madsen, 2004).

Denmark has traditionally addressed the negative impacts associated with workers' economic security through the provision of income security for those experiencing unem-ployment. The inability of this trade-off to prevent dilemmas associated with high levels of structural unemployment and welfare "dependency" (Andersen & Svarer, 2007) led to the adoption of active labour market policies (ALMPs) in 1993. These reforms intensified investments in education and skills training programs, reduced the duration of unem-ployment insurance benefits, and made benefit eligibility conditional upon participation in reintegrating strategies. In effect, these reforms coordinated the welfare state, labour market, and ALMPs into a tripartite arrangement that has been labelled the "golden tri-angle" (Wilthagen & Tros, 2004). As the flexicurity literature repeatedly points out, the formation and administration of this employment system rely heavily upon the distinctive

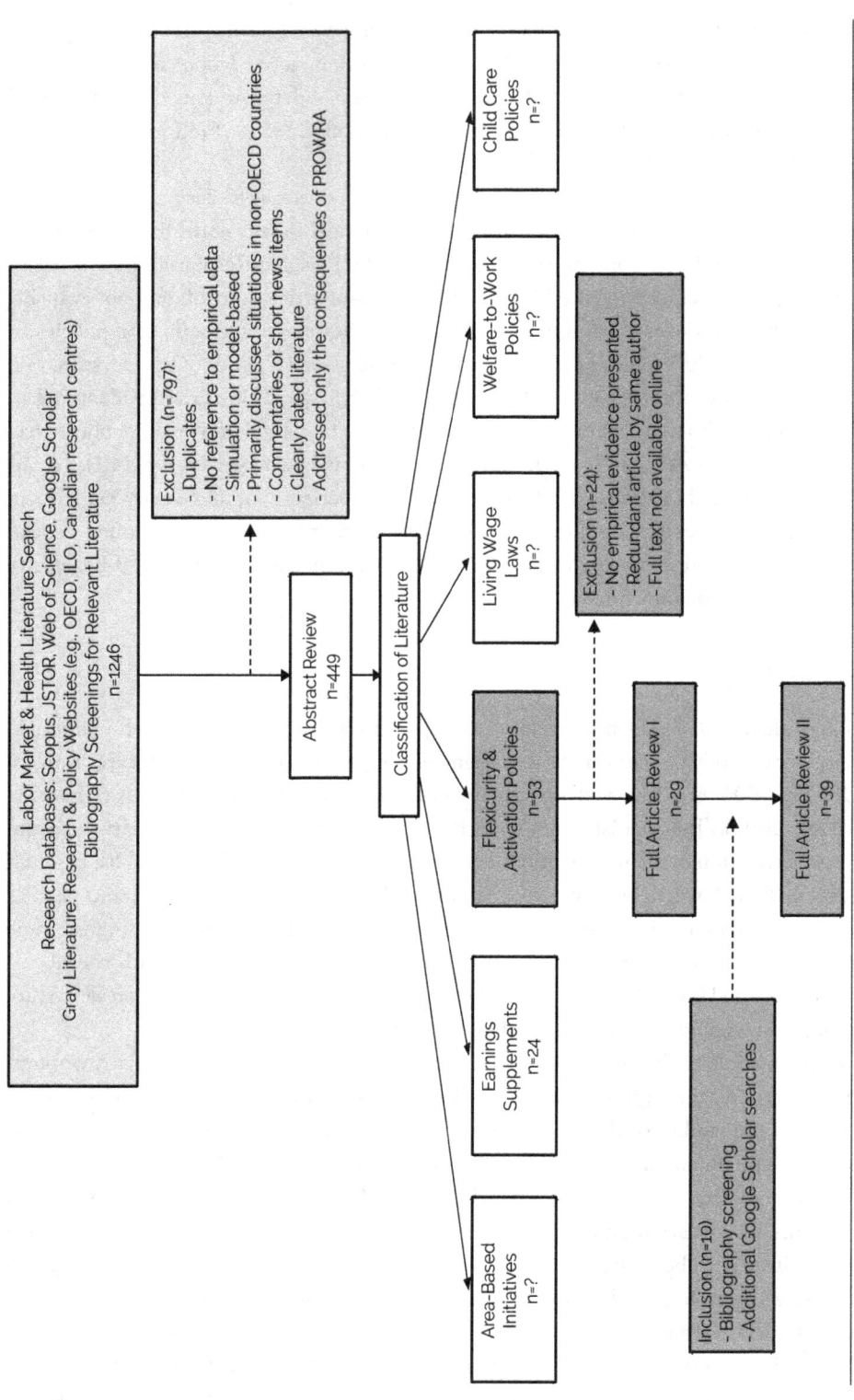

Figure 14.1: Selection of Literature

corporatist tradition of labour market regulation (Bredgaard, Larsen, & Madsen, 2006; Madsen, 2004). This corporatist tradition serves as a precondition for flexicurity success, emphasizing mutual trust, cooperation, and consensus-based social dialogue in relationships between the state, employer organizations, and social partners.

Denmark's labour market performance since the mid-1990s serves as a case study of a small country that successfully confronts, adopts, and grows during rapid globalization. According to a 2004 European survey, Denmark had the highest employment rate in the European Union, with more than 75 percent of people aged 15–65 participating in the labour force (IndexMundi, n.d.). Similarly, Bredgaard and colleagues note that the registered unemployment rate in 2001 reached its lowest level since 1974, representing nearly half of the 1994 rate (Bredgaard & Larsen, 2006; Bredgaard, Larsen, & Madsen, 2005). Much of the literature is careful not to attribute this largely positive labour market performance solely to labour market reforms in the mid-1990s (Andersen & Svarer, 2007; Bredgaard & Larsen, 2006; Bredgaard, Larsen, & Madsen, 2006). Other explanations emphasize the role of economic growth and Denmark's ability to align itself with global trends towards low inflation. Such an alignment was made possible by the 1987 declaration of social partners to "negotiate wage increases below international wage inflation in order to improve the competitiveness of Danish industry" (Madsen, 2004, p. 201).

The literature highlights the changing characteristics of the following pillars that constitute the flexicurity model. Denmark operates a two-tiered system of unemployment compensation: (a) the unemployment insurance fund, which is based on voluntary membership, and (b) the social assistance program, which provides coverage for everyone else. Denmark's level of income-benefit replacement rate is significantly higher than that of other OECD countries. Whereas the average unemployed production worker was compensated for 70 percent of his or her previous salary at the start of the century, the replacement rate for low-income individuals was actually higher (Madsen, 2004). Although the adoption of labour market policies restructured the Danish welfare state in ways that increased the employment incentive, these policies did not initially reduce benefit levels. Since these reforms, welfare state restructuring has continued in the direction of tightening eligibility criteria for obtaining unemployment insurance and reducing duration of the passive benefit period. For example, the time before participation in activation programs became mandatory, and this period was shortened from four to two years in 1996 (Andersen & Svarer, 2007) and further reduced to one year for adult unemployed persons in 1999 (Madsen, 2004).

Denmark's "exceptionally large commitment to ALMPs" (Schmitt, 2011) translated into a 70 percent increase in these expenditures from 1994 to 2004 (Andersen & Svarer, 2007). Researchers note that Danish policy-makers have increasingly prioritized investments in private job training while reducing educational initiatives (Andersen & Svarer, 2007; Bredgaard, Larsen, & Madsen, 2006; Hansen, 2007). The high cost of administration and programming has raised concerns about the efficiency and cost-effectiveness of these policies (Madsen, 2004; Zhou, 2007). Some researchers have rationalized these expenses on the basis that ALMPs are "investments in a mobile and flexible labour market," facilitate numerical flexibility, and contribute to functional flexibility by ensuring "adequate and high-quality training and education of the workforce" (Bredgaard, Larsen, & Madsen, 2006, p. 70). In a similar vein, Andersen and Svarer argue that although ALMPs are "resource demanding," their cost-effectiveness ratio has significantly improved relative to past policies (Andersen & Svarer, 2007). These authors recommend the adoption of measures that involve a greater emphasis on private job training programs, as well as increased sanctioning and monitoring of the unemployed through cancellation of unemployment insurance benefits (Andersen & Svarer, 2007). This approach has played a significant role in Danish employment policy-making since the 1990s. While Danish activation strategies have always been composed of "both social disciplining and social integration" (Bredgaard, Larsen, & Madsen, 2006), it is clear that motivation and discipline were increasingly given a prominent position in the design of employment policies.

THE POTENTIAL IMPACT OF FLEXICURITY ON HEALTH AND WELL-BEING

To date, discussions on the effect of flexicurity on workers' health and well-being have been limited to untested claims. Given the dearth of research on the health-related effects of flexicurity, we are limited to making inferences on their potential value and impact. On one hand, the negative effects of limited employment protection in Denmark are readily apparent. For example, the average job tenure is short (Andersen & Svarer, 2007; Bredgaard & Larsen, 2007), worker turnover is high (Madsen, 2004), and short-term unemployment rates are near record highs among European nations (Andersen & Svarer, 2007; Bredgaard & Larsen, 2007). On the other hand, a low EPL index does not appear to have resulted in "excessive employment volatility" (Andersen & Svarer, 2007) or perceptions of low job security (Bredgaard & Larsen, 2007; Bredgaard, Larsen, & Madsen, 2006; Madsen, 2004). Rather, a low EPL index has contributed to a high degree of job mobility in Denmark, which is consistent with the preferences of Danish workers, 70 percent of whom think that "changing jobs every few years is good" (Bredgaard & Larsen, 2007, p. 11). In conjunction with feelings of high job security, Danish workers report lower perceptions of labour market risks compared to their counterparts in other European countries (Andersen & Svarer, 2007).

Using data from the 2005 European Working Conditions Survey and the 2006 European Social Survey, Burchell (2009) used individual-level data to rank countries based on the strength of association between perceived job insecurity and well-being. Results found "no evidence of any systematic differences between countries in [this] relationship" and a lack of correlation with any indices of flexicurity (Burchell, 2009, p. 5). Flexicurity policies promise to normalize atypical employment relations by balancing characteristics of flexibility with elements of security. Rather than investigating whether this promise is fulfilled in practice, the literature on flexicurity has given "cursory attention" to those atypically employed (Seifert & Tangian, 2006) and tends to assume that "workers are in regular open-ended contracts, or, if not, that part-time or temporary contracts can be considered equivalent to regular employment" (Bredgaard, Larsen, Madsen, & Rasmussen, 2009, p. 4). Our review of the evidence on flexible employment, job insecurity, and health (Kim et al., 2012) finds that associations between flexible employment, job insecurity, and ill health are less likely to be reported in countries with strong welfare regimes such as Denmark. Despite valid reasons for rising rates in sickness absenteeism (Bredgaard & Larsen, 2006), it seems that the "ever-faster pace and productivity demands in the labour market" play an important role (Bredgaard, Larsen, & Madsen, 2006, p. 73). Not surprisingly, there has been a corresponding increase in the number of people on sickness benefits in Denmark (Bredgaard & Larsen, 2006).

CONCLUSION

Ascertaining the overall effectiveness and health consequences of Denmark's social and labour market policies is a difficult challenge. At least until the post-2008 recession, Denmark may have been the labour market with the best performance among all OECD countries (Schmitt, 2011) given the country's performance in avoiding the creation of a low-wage, marginalized segment of the labour market (Viebrock & Clasen, 2009) and in maintaining overall and youth unemployment rates considerably lower than Canada and the OECD average. However, it should be noted that Denmark's ability to maintain fewer low-wage jobs compared to other high-income countries long preceded the implementation of flexicurity reforms (Mason & Salverda, 2010). Although Denmark's unemployment rate is lower than the European Union average, it has increased more steeply in recent years compared to other countries, rising from 4.0 percent to 7.0 percent between 2007 and 2010 (Schmitt, 2011). Even before the financial crisis, the influence of trade unions on social and labour market policies was declining (Jørgensen & Schulze, 2011). Unions responded to the post-crisis climate and their reduced power in the flexicurity model by organizing open protests and demonstrations (Jørgensen, 2011).

The impact of flexicurity in Denmark must be understood within a wider labour and economic context that includes a 69 percent union membership rate, which is twice as high as Canada's, and government revenues that have never dropped below 45 percent of gross domestic product since the early 1980s. In contrast, Canada's total government revenues peaked at 37 percent of gross domestic product in 1997 and have been declining steadily since. This does not suggest that social and labour market policies are not effective interventions to reduce health inequalities by way of social determinants of health. Quite the opposite—the example of Denmark demonstrates the potential of flexicurity to promote the public's health. Our concern is rather with efforts to "export" particular policy nostrums, like flexicurity, without necessary attention to a variety of other policy options and entry points. For example, a policy conundrum that has been on Ontario's agenda for decades is the so-called welfare wall. Despite the availability of Canada's universal health care system, low-income individuals with children on social assistance may experience greater losses, in the form of affordable childcare and drug and dental benefits, than potential gains from entering the labour market, becoming employed, and earning a wage (Subcommittee on Cities of the Standing Senate Committee on Social Affairs, Science and Technology, 2009). Childcare and parenting policies deserve special attention (Heymann, 2006) as there is a very small number of regulated child care spaces for children under 12 in Ontario, and thus waiting lists for subsidized child care are typically very long in Ontario (Family Service Toronto, 2010). Rather than redesigning Ontario's labour market arrangements to be more flexible and secure, the need is to ensure that the impact of negative determinants of health is minimized, while recognizing that this may mean increasing rather than reducing welfare generosity levels and raising the necessary revenues.

GLOSSARY

Flexicurity: A labour market institution characterized with high levels of employer flexibility with regard to hiring and firing workers combined with strong social protection (e.g., pensions, health care, unemployment insurance, active labour market policies).

DISCUSSION QUESTIONS

1. How do you think Canadian political parties would apply the flexicurity idea to the Canadian context?
2. How can flexicurity impact the health of Canadian populations negatively? What groups could suffer most from these aspects?
3. How can flexicurity impact the health of Canadian populations positively? What groups could benefit most from these aspects?
4. Design your ideal flexicurity policies for the Canadian labour market.

REFERENCES

Andersen, T. M., & Svarer, M. (2007). Flexicurity: Labour market performance in Denmark. *CESifo Economic Studies, 53*, 389–429.

Arksey, H., & O'Malley, L. (2005). Scoping studies: Towards a methodological framework. *International Journal of Social Research Methodoogy, 8*, 19–32.

Benach, J., Muntaner, C., Haejoo, C., Solar, O., Santana, V., Friel, S., Marmot, M. (2010a). Reducing the health inequalities associated with employment conditions. *BMJ, 340*, 1392–1395.

Benach, J., Solar, O., Vergara, M., Vanroelen, C., Santana, V., Castedo, A., Muntaner, C. (2010b). Six employment conditions and health inequalities: A descriptive overview. *International Journal of Health Services, 40*, 269–280.

Bredgaard, T., & Larsen, F. (2006). *The transitional Danish labour market: Understanding a best case, and policy proposals for solving some paradoxes.* Denmark: University of Aalborg, Centre for Labour Market Research (CARMA).

Bredgaard, T., & Larsen, F. (2007). *Comparing flexicurity in Denmark and Japan.* Denmark: University of Aalborg, Centre for Labour Market Research (CARMA). Retrieved from http://vbn.aau.dk/files/8320939/JILPT_report-final_1_.pdf

Bredgaard, T., Larsen, F., & Madsen, P. K. (2005). *The flexible Danish labour market: A review.* Denmark: University of Aalborg, Centre for Labour Market Research (CARMA).

Bredgaard, T., Larsen, F., & Madsen, P. K. (2006). Opportunities and challenges for flexicurity: The Danish example. *Transfer: The European Review of Labour and Research, 12,* 61–82.

Bredgaard, T., Larsen, F., Madsen, P. K., & Rasmussen, S. (2009). *Flexicurity and atypical employment in Denmark.* Denmark: University of Aalborg, Centre for Labour Market Research (CARMA). Retrieved from http://www.epa.aau.dk/fileadmin/user_upload/conniek/Dansk/Research_papers/2009-1-Kongshoej_m-fl.pdf

Burchell, B. (2009). Flexicurity as a moderator of the relationship between job insecurity and psychological well-being. *Cambridge Journal of Regions, Economy and Society, 2,* 365–378.

Commission on Social Determinants of Health. (2008). *Closing the gap in a generation: Health equity through action on the social determinants of health.* Final report. Geneva: World Health Organization.

European Expert Group on Flexicurity. (2007). *Flexicurity pathways: Turning hurdles into stepping stones.* Retrieved from http://ec.europa.eu/social/main.jsp?catId=117&langId=en

Family Service Toronto. (2010). *2010 report card on child & family poverty in Ontario poverty reduction: Key to economic recovery for Ontario families.* Ontario Campaign 2000. Retrieved from http://www.campaign2000.ca/reportCards/provincial/Ontario/2010OntarioReportCardEnglish.pdf

Fuller, S., & Vosko, L. (2008). Temporary employment and social inequality in Canada: Exploring intersections of gender, race and immigration status. *Social Indicators Research, 88,* 31–50.

Greenhalgh, T., Humphrey, C., Hughes, J., Macfarlane, F., Butler, C., & Pawson, R. (2009). How do you modernize a health service? A realist evaluation of whole-scale transformation in London. *Milbank Quarterly, 87,* 391–416.

Hansen, L. L. (2007). From flexicurity to flexicarity? Gendered perspectives on the Danish model. *Journal of Social Sciences, 3,* 88–93.

Heymann, J. (2006). *Forgotten families: Ending the growing crisis confronting children and working parents in the global economy.* New York: Oxford University Press.

IndexMundi. (n.d.). *Denmark unemployment rate.* Retrieved from http://www.indexmundi.com/denmark/unemployment_rate.html

Jørgensen, H. (2011). Danish "flexicurity" in crisis—or just stress-tested by the crisis? Stockholm: Friedrich Ebert Stiftung. Retrieved from http://library.fes.de/pdf-files/id/07911.pdf

Jørgensen, H., & Schulze, M. (2011). Leaving the Nordic path? The changing role of Danish trade unions in the welfare reform process. *Social Policy & Administration, 45,* 206–219.

Kim, I. H., Muntaner, C., Vahid Shahidi, F., Vives, A., Vanroelen, C., & Benach, J. (2012). Welfare states, flexible employment, and health: A critical review. *Health Policy, 104,* 99–127.

Lewchuk, W., Clarke, M., & De Wolff, A. (2011). *Working without commitments*. Montreal: McGill-Queen's University Press.

Madsen, P. K. (2004). The Danish model of 'flexicurity': Experiences and lessons. *Transfer: The European Review of Labour and Research, 10*, 187–207.

Mason, G., & Salverda, W. (2010). Low pay, working conditions, and living standards. In J. Gautié and J. Schmitt (eds.), *Low-wage work in the wealthy world* (pp. 35–90). New York: Russell Sage Foundation.

Muntaner, C., Solar, O., Vanroelen, C., Martinez, J. M., Vergara, M., Santana, V., Benach, J. (2010). Unemployment, informal work, precarious employment, child labor, slavery, and health inequalities: Pathways and mechanisms. *International Journal of Health Services, 40*, 281–295.

Ontario Progressive Conservative Caucus. (2012). *Paths to prosperity: Flexible labour markets*. Toronto: Ontario Progressive Conservative Caucus. Retrieved from http://pettapiece.ca/wp-content/uploads/2012/12/PtP-Health-care.pdf

Schmitt, J. (2011). *Labor market policy in the great recession: Some lessons from Denmark and Germany*. Washington, D.C.: Center for Economic and Policy Research.

Seifert, H., & Tangian, A. (2006). Globalization and deregulation: Does flexicurity protect atypically employed? *EconPapers, 143*. Retrieved from http://econpapers.repec.org/paper/zbwwsidps/143.htm

Subcommittee on Cities of the Standing Senate Committee on Social Affairs, Science and Technology. (2009). *In from the margins: A call to action on poverty, housing and homelessness*. Retrieved from http://www.parl.gc.ca/Content/SEN/Committee/402/citi/rep/rep02dec09-e.pdf

Viebrock, E., & Clasen, J. (2009). *Flexicurity: A state-of-the-art review*. Edinburgh: RECWOWE Dissemination and Dialogue Centre. Retrieved from http://ssrn.com/paper=1489903

Vosko, L. (ed.). (2006). *Precarious employment: Understanding labour market insecurity in Canada*. Montreal: McGill-Queen's University Press.

Wilthagen, T., & Tros, F. (2004). The concept of "flexicurity": A new approach to regulating employment and labour markets. *Transfer: The Euopean Review of Labour and Research, 10*, 166–186.

Wilthagen, T. C., Tros, F. H., & Van Lieshout, H. (2003). *Towards 'flexicurity'? Balancing flexibility and security in EU member states*. Retrieved from https://papers.ssrn.com/sol3/papers =1133940

Zhou, J. (2007). *Danish for all? Balancing flexibility with security: The flexicurity model*. International Monetary Fund Working Papers. Retrieved from http://ssrn.com/paper=967877

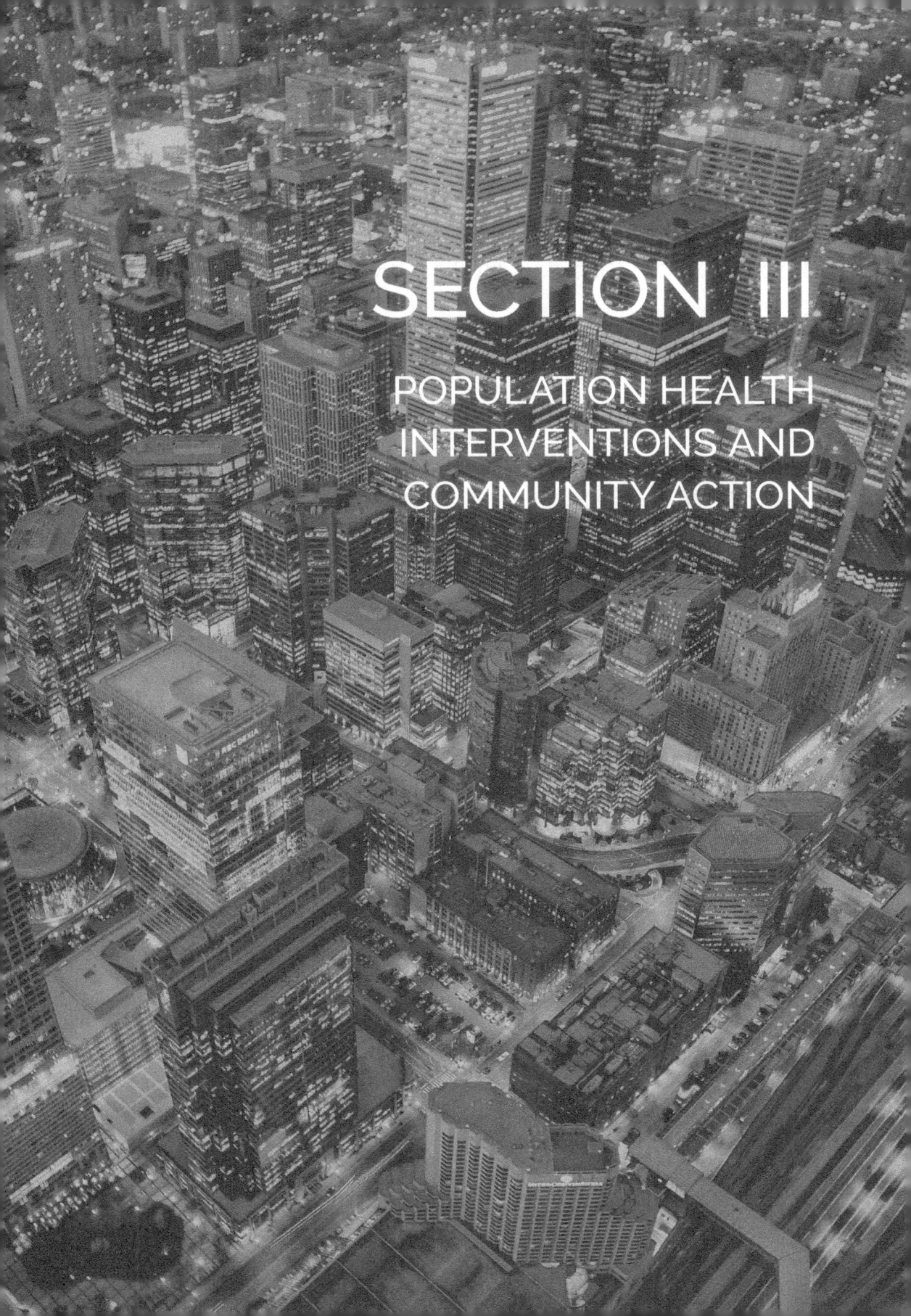

SECTION III

POPULATION HEALTH INTERVENTIONS AND COMMUNITY ACTION

CHAPTER 15

Knowledge Translation for Intersectoral Action: The Case of Canada's Building Codes

Nancy C. Edwards

TAKE-HOME MESSAGE

- To successfully communicate research evidence to policy-makers in different sectors, an understanding of values and perspectives about the role of policy and regulations in those sectors is necessary.

INTRODUCTION

The built environment is recognized as a key determinant of health (PHAC [Public Health Agency of Canada], 2013). It is omnipresent in our day-to-day lives and can directly or indirectly increase or mitigate injury and disease risks. However, the built environment is largely influenced through non-health sectors such as housing and transportation. Successful knowledge translation from health to other sectors requires an understanding of the perspectives of those in non-health disciplines.

Building codes are an important regulatory base for the built environment. Thus, an examination of the process for making revisions to model codes in Canada is a pertinent case for consideration. The introduction of performance-based codes has reinforced the need for monitoring systems that capture diverse outcomes bridging health, business, construction, and social welfare sectors (Meacham, Bowen, Traw, & Moore, 2005), illustrating the importance of a knowledge translation approach that connects sectors. But there are substantial differences in views between health and other sectors regarding the weight of factors that should be considered in proposing modifications to building codes. Before discussing key intersectoral differences, I review the building code revision processes in Canada.

BUILDING CODE REVISIONS IN CANADA

Building codes stipulate minimum requirements for the construction of both residential homes and public buildings. Revisions are the product of a two-part process. Model codes are developed at the national level, and then provinces and territories choose whether or not to adopt these recommendations in their legislation.

Creating model codes is the responsibility of the Canadian Commission on Building and Fire Codes (Clemmensen, 2003). Composed of volunteers, approximately one-third of the Commission's members are from the building industry; another third are building regulators; and the final third come from sectors including municipal affairs, consumer and safety groups, and emergency services (NRCC [National Research Council Canada], 2014). This composition reflects the fact that civil engineers, home builders, and architects have historically been the primary proponents for modifications to building codes in Canada. National code changes in Canada are established through a multi-stage consensus process with revision cycles of five years.

Groups involved in the review of code changes are the Provincial/Territorial Policy Advisory Committee on Codes, composed of ministerial representatives; standing committees responsible for developing the technical content of the codes; and task groups providing input on specific code elements. Task groups and standing committees consider laboratory and community-based research evidence, codes from other jurisdictions, input from the public and Canadian industries, and congruence between different code sections.

Revising codes involves an intricate process of consensus building and decision making over a lengthy time period. A wide range of interdisciplinary evidence, from laboratory, human factors, and population health research is needed to inform code development. Knowledge translation approaches must integrate evidence from all these fields of research. Furthermore, prominent intersectoral debates regarding changes to building codes, such as those outlined below, must be understood.

INTERSECTORAL DEBATES

While strong public safety arguments have resulted in more stringent codes for public buildings, similar requirements for private dwellings have been described as government intruding into homeowners' property rights. While public health professionals may consider regulations to be a critical means to achieve health improvements (e.g., tobacco control and injuries) (Bunnell et al., 2012; Koh et al., 2010), those in other sectors may prefer voluntary alternatives, such as encouraging insurance industry incentives or making a wider range of manufactured products available for optional installation by homeowners (e.g., handrails for stairs). Reconciling divergent viewpoints about the role of government regulation across sectors will be a key issue in discussions about how and whether to use building code legislation as a lever for health improvements.

The second debate concerns universal access—the accessibility of the built environment for people with varying levels of physical ability. In the Canadian model codes there are two separate standards for the built environment: universal access requirements and residential home requirements. Currently, the model codes specify that universal access requirements are applicable only for buildings so designated;

they do not apply for general housing stock. Proponents of the status quo argue that accessible design should be optional rather than imposed, since it increases construction costs, places limitations on architectural design, and may be associated with the stigma of disability.

This position is beginning to shift, with growing public concerns about home visitability (CMHC, 2008) and supportive housing needs alongside government policy directives for aging in place. Human rights commissions have also called for more accessible residential homes (OHRC [Ontario Human Rights Commission], 2013). Building homes with universal access features costs less at the time of construction than during retrofitting. Thus, those who are physically challenged would benefit from universal access requirements but the public at large would have to bear the additional cost of universal design features in residential homes. Moving in the direction of more universal access, the Ontario government has introduced amendments to the building code that require higher standards of accessibility in new buildings (OMMAH [Ontario Ministry of Municipal Affairs and Housing], 2014).

The third debate is about which sector bears cost expenditures and which sector achieves savings. Health care savings would be accrued through safer, injury-reducing built environments. However, the housing sector and construction industry, and subsequently home buyers, would bear the direct costs of more stringent codes. As an example, manufacturers cite potential financial and job losses that may result when stricter regulations no longer permit them to sell pre-fabricated products such as stairs or handrails.

These lines of debate are important for health professionals to understand if they are going to act as knowledge translators for building code revisions. Values underlie these debates and frame how evidence is used and what options for change are considered viable. These debates also play out in the public arena. Since public input is considered a critical part of the consensus-building process to update Canada's model codes, it is important to understand how different disciplines and sectors prioritize and engage community stakeholders.

PRINCIPLES FOR INTERSECTORAL KNOWLEDGE TRANSLATION

Several principles for intersectoral knowledge translation arise from the preceding debates. Research evidence must be understood and conveyed in a way that explicitly acknowledges what shapes interdisciplinary perspectives and drives intersectoral decision making. Those engaged in knowledge translation must be prepared to fully discuss options for building code revisions from different disciplinary and ideological stances with those directly involved (e.g., internal committees) and indirectly involved (e.g., the public) in the process. Finally, if health professionals and non-governmental organizations are to effectively support the application of research evidence to building code revisions, they too must be made aware of fundamental differences and similarities in the intersectoral debates about revisions.

CONCLUSION

While evidence is a key input for knowledge translation, the process of revising building codes highlights other major considerations that must be taken into account. A better awareness of core debates from the perspective of different sectors may also inform the development of a more robust evidence base for decision making about code changes. This discussion has focused on building codes, but it is likely that the principles outlined above are pertinent to other arenas of intersectoral policy change.

GLOSSARY

Aging in place: The ability to live in one's own home and community safely, independently, and comfortably, regardless of age, income, or ability level.

Built environment: The part of the physical environment that human activity has created.

Determinants of health: Factors that change the status of a person's health.

Home visitability: The concept of designing and building homes with basic accessibility, providing easy access on the main level for visitors of all ages and mobility levels.

Insurance industry incentives: Conscious use of rewards and penalties in the cost of insurance to encourage good practices.

Knowledge translation: The synthesis, dissemination, exchange, and application of knowledge.

Performance-based codes: Building codes that specifically state their safety goals, and reference-approved methods that can be used to demonstrate compliance with their requirements.

Supportive housing: Housing for seniors and people with disabilities that require some assistance to continue to live independently.

Universal access: Accessibility of the built environment for people with varying levels of physical ability.

DISCUSSION QUESTIONS

1. What different perspectives about building codes are described in this paper?
2. Why is it important to understand how perspectives about regulatory action in housing differ across stakeholder groups?
3. How can knowledge of these perspectives inform strategies to encourage the use of research evidence to inform building codes?

REFERENCES

Bunnell, R., O'Neil, D., Soler, R., Payne, R., Giles, W., Collins, J., & Bauer, U. (2012). Fifty communities putting prevention to work: Accelerating chronic disease prevention through policy, systems and environmental change. *Journal of Community Health, 37*(5), 1081–1090.

Clemmensen, B. (2003). Building codes – a good tool in the right context. Paper presented at the Global Summit on Performance-based Building Codes, Washington, DC, Nov 3–5. Retrieved from www.nationalcodes.ca/ccbfc/toolcontext_e.pdf

CMHC (Canada Mortgage and Housing Corporation). (2008). *Understanding the status of visibility in Canada.* Retrieved from http://www.measureupthenorth.com/UserFiles/Research%20Highlight%20Visitable%20Housing.pdf

Koh, H., Oppenheimer, S., Massin-Short, S., Emmons, K., Geller, A., & Viswanath, K. (2010). Translating research evidence into practice to reduce health disparities: A social determinants approach. *American Journal of Public Health, 100*(S1), S72–S80.

Meacham, B., Bowen, R., Traw, J., & Moore, A. (2005). Performance-based building regulation: Current situation and future needs. *Building Research & Information, 33*(2), 91–106.

NRCC (National Research Council Canada). (2014). *Canadian Commission on Building and Fire Codes.* Retrieved from http://www.nationalcodes.nrc.gc.ca/eng/ccbfc/commission.html

OHRC (Ontario Human Rights Commission). (2013). *OHRC submission to the MMAH on proposed changes to the Ontario Building Code.* Retrieved from http://www.ohrc.on.ca/en/ohrc-submission-mmah-proposed-changes-ontario-building-code

OMMAH (Ontario Ministry of Municipal Affairs and Housing). (2014). *New accessibility amendments to Ontario's Building Code.* Retrieved from http://www.mah.gov.on.ca/Page10546.aspx

PHAC (Public Health Agency of Canada). (2013). *What makes Canadians healthy or unhealthy?* Retrieved from http://www.phac-aspc.gc.ca/ph-sp/determinants/determinants-eng.php#physenviron

Srinivasan, S., O'Fallon, L., & Dearry, A. (2003). Creating healthy communities, healthy homes, healthy people: Initiating a research agenda on the built environment and public health. *American Journal of Public Health, 93*(9), 1446–1450.

CHAPTER 16

Who Says What? Tobacco Control Interest Groups' Activities as Portrayed in a Canadian Newspaper from 1993 to 2004

Adenike Y. Rowaiye, Anita Kothari, and Dana Gore

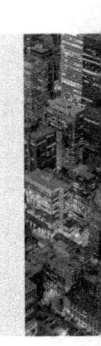

TAKE-HOME MESSAGE

- Tobacco control interest groups use the media to discuss tobacco issues.
- Anti-tobacco organizations use the media more than health advocacy groups and health professional groups, and all groups use the media to talk about legislation.
- Using the media is a strategy to influence policy and public opinion, but we don't know if tobacco control interest groups' use of the media has been effective.

INTRODUCTION

Tobacco is a well-known major health hazard to smokers and to society at large. As a result, Canadian tobacco control interest groups (organizations committed to reducing the cultural acceptability of tobacco use) have become extremely vocal, using information and resources to change social norms regarding smoking and policy decisions. Tobacco control interest groups differ in their messaging strategies depending on the orientation of the group, the resources at their disposal, and the outlet or means they select to air their views.

A study by Rowaiye examined the content of tobacco-related newspaper coverage in the *Globe and Mail*, a Canadian media source (Rowaiye, 2007). The findings identified the dominant tobacco control interest groups in the *Globe and Mail* newspaper and their key messages over the course of a decade (1993–2004) through the examination of their direct quotes.

METHODS

A set of tobacco-related newspaper articles (n=653) was identified from the *Globe and Mail*. Direct quotations attributed to tobacco control interest groups were extracted and analyzed using content analysis. The source of the quotes was classified into one of three categories: (1) anti-tobacco organizations, non-governmental health organizations committed exclusively to promoting public health by eliminating illness and death caused by tobacco, including second-hand smoke; (2) health advocacy groups, organizations committed to health promotion in a broader sense as well as health issues related to tobacco use; and (3) professional (medical) organizations, composed of and committed to the general advancement of health care professionals, such as the Canadian Medical Association.

To identify larger themes represented by the quotes, the content analysis instrument by Clegg-Smith et al. (2002) was piloted and adapted for use in this study. The final instrument included 21 tobacco-related thematic categories, such as: tobacco advertising, economics, addiction and quitting, and promotion and sponsorship. Once all the quotes were coded into categories, the data were entered and analyzed using Statistical Package for Social Sciences (SPSS).

RESULTS

Sources of quotes: A total of 370 quotes were retrieved from 653 tobacco-related articles from January 1993 to June 2004 in the *Globe and Mail.* Anti-tobacco organizations had the highest number of quotes (N= 272, 73.5%), followed by health advocacy groups (N= 78, 21.1%) and professional (medical) organizations (N=20, 5.4%). The Non-Smokers' Rights Association (NSRA) had the highest number of quotes (N=186, 50.3%), followed by Physicians for a Smoke-Free Canada (PSC) (N=69, 18.6%).

Key messages of quotes: "Bills/legislation" were the most talked about theme (N=50, 13.5%), followed by "economics" (N= 41, 11.1%), "tobacco industry" (N=39, 10.5%), and "government" (N=38, 10.3%). Second-hand smoke and related smoke-free policies were rarely referenced; only two organizations were quoted on these themes.

Timing of the messages: In terms of how the themes changed over time, each theme experienced some variations throughout the study period. The variations experienced in the themes of bills/legislation, economics, government and tobacco advertising, promotion, and sponsorship were not random, statistically speaking, which means that there might be specific trigger events responsible for the observed patterns.

DISCUSSION

Who Is Getting the Most Attention from the Media and Why?

Anti-tobacco organizations, especially the Non-Smokers' Rights Association (NSRA) and Physicians for a Smoke-Free Canada (PSC), were the most heavily quoted tobacco control interest groups in this study. A potential explanation for this lies in the fact that these groups have specific goals to fight tobacco use through political action, and the NSRA in particular has a reputation for taking a major leadership role in the fight against tobacco use

(Cunningham, 1996; Studlar, 2002). This could suggest that groups that are committed to political action and whose primary objective is to decrease the adverse effects of tobacco use are using the media the most. They also may have more experience working with the media, and as such, anti-tobacco organizations could be a more obvious resource for journalists to turn to for comments than health advocacy groups or professional organizations.

However, an interesting question to consider is how much the quantity of quotes that an organization has in a newspaper influences the shaping of public opinion and policy. Is the group that takes up the most media space the same group that is leading the fight against tobacco in all other important aspects, such as direct lobbying efforts? In the event that an exclusive focus on tobacco control does contribute to more media space and anti-tobacco messaging, other health groups and professional organizations might also consider forming similar subgroups that are able to concentrate solely on tobacco control.

What Are the Tobacco Control Interest Groups Talking About?

Bills and legislation were the most dominant theme in the *Globe and Mail*, perhaps due to legislative events that occurred during that period. For example, the federal law raised the legal age for buying tobacco products from 16 to 18 years and imposed fines of up to $50,000 on those selling the product to persons below 18 (Dunsmuir, Blanchette, Dupus, & Chenier, 1998; Studlar, 2002). By focusing on the bills and legislation, tobacco control interest groups could be demonstrating that they are more interested in influencing legislators and the public than in other methods used for reducing the cultural acceptability of tobacco use. Alternatively, the high number of quotes could be a reaction to the legislative changes at that time, and not necessarily representative of general messaging strategies.

A small portion (4 percent) of the quotes attributable to tobacco control interest groups discussed the theme of the health effects of smoking, which is consistent with what has been found in previous studies on reporting of negative effects of smoking (Clegg-Smith et al., 2002; Clegg-Smith & Wakefield, 2005; Durrant et al., 2003; Lima & Siegel, 1999; Long, Slater, & Lysengen, 2006). This may suggest that the theme is no longer seen as controversial or that tobacco control interest groups no longer see the need to emphasize it. However, this could also point to distinct messaging strategies for different aspects of tobacco use. For example, perhaps tobacco control interest groups feel that direct education campaigns would be a better medium through which to shape public opinion about the adverse health effects of tobacco.

What Were the Patterns in Messaging Over Time?

There was considerable variation in the themes used by tobacco control interest groups between 1993 and 2004, which could be due to a number of reasons. It could be that the limited amount of time or space for health news in the print media forces journalists to constantly introduce new issues in order to maintain the interest of the readers (Downs,

1972). The variation could also reflect demand for a policy option (a proactive messaging strategy) or may be in response to policy already enacted (a reactive strategy), such as the smoke-free bans that came into effect in 2003 (Borio, n.d.; Wallack, Dorfman, Jernigan, & Themba, 1993; Ziegler & Huelshoff, 1980). The fact that the themes were not generally consistent could be problematic; messages by the tobacco industry have been consistent, powerful, and compelling over time (Menashe & Siegel, 1998), and consequently tobacco control interest groups may need to respond in a similar fashion to be most effective.

A number of limitations must be considered when drawing conclusions from this study: the results do not present a comprehensive analysis of all print media in Canada, and the *Globe and Mail* caters to a specific readership. Additionally, the study did not assess the accuracy of the quotes; hence, they might have been taken out of context to suit the journalist's or editor's position. Most importantly, this type of analysis does not take into account enough of the relevant context (e.g., history, policy changes, media selection of quotes) to provide definitive answers about the messaging strategies of tobacco control interest groups.

However, this study does raise some interesting questions regarding the use of quotes by tobacco control interest groups in the *Globe and Mail*. Does the fact that tobacco control interest groups focus on a variety of themes reflect a lack of cohesion in the messages they intend to send, or is it done purposefully in order to draw attention to various aspects of tobacco use? How representative are newspaper quotes of a tobacco control group's actual messaging strategy to policy-makers and the public, considering that they use a variety of advocacy strategies outside of the *Globe and Mail* and that only a fraction of what is said during an interview is quoted and published? How much of what is quoted depends on the context of current political or policy events, the political persuasions of the newspaper in question, or even the direction of the article itself? Future research might be crafted to answer some of these questions.

CONCLUSION

Tobacco control interest groups have an important role to play in the fight against tobacco and related health effects. They can help to inform and shape the views of both the public and policy-makers about tobacco. This study raises further questions that might be compelling for tobacco control interest groups to consider. For instance, it provides a starting point for thinking about the quantity, thematic content, and diversity of their quotes in a major newspaper outlet. This could be used to fuel further discussion on how to approach changing public opinion and policy (e.g., through which representatives, through what avenues, and with what messages).

GLOSSARY

Tobacco control interest groups: Organizations committed to reducing the cultural acceptability of tobacco use.

DISCUSSION QUESTIONS

1. Should tobacco control interest groups continue to produce broad and varied media messaging or is a common media message more effective? Why?
2. What are other ways that tobacco control interest groups can promote the development of tobacco control policies?
3. Why do you think that tobacco control has had success developing policies (as a population-level intervention) compared to other areas of health promotion?

REFERENCES

Borio, G. (n.d.) Tobacco timeline: The twenty-first century — the new millennium. In G. Borio (ed.), *Tobacco timeline*. Retrieved from http://archive.tobacco.org/History/Tobacco_History.html

Clegg-Smith, K., & Wakefield, M. (2005). Textual analysis of tobacco editorials: How are key media gatekeepers framing the issues? *American Journal of Health Promotion, 19,* 361–368.

Clegg-Smith, K., Wakefield, M., Siebel, C., Szczypka, G., Slater, S., Terry-McElrath, Y., Chaloupka, F. J. (2002). Coding the news: The development of a methodological framework for coding and analyzing newspaper coverage of tobacco issues. *ImpacTeen*. Retrieved from http://www.impacteen.org/ab_RPNo21_2002.htm

Cunningham, R. (1996). *Smoke and mirrors: The Canadian tobacco war.* Ottawa: International Development Research Centre (IDRC).

Downs, A. (1972). Up and down with ecology: The "issue-attention cycle." *Public Interest, 28,* 38–50.

Dunsmuir, M., Blanchette, C., Dupus, J., & Chenier, N. M. (1998). *Tobacco and health: Government responses.* Parliamentary Research Branch. Retrieved from http://dsp-psd.pwgsc.gc.ca/Collection-R/LoPBdP/modules/prb98-8-tobacco/index-e.htm

Durrant, R., Wakefield, M., McLeod, K., Clegg-Smith, K., & Chapman, S. (2003). Tobacco in the news: An analysis of newspaper coverage of tobacco issues in Australia. *Tobacco Control, 12,* ii75–ii81.

Lima, J. C., & Siegel, M. (1999). The tobacco settlement: An analysis of newspaper coverage of a national policy debate, 1997-98. *Tobacco Control, 8,* 247–253.

Long, M., Slater, M. D., & Lysengen, L. (2006). US news media coverage of tobacco control issues. *Tobacco Control, 15,* 367–372.

Menashe, C. L., & Siegel, M. (1998). The power of a frame: An analysis of newspaper coverage of tobacco issues—United States, 1985–1996. *Journal of Health Communication, 3,* 307–325.

Rowaiye, A. (2007). *Interest groups, the print media and policy formulations: The case of tobacco control.* Master's Thesis. University of Western Ontario.

Studlar, D. T. (2002). *Tobacco control: Comparative politics in United States and Canada.* Peterborough, ON: Broadview Press.

Wallack, L., Dorfman, L., Jernigan, D., & Themba, M. (1993). *Media advocacy and public health: Power for prevention.* Newbury Park: Sage Publications.

Ziegler, H., & Huelshoff, M. (1980). Interest groups and public policy. *Policy Studies Journal, 9,* 439–488.

CHAPTER 17

Walking, Walkability, and Health Disparities: Condensed Review Summary and Update

Theresa Grant

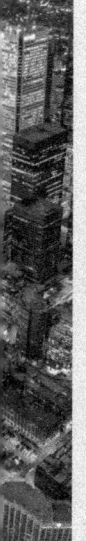

TAKE-HOME MESSAGE

- Environments that invite people to walk have multiple associated health benefits, such as increased levels of physical activity, lower rates of diabetes and obesity, and lower incidence of childhood asthma.
- There is evidence that socially disadvantaged groups often live in places with higher levels of traffic, lower-quality pedestrian infrastructure, and poor connections with public transit. These are all features of the built environment that make walking more difficult and unpleasant.
- This chapter summarizes the findings of a literature review on inequalities of walking conditions and provides some insight on the reasons that these differences exist. Creating more walkable environments in the future means thinking about the impact of planning decisions to ensure that vulnerable pedestrians such as older people, those living in low-income neighbourhoods, and persons with disabilities are not unfairly disadvantaged.

INTRODUCTION

Rising rates of obesity and diabetes in Canadian cities, as well as growing concern regarding environmental sustainability, have prompted societal attention towards the importance of creating walkable environments. It is especially important in Ontario, where both the population (Ontario Ministry of Finance, 2010) and greenhouse gas emissions (Neptis Foundation, 2006) are growing and are projected to continue to do so. A review by Grant (2011) described the connections between walking, municipal environments, and socio-economic disparities. This chapter summarizes literature and recommendations made in the review as well as referencing recently published tools pertinent to the creation of more walkable urban environments in Ontario.

BENEFITS OF WALKABLE ENVIRONMENTS

Walking is the most common and preferred physical activity among Canadian adults, with 81 percent of people reporting that they walk at least occasionally (Canadian Fitness and Lifestyles Research Institute, 1998). Lack of physical activity has been estimated to contribute to 21,000 premature deaths in a single year and 5.3 billion in annual health care expenditures (Katzmarzyk, Gledhill, & Shephard, 2000). Many Canadians have indicated that they would like to become more physically active but are deterred largely by concerns around the convenience of getting more exercise (Spence, Shephard, Craig, & McGannon, 2011), particularly in Ontario and Nova Scotia (Canadian Fitness and Lifestyles Research Institute, 2007). Creating more walkable environments can support the ability of Canadians to incorporate more physical activity into their daily lives by using walking as a mode of transport. In addition to increasing levels of physical activity, creating walkable environments in combination with enhancing public transit is an essential component of addressing the environmental effects of widespread automobile use. These effects include poor air quality, threats to water quality due to salt use and drainage problems, and casualties/injuries associated with collisions—all of which have negative implications for human health (Bray, Elliott, Vakil, & Abelsohn, 2005; Frumkin, 2002).

There is extensive evidence indicating that people walk more for transport in environments characterized by compact land development (i.e., medium to high dwelling densities), interconnected city blocks, and mixed land-use (Badland & Schofield, 2008; Berke et al., 2007; Clark et al., 2009; Duncan et al., 2010; Ewing, Meakins, Hamidi, & Nelson, 2014; Frank & Engelke, 2001; Frank, Saelens, Powell, & Chapman, 2007; Frank et al., 2005; Gauvin et al., 2008; King et al., 2005; Owen et al., 2007; Saelens, Sallis, & Frank, 2003). These studies have used both self-reported walking levels and pedometer readings as outcome variables. Areas of urban sprawl (i.e., low density, homogeneous land-use development) are associated with higher levels of automobile dependence and overweight populations than cities with more compact building development (Ewing, Meakins, Hamidi, & Nelson, 2014; Frank, Andresen, & Schmid, 2004; Saelens, Sallis, & Frank, 2003). In other words, there is no shortage of proof that people will walk for transportation more often when it is feasible to do so.

In addition to the characteristics of dwelling density, mixed-land use, and street pattern connectivity, other studies have documented the importance of safety, pleasant surroundings, sidewalks, and accessible recreational facilities such as parks and walking trails (Booth et al., 2000; Fisher, Li, Michael, & Cleveland, 2004; King, 2008; Li et al., 2005). Based on a large American study done in five states, the Centers for Disease Control concluded that people who perceived their neighbourhoods as unsafe were significantly more likely to be physically inactive (Weinstein et al., 1999). The level of influence that neighbourhood attributes have on walking for recreation or leisure walking can vary according to the place in which they are studied (Van Dyck et al., 2013a, 2013b).

Recent studies done in Toronto found that not only did people walk and cycle more in walkable neighbourhoods but that walkable neighbourhoods also had:

- lower rates of diabetes (Booth et al., 2013; Glazier et al., 2014; Glazier & Booth, 2007);
- lower rates of obesity (Glazier et al., 2014); and
- lower incidence of childhood asthma (Simons, Dell, Moineddin, & To, 2014).

QUALITY OF NEIGHBOURHOOD ENVIRONMENTS: EVIDENCE OF DISPARITY

People are less likely to be active in an environment that is hazardous or unappealing. Not being able to afford a gym membership or a car to travel to a more inviting environment means that many people living on low incomes are less likely to engage in sufficient physical activity in socially disadvantaged places in the limited hours they have to do so. There is growing evidence suggesting that the quality of neighbourhood environments is less supportive of physical activity in socially disadvantaged places than in socially advantaged places (Aytur et al., 2008; Crawford et al., 2008; Estabrooks, Lee, & Gyurcsik, 2003; Grant et al., 2010; Hajat et al., 2013; Hillsdon, Panter, Foster, & Jones, 2007; Lovasi, Hutson, Guerra, & Neckerman, 2009; Northridge, & Freeman, 2011; Timperio et al., 2007). These differences include higher levels of traffic, lack of high-quality pedestrian infrastructure, and poor connections with public transit in lower-income neighbourhoods (Balfour & Kaplan, 2002; Clark et al., 2009; Giles-Corti & Donovan, 2002; Grant et al., 2010; Kelly et al., 2007; Leslie et al., 2005; Wilson, Kirtland, Ainsworth, & Addy, 2004). Residents of lower-income neighbourhoods most definitely experience a much higher risk of pedestrian injury (Lord et al., 2010).

In summary, environments that limit walking:

- provide unequal transportation opportunities for those who cannot drive;
- limit access to safe and enjoyable walking experiences; and
- pose injury risks and hardship in accessing walking infrastructure.

The body of research on disparities in walking conditions highlights the issue of resource distribution and necessitates consideration of whether the processes driving unequal distribution of walking amenities are fair.

WALKABILITY, DISPARITIES, AND SOCIO-POLITICAL INFLUENCES

The way that a society organizes itself and the decisions that governments make end up shaping the environments in which we live. These socio-political influences on walkability have resulted in different kinds of disparities. The first type of disparity has meant that most environments in North America are more conducive to driving rather than walking. In other words, people who are unable or do not want to drive face a transportation disadvantage.

The second type of disparity with regards to walking conditions concerns the differences between socially advantaged and disadvantaged places. This means that people living in higher-income neighbourhoods can generally have safer and more enjoyable walking experiences compared to people living in lower-income neighbourhoods.

A third type of disparity arises when the needs of vulnerable pedestrians such as children, the elderly, and people with disabilities are not considered when pedestrian infrastructure is built. This means that these pedestrians either cannot access the infrastructure or face greater risk or hardship when they do, as evidenced by the overrepresentation of children in pedestrian vehicle collisions as well as a disproportionate level of injury and death among older pedestrian victims (Campbell, Zegeer, Huang, & Cynecki, 2014; Lord et al., 2010).

The larger review by Grant (2011) summarized research explaining factors that contribute to disparities in environmental conditions. These include historical factors that perpetuate auto-oriented development as well as explain why higher-income neighbourhoods are in a better position to advocate for improved walking conditions. For example, higher-income neighbourhoods often have:

- larger property-owner groups that have clout with local governments in advocating for neighbourhood improvements;
- more stable populations, meaning that there are more long-term residents who have accumulated knowledge about how best to advocate for improvements;
- higher numbers of people with the resources (e.g., time, money, education) to address neighbourhood problems; and
- higher likelihood that a political representative lives in the same neighbourhood.

Lessons learned from the environmental justice movement in the United States have taught us that disparities between environmental conditions in socially disadvantaged neighbourhoods represent more than just material differences (Bullard & Johnson, 2000; Rhodes, 2003). Instead they often represent decisions, policies, and enforcement strategies that unfairly disadvantage the most vulnerable members of society.

The reduction of health disparities and the conditions that support them has been identified as a priority by the Chief Medical Officers of Health for both Ontario (Basrur, 2004; Ontario Health Leadership Council, 2013) and Canada (Chief Medical Officer of Health, 2008). Creating walkable places is an important part of addressing the problem of health disparities, since lower-income and vulnerable groups rely on walking to get around and are over-exposed to the hazards of auto-oriented development.

Creating walkable places means more than building wider sidewalks. It involves making walking a legitimate form of travel and ensuring that this legitimacy is reflected in funding decisions, planning processes, and legislative frameworks.

RECOMMENDATIONS

Detailed report recommendations are summarized here:

- Develop and coordinate growth management plans that include active transport and public transit infrastructure.
- Ensure that municipalities have the tools and the funding to update institutional procedures; and develop, enhance, and implement active transportation infrastructure and pedestrian and cycling plans.
- Ensure that both public transportation and active transportation infrastructure, along with their connections, are safe, efficient, and accessible for all population groups including people with disabilities, seniors, and children.
- Ensure that built environment accessibility standards address the outdoor mobility needs of disabled persons; and support the implementation of these standards across private and public sectors.
- Redistribute the costs of vehicular use more equitably.
- Support traffic-calming strategies and car-sharing programs, and reduce standard vehicular speeds on shared streets.
- Consider how provisions to the Highway Traffic Act may provide greater safety and legitimacy for pedestrians, and adopt legislation that requires transportation equity spending on active transportation infrastructure.
- Ensure that environmental protection, accessibility, and land use laws are enforced equally well in socially advantaged and disadvantaged places.
- Develop mechanisms to promote intersectoral collaboration among government departments both vertically and horizontally.
- Integrate a health-impact assessment into municipal land-use and transportation planning procedures.
- Support planning approaches that are place-centred and involve ongoing public consultation.
- Develop mechanisms for meaningful public engagement with a focus on vulnerable pedestrians.
- Support public efforts to adopt pedestrian charters.
- Support community development resources, particularly for socially disadvantaged areas.
- Monitor and reduce disparities in walking conditions and access to public transit that occur among socially advantaged and disadvantaged neighbourhoods.
- Take action to ensure that public resources are distributed in a way that benefits everyone.

SELECTED RESOURCES FOR TAKING ACTION

New resources and reports supporting the creation of more walkable environments have been published since the 2011 review that this chapter is based on. The following list represent selected resources that are particularly pertinent for Ontario stakeholders interested in creating more walkable environments:

- Centers for Disease Control and Prevention. (2013). *Healthy communities program*. Retrieved from http://www.cdc.gov/nccdphp/dch/programs/healthycommunitiesprogram/index.htm
- Jane's Walk Project. (2017). *Walkability checklist*. Retrieved from http://janeswalk.org/files/4514/5331/5868/2010_walkability_checklist_janes_walk.pdf
- Toronto Public Health (2012). The *walkable city: Neighbourhood design preferences, travel choices and health*. Retrieved from https://www1.toronto.ca/city_of_toronto/toronto_public_health/healthy_public_policy/hphe/files/pdf/walkable_city.pdf
- World Health Organization (2012). *Addressing the social determinants of health: The urban dimension and the role of government*. Retrieved from http://www.euro.who.int/en/publications/abstracts/addressing-the-social-determinants-of-health-the-urban-dimension-and-the-role-of-local-government

GLOSSARY

Built environment: Aspects of the physical environment that have been designed with patterns of human activity in mind, including urban design elements, land use, and transportation systems.

Walkability: The extent to which the built environment supports pedestrian comfort, convenience, enjoyment, and safety.

DISCUSSION QUESTIONS

1. Traditional measures of walkability have focused on dwelling density, mixed-land use, and street pattern connectivity. Discuss why these characteristics of the built environment support walking. Are there situations where all these characteristics may be present but yet an area is still unfriendly to pedestrians?
2. Creating more walkable places involves many stakeholders and multiple sectors of society, including the public (e.g., community groups), municipal governments, provincial governments, the private sector, and the transportation sector. Use the walkability checklist provided by Jane's Walk (included in the resource list above) to conduct an audit of your neighbourhood. Determine who the key stakeholders are in the

area where you live and what role each can play for improving walkability. Consider the interest of each stakeholder as well as potential social and economic barriers to action. Consult the Toronto Public Health (2012) report listed in the resources above to guide your consideration of the role that various stakeholders may play.

3. This chapter makes reference to the American environmental justice movement, which arose in response to practices and policies that resulted in disproportionate environmental exposures and adverse health outcomes in low-income and racial minority neighbourhoods. The cited article by Bullard & Johnson (2000) gives a historical overview of this movement and mentions a landmark national study (United Church of Christ, 1987) that examined the correlation between toxic waste sites and population demographics. Why was this study important to the environmental justice movement? What does it tell us about the urban planning process?

REFERENCES

Aytur, S., Rodriguez, D., Evenson, K., Catellier, D., & Rosamond, W. (2008). The sociodemographics of land use planning: Relationships to physical activity, accessibility, and equity. *Health Place, 14*, 367–385.

Badland, H. M., & Schofield, G. M. (2008). Understanding the relationships between private automobile availability, overall physical activity, and travel behavior in adults. *Transportation, 35*, 363–374.

Balfour, J., & Kaplan, G. (2002). Neighborhood environment and loss of physical function in older adults: Evidence from the Alameda County Study. *Journal of Epidemiology, 155*, 507–515.

Basrur, S. (2004). *Chief Medical Officer of health report: Healthy weights, healthy lives*. Toronto: Ontario Ministry of Health and Long-Term Care.

Berke, E. M., Koepsell, T. D., Moudon, A. V., Hoskins, R. E., & Larson, E. B. (2007). Association of the built environment with physical activity and obesity in older persons. *American Journal of Public Health, 97*, 486–492.

Booth, G., Creatore, M., Moineddin, R., Gozdyra, P., Weyman, J., Matheson, F., & Glazier, R. H. (2013). Unwalkable neighborhoods, poverty, and the risk of diabetes among recent immigrants to Canada compared with long-term residents. *Diabetes Care, 36*, 302–308.

Booth, M. L., Owen, N., Bauman, A., Clavisi, O., & Leslie, E. (2000). Social-cognitive and perceived environment influences associated with physical activity in older Australians. *Preventive Medicine, 31*, 15–22.

Bray, R., Elliott, D., Vakil, C., Abelsohn, A. (2005). *Report on urban sprawl and public health in Ontario: A review of the pertinent literature*. Toronto: Ontario College of Family Physicians.

Bullard, R., & Johnson, G. (2000). Environmental justice: Grassroots activism and its impact on public policy decision making. *Journal of Social Issues, 56*(3) 555–578.

Campbell, B., Zegeer, C., Huang, H., & Cynecki, M. (2014). A review of pedestrian safety research in the United States and abroad. Washington, DC: U.S. Department of Transportation, Federal Highway Administration.

Canadian Fitness and Lifestyles Research Institute. (1998). *Popular physical activities*. Ottawa: Canadian Fitness and Lifestyles Research Institute.

Canadian Fitness and Lifestyles Research Institute. (2007). *Changing the Canadian landscape... one step at a time: Results of the Physical Activity Monitor 2007*. Ottawa: Canadian Fitness and Lifestyles Research Institute.

Chief Medical Officer of Health. (2008). *The state of public health in Canada: Addressing health inequalities*. Ottawa: Public Health Agency of Canada.

Clark, C., Kawachi, I., Ryan, L., Ertel, K., Fay, M., & Berkman, L. (2009). Perceived neighborhood safety and incident mobility disability among elders: The hazards of poverty. *BMC Public Health, 9*, 162.

Crawford, D., Timperio, A., Giles-Corti, B., Ball, K., Hume, C., Roberts, R., Salmon, J. (2008). Do features of public open spaces vary according to neighbourhood socio-economic status? *Health Place, 14*, 889–893.

Duncan, M. J., Winkler, E., Sugiyama, T., Cerin, E., Dutoit, L., Leslie, E., & Owen, N. (2010). Relationships of land use mix with walking for transport: Do land uses and geographical scale matter? *Journal of Urban Health, 87*(5), 782–795.

Estabrooks, P., Lee, R., & Gyurcsik, N. (2003). Resources for physical activity participation: Does availability and accessibility differ by neighborhood socioeconomic status? *Annals of Behavioral Medicine, 25*, 100–104.

Ewing, R., Meakins, G., Hamidi, S., & Nelson, A. (2014). Relationship between urban sprawl and physical activity, obesity, and morbidity — Update and refinement. *Health & Place, 26*, 118–126.

Fisher, K. J., Li, F., Michael, Y., & Cleveland, M. (2004). Neighborhood-level influences on physical activity among older adults: A multilevel analysis. *Journal of Aging and Physical Activity, 12*, 45–63.

Frank, L. D., Andresen, M. A., & Schmid, T. L. (2004). Obesity relationships with community design, physical activity, and time spent in cars. *American Journal of Preventive Medicine, 27*, 87–96.

Frank, L. D., & Engelke, P. O. (2001). The built environment and human activity patterns: Exploring the impacts of urban form on public health. *Journal of Planning Literature, 16*, 202–18.

Frank, L. D., Saelens, B. E., Powell, K. E., & Chapman, J. E. (2007). Stepping towards causation: Do built environments or neighborhood and travel preferences explain physical activity, driving, and obesity? *Social Science & Medicine, 65*, 1898–1914.

Frank, L. D., Schmid, T. L., Sallis, J. F., Chapman, J., & Saelens, B. E. (2005). Linking objectively measured physical activity with objectively measured urban form: Findings from SMARTRAQ. *American Journal of Preventive Medicine, 28*(2 Suppl. 2), 117–125.

Frumkin, H. (2002). Urban sprawl and public health. *Public Health Reports, 117*, 201–217.

Gauvin, L., Riva, M., Barnett, T., Richard, L., Craig, C. L., Spivock, M., Gagné, S. (2008). Association between neighborhood active living potential and walking. *American Journal of Epidemiology, 167*, 944–953.

Giles-Corti, B., & Donovan, R. (2002). Socioeconomic status differences in recreational physical activity levels and real and perceived access to a supportive physical environment. *Preventive Medicine, 35*, 601–611.

Glazier, R., & Booth, G. (2007). *Neighbourhood environments and resources for healthy living: A focus on diabetes in Toronto.* Toronto: Institute for Clinical Evaluative Sciences.

Glazier, R. H., Creatore, M. I., Weyman, J. T., Fazli, G., Matheson, F. I., Gozdyra, P., Booth, G. L. (2014). Density, destinations or both? A comparison of measures of walkability in relation to transportation behaviors, obesity and diabetes in Toronto, Canada. *PLoS One, 9*(1), e85295.

Grant, T. (2011). *Walking, walkability and health disparities: A review of the evidence and directions for actions in Ontario.* Ottawa: Population Health Improvement Research Network.

Grant, T., Edwards, N., Sveistrup, H., Andrew, C., & Egan, M. (2010). Inequitable walking conditions among older people: Examining the interrelationship of neighbourhood socio-economic status and urban form using a comparative case study. *BMC Public Health, 10*, 677.

Hajat, A., Diez-Roux, A., Adar, S., Auchincloss, A., Lovasi, G., O'Neill, M., Kaufman, J. D. (2013). Air pollution and individual and neighborhood socioeconomic status: Evidence from the Multi-Ethnic Study of Atherosclerosis (MESA). *Environmental Health Perspectives, 121*, 11–12.

Hillsdon, M., Panter, J., Foster, C., & Jones, A. (2007). Equitable access to exercise facilities. *Journal of Preventive Medicine, 32*, 506–508.

Katzmarzyk, P., Gledhill, N., & Shephard, R. (2000). The economic burden of physical inactivity in Canada. *Canadian Medical Association Journal, 163*, 1435–1440.

Kelly, C., Schootman, M., Baker, E., Barnidge, E., & Lemes, A. (2007). The association of sidewalk walkability and physical disorder with area-level race and poverty. *Journal of Epidemiology, 61*, 978–983.

King, D. (2008). Neighborhood and individual factors in activity in older adults: Results from the neighborhood and senior health study. *Journal of Aging and Physical Activity, 16*, 144–170.

King, W., Belle, S., Brach, J., Simkin-Silverman, L., Soska, T., & Kriska, A. (2005). Objective measures of neighborhood environment and physical activity in older women. *American Journal of Preventive Medecine, 28*, 461–469.

Leslie, E., Saelens, B., Frank, L., Owen, N., Bauman, A., Coffee, N., & Hugo, G. (2005). Residents' perceptions of walkability attributes in objectively different neighbourhoods: A pilot study. *Health Place, 11*, 227–236.

Li, F., Fisher, K. J., Bauman, A., Ory, M. G., Chodzko-Zajko, W., Harmer, P., Cleveland, M. (2005). Neighborhood influences on physical activity in middle-aged and older adults: A multilevel perspective. *Journal of Aging and Physical Activity, 13*, 87–114.

Lord, S., Hameed, S., Schuurman, N., Bell, N., Simons, R., & Chir, B. (2010). Vulnerability to pedestrian trauma: Demographic, temporal, societal, geographic, and environmental factors. *BC Medical Journal, 53*, 136–143.

Lovasi, G., Hutson, M., Guerra, M., & Neckerman, K. (2009). Built environments and obesity in disadvantaged populations. *Epidemiologic Reviews, 31*(1), 7–20.

Neptis Foundation. (2006). *Commentary on the Ontario government's proposed growth plan for the Greater Golden Horseshoe.* Toronto: Nepis Foundation.

Northridge, M., & Freeman, L. (2011). Urban planning and health equity. *Journal of Urban Health, 88*, 582–597.

Ontario Health Leadership Council. (2013). *Make no little plans.* Toronto: Ontario Ministry of Health.

Ontario Ministry of Finance. (2010). *Ontario population projections update.* Toronto: Ontario Ministry of Finance.

Owen, N., Cerin, E., Leslie, E., duToit, L., Coffee, N., Frank, L. D., Salis, J. F. (2007). Neighborhood walkability and the walking behavior of Australian adults. *American Journal of Preventive Medicine, 33,* 387–395.

Rhodes, E. (2003). *Environmental justice in America.* Bloomington: University of Indiana Press.

Saelens, B. E., Sallis, J. F., & Frank, L. D. (2003). Environmental correlates of walking and cycling: Findings from the transportation, urban design, and planning literatures. *Annals of Behavioural Medicine, 25,* 80–91.

Simons, E., Dell, S., Moineddin, R., & To, T. (2014). Longitudinal associations between neighbourhood walkability and incident childhood asthma. *Allergy, Asthma & Clinical Immunology, 10*(Suppl. 1): A8.

Spence, J., Shephard, R., Craig, C., & McGannon, K. (2011). *Compilation of evidence of effective active living interventions: A case study approach.* Toronto: Canadian Consortium of Health Promotion Research.

Timperio, A., Ball, K., Salmon, J., Roberts, R., & Crawford, D. (2007). Is availability of public open space equitable across areas? *Health Place, 13,* 335–340.

United Church of Christ, Commission for Racial Justice. (1987). *Toxic wastes and race in the United States: A national report on the racial and socio-economic characteristics of communities with hazardous waste sites.* Public Data Access, Inc.

Van Dyck, D., Cerin, E., Conway, T. L., De Bourdeaudhuij, I., Owen, N., Kerr, J., Sallis, J. F. (2013a). Interacting psychosocial and environmental correlates of leisure-time physical activity: A three-country study. *Health Psychology, 33*(7), 699–709.

Van Dyck, D., Cerin, E., Conway, T. L., De Bourdeaudhuij, I., Owen, N., Kerr, J., Sallis J. F. (2013b). Perceived neighborhood environmental attributes associated with adults' leisure-time physical activity: Findings from Belgium, Australia and the USA. *Health Place, 19,* 59–68.

Weinstein, A., Feigley, P., Pullen, P., Mann, L., & Redman, L. (1999). Neighborhood safety and the prevalence of physical inactivity – selected states, 1996. *Journal of the American Medical Association, 281,* 1373.

Wilson, D., Kirtland, K., Ainsworth, B., & Addy, C. (2004). Socioeconomic status and perceptions of access and safety for physical activity. *Annals of Behavioural Medicine, 28,* 20–28.

CHAPTER 18

Local Food Charters and Policies in Canada

Vivien Runnels

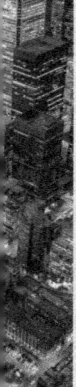

TAKE-HOME MESSAGE

- Developing food policies, conducting analyses, and implementing associated tasks with policy development is not easy to carry out given the complexities of food systems and the myriad of interests.
- The tool for food policy/food charter analysis was intended as a helpful resource for individual members of the public, local government decision-makers, community-based organizations, and other stakeholders who are interested in local food policy and may be either pondering the purpose, development, and implementation of their own food policy or considering revisiting and revising older policies.

INTRODUCTION

Following the theme of improving population health in Ontario, PHIRN looked at certain determinants of health, those conditions that impact or contribute to a population's health status. Food and its nutritional qualities are a critical determinant of health, a message that bears repeating in food policies and food charters. Although PHIRN's focus was on population health in Ontario, this study and analysis of the content of local food policies and food charters, and their direct and indirect concerns for health, has some lessons for all of Canada.

The ways in which Canadians think about food in their daily lives are being challenged with new knowledge, raising questions about aspects of food access and availability, as well as affordability and acceptability. New tastes and products have become available as a result of globalization and immigration. Terms such as *food systems, the 100-mile diet, food security, food insecurity* and *food sovereignty* are widely used. This new complexity around food consumption (and the inclusion of food waste disposal) also means that many consumers are increasing their knowledge and understanding of food systems, and developing a greater sense of responsibility in relation to food.

In recent years, concerned citizens and community organizations have increasingly become engaged in food-related action and the development of food-related statements at the local level. These statements, referred to as food charters and policies, are often written for citizens, designed to serve them and to improve their food security. Some statements have been developed outside formal structures of local government, although some of these are intended for acceptance and formalization. They are written with the understanding that policies and by-laws that affect food production and food availability can have an impact on local food systems and food security, and may also have the potential to affect food security and the nutritional status of the local population, communities, neighbourhoods, and individuals and their families.

Local governments have jurisdiction to set policies at the local level that can affect local food systems and impact food production and food availability, with potential for effects on citizen food security and nutritional status. Some of the policy types that local governments in Canada have jurisdiction over include planning and zoning (although subject to modification by provincial authorities). Planning, for example, can determine the presence, location, and size of food retail outlets, community gardens, and urban farmers' markets. Zoning can be used to preserve or protect food-producing agricultural land. Other types of policy related to food at the local level can include promoting health and influencing what people eat (e.g., through departments of health), determining what types of food are available to the public (e.g., through the licensing specifications of mobile food trucks), and institutional purchasing policies that can determine from where food is sourced. Local governments can also provide community grants programs to support community-based initiatives around food security (Enns, Rose, de Vries, & Hayes, 2008).

In response to a local health department's request for information on local food policy, PHIRN undertook a search and collection of existing Canadian food policies, and developed a tool for analyzing their content so that individuals and groups who are involved in thinking about local food policy and health can critically assess other policies. By providing a basis for discussing food policy that is targeted and tailored to their own local context, individuals and groups can make informed decisions as to what is important for their own food policy or charter.

We started our task with a search and collection of all the food policies and charters we could locate in Canada. At the time of the search (2013), we found 31 policies. Gathered into one collection, these policies serve as a demonstration of the amount of interest and work related to food and food security that had taken place in Canada up to that point in time.

A TOOL FOR FOOD POLICY/FOOD CHARTER ANALYSIS

Developing food policies, conducting analyses, and implementing associated tasks with policy development (which may include knowledge transfer, lobbying, and/or advocacy) is not easy to carry out given the complexities of food systems and the myriad of interests involved. The tool for food policy/food charter analysis was intended as a helpful resource for individual members of the public, local government decision-makers, community-based organizations, and other stakeholders who are interested in local food policy and may be either pondering the purpose, development, and implementation of their own food policy, or considering revisiting and revising older policies. The tool we developed was designed as a set of questions to be applied to food policies, helping users to unpack their origins and contents, and the reasons, purposes, and accountabilities for the policies. Also included in the tool were questions that probe for assessment of benefit and costs of food policy components. These are both fundamental and critical approaches to policy assessment.

The set of questions is not intended for users to determine which policies are good or bad: after all, it is for citizens and the decision-makers whom they appoint or elect to decide the focus of a policy and the values expressed through it. The tool is therefore designed for policy amateurs and others to help them consider the many aspects of policy content—its underlying values, intentions, and potential outcomes—as well as policy development and uptake, including considerations of institutional structures, the processes of decision making, and the power and influence of those who can bring about change. The tool consists of 16 questions. The first section (questions 1 to 3) largely provides a description of the policy. Questions 4 and 5 draw attention to the relationship of health and food-related issues, which will be of major interest to some groups, such as local public health units. Question 6 specifically asks for any evidence of public involvement, because public participation is considered to be essential for public policy in which members of the public are directly affected; public participation also includes the notion of the use of public knowledge. Questions 7 and 8 concern the targeting of the policy, specifically the individuals for whom the policy document is tailored. Questions 9 to 15 try to get at fundamental issues regarding the distribution of benefit and the allocation of power related to implementing and monitoring the policy. Question 16 is an informational question as to where the document can be found, but can also raise issues of access. The full tool to assist in developing and assessing food policy for the local level in Canada can be found in the appendix at the end of this chapter. The whole tool with explanatory notes for each question, along with examples, is available in the full report "Local Food Policies and Charters in Canada: A Collection and Guide for Analysis" (Runnels, 2013).

SUMMARIZING THE CONTENTS OF EXISTING FOOD POLICIES IN CANADA

Our analysis of 31 policies revealed a number of characteristics:

- Most policies included a description of the means to achieve food security or other goals and made policy recommendations to achieve these goals.
- Intended audiences included regional or municipal governments, federal or provincial governments, and local residents.

- Often, the reasons why the policies were created are described in a positive light; for example, the policy may be placed within the context of human rights, rather than given as a means to address a specific problem.
- A majority of policies contained a direct reference to health, sometimes featuring references to a healthy environment and associated themes. Many policies contained both direct and indirect references to citizen health and nutrition.
- An analysis of policy readability found that, while some policies could be easily read by members of the general public, others were written in highly technical language. Readability was not always aligned with the intended audience.
- While policies were not assessed for accessibility for the purposes of this project, we stress the importance of ensuring that documents are accessible to all, including people with disabilities and people with age-related impairments.
- How to achieve the goals or ends of the policy, or the means of change, were sometimes difficult to determine.
- Only one policy included a discussion of the costs of implementing any of the proposed plans.
- Most policies were unclear about who would be responsible for implementation.

CONCLUSION

The analytic tool we suggest will be helpful for food policy development, although in trying to answer the tool's questions a number of additional questions are likely to be raised. Through the tool, we hope to encourage individuals and groups that are involved in thinking about food policy and health to critically assess other policies and be able to make some decisions about what is important for their own policies.

GLOSSARY

Food charter: Food-related action and development of food-related statements written for citizens, designed to serve them and to improve their food security

DISCUSSION QUESTIONS

1. What are some of the key deficiencies in existing Canadian food policies?
2. What are the potential consequences of not addressing these issues with respect to the possibility of acceptance and implementation by local governments?

REFERENCES

Enns, J., Rose, A., de Vries, J., & Hayes, J. (2008). *A seat at the table: Resource guide for local governments to promote food secure communities.* Vancouver: Provincial Health Services

Authority. Retrieved from http://www.phsa.ca/Documents/aseatatthetableresourceguide-forlocal governmentstop.pdf

Runnels, V. (2013). *Local food policies and charters in Canada: A collection and guide for analysis.* PHIRN Working Paper Series. Ottawa: Institute of Population Health, University of Ottawa. Retrieved from http://rrasp-phirn.ca/images/stories/formated_paper.pdf

APPENDIX 18.1: A TOOL TO ASSIST IN DEVELOPING AND ASSESSING FOOD POLICY FOR THE LOCAL LEVEL IN CANADA

Instructions: Please use the tool's questions either to discuss other food policies, or as a guide to develop your own. Please keep notes as your group discusses the different items.

1. What is the (organizational) source of the document or set of documents?
2. Who is/are the authors of the food policies/charters? How did the policy document come into being?
3. What is the format of the document (does it contain a values statement, discussion paper, policy directions, etc.), and why was this particular format chosen?
4. What is/are the stated and/or implied problems the food policies/charters are addressing (e.g., origin, historical or current events, lack of food, distribution, economic development, globalization)?
5. What is the content of the document that relates directly to health? Relates indirectly to health? AND/OR What are the references in the policy that relate directly to health? Relate indirectly to health?
6. What, in the document, suggests public involvement or engagement in the development, adoption, and implementation of the policy (e.g., democratic intentions, incorporation of whose knowledge, community and expert knowledge)?
7. Who is the intended target audience for the document (e.g., if the audience is government, what level(s) of government is targeted? What about the level of language and for whom the document is accessible?)
8. Whose interests are addressed in the policies/charters? (Who are the beneficiaries? What goals/values are sought and by whom?)
9. What is the (implied) means (theory logic or theory of change) that will address the problems?
10. What outcomes (ends) are projected for the implementation of the policies/charters?
11. What are the major policy recommendations (if any) proposed/set out in the document?
12. Who is allocated responsibility for implementing the policies/charter (What body is responsible for enacting policy)?
13. Who is allocated responsibility for monitoring implementation of and compliance with the it?

14. What are the costs (if any) associated with the implementation of the policies/charter?
15. Where can the document be found? Where can other information/resources for the policy/charter be found?

CHAPTER 19

Social Entrepreneurship and Services for Marginalized Groups*

Sean Kidd and Kwame McKenzie

TAKE-HOME MESSAGE

- Effective services for marginalized groups in high-income contexts are highly embedded in the communities that they serve.
- Underlying the term *social entrepreneurship* in this area is a complex and strategic approach, at least considering highly successful examples.
- In a field where very little strategy is documented, there is a need to capture successful approaches to increase the success rate and viability of new endeavours.

BACKGROUND

Mental health services across the world face the twin challenges of tight fiscal governance while delivering equitable services for increasingly diverse populations (Standing Senate Committee, 2006; Department of Health UK, 2005, 2009; Mental Health Commission of Canada, 2012). In this context, marginalized groups face greatly heightened morbidity and mortality as a function of poor mental health (Cochran & Mays, 2009; Kirmayer et al., 2007; Roy et al., 2004) and there are indications of heightened risk among immigrant groups, particularly visible minority migrants (Cantor-Graae & Selton, 2005).

Such findings, while reflective of the many determinants of health that lead to differing needs and poorer outcomes, also reflect the shortcomings of service systems (Department of Health UK, 2005). Mainstream services have struggled to develop an effective service response to diversity and marginalization despite substantial service, policy, research, and personal resources expended (Committee, 2006; Department of Health UK, 2005; Department of Health UK, 2009; Mental Health Commission of Canada 2012). Clinical trials are scarce (Aisenberg, 2008), and the evidence for some of the most

* This chapter first appeared as an article in 2014 in *Ethnicity and Inequalities in Health and Social Care*, Volume 7, Issue 1. It is reproduced with permission from Emerald Group Publishing Limited.

commonly discussed interventions, such as cultural competence training, is modest (Bhui et al., 2007).

One strategy for trying to deal with the challenge of improving services without significantly increasing costs is for mainstream providers to support local communities to develop and deliver better supports. For instance, in the UK, the Big Society is a centrepiece policy idea. The UK government's stated aim is to create a climate that empowers local people and communities: "Only when people and communities are given more power and take more responsibility can we achieve fairness and opportunities for all" (Cabinet Office, 2010, p. 1). The priorities are to give communities more powers, encourage people to take an active role in their communities, transfer power from central to local government, and to support co-ops, charities, and social enterprises (Cabinet Office, 2010).The Canadian mental health strategy echoes these themes by calling for mainstream services to "support immigrant, refugee, ethnocultural and racialised community organisations in assessing local mental health needs and strengths and in taking action on local priorities, in collaboration with mental health and other service systems." (Mental Health Commission of Canada, 2012, p. 87).

There may be concerns about whether hard-pressed marginalized communities have the capacity to develop the resources to build the required services. In addition, those who develop services in marginalized groups often do not document their models, processes, and outcomes, which makes them hard to evaluate and less attractive to systems that are invested in offering high-quality evidence-based interventions (Drake et al., 2001). Furthermore, services developed by community groups may have modest longevity. However, at least anecdotally, many service providers, clients, and families can readily identify a provider, program, or service that has very effectively addressed the mental health needs of a marginalized community. These are providers have found innovative ways to engage communities and groups that experience mental health inequity, successfully navigating the complexity of the individual, social, and political problems faced with few resources and, in some cases, active opposition to their efforts.

Social Entrepreneurship

The challenge for those aiming to develop practices and policies that feature collaboration with marginalized community groups is to be able to identify partnerships that are more likely to be effective and sustainable. The literature on initiating and sustaining specific mental health services for marginalized populations by non-profits is not well developed. One way of considering the attributes of non-profit organizations that have succeeded in delivering services to marginalized groups despite limited resources is to use the lens of social entrepreneurship.

Social entrepreneurs are "people with new ideas to address major problems who are relentless in the pursuit of their visions, people who simply will not take 'no' for an answer, who will not give up until they have spread their ideas as far as they possibly can" (Bornstein, 2007, p. 1). The concept of social entrepreneurship (SE) emerged in the early 1980s, growing largely out of Bill Drayton's work in identifying and supporting individuals who were addressing major social problems in developing countries (Bornstein, 2007).

He and others sought to identify persons who had developed innovative ways of unraveling complex systems of oppression, apathy, and dependency to mobilize communities and effect change. These were persons who employed highly leveraged approaches, having identified a focused effort that might yield large systemic change.

While there is some contention as to the meaning of SE, it is generally taken to be the equivalent of a business entrepreneur that focuses on creating social value in their efforts rather than financial gain. These are individuals and groups who (i) identify and develop a solution that addresses an unmet need; (ii) are relentless in their effort to create social value; (iii) are continuously engaged in innovation and modification and act despite adversity and few resources; (iv) are highly embedded in the communities and networks related to their work; (v) generate social capital; and (v) have developed sustainable and transferable solutions (Paredo & McLean, 2006; Myers & Nelson, 2011; Shaw & Carter, 2007).

Social Entrepreneurship and Health

There have been several recent calls for the use of the SE framework to address health equity (e.g., Drayton, Brown, & Hillhouse, 2006; Germak & Singh, 2010; Savaya, Packer, Stange, & Namir, 2008; Wei-Skillern, 2011), in large part driven by its applicability to the problems underlying health inequity. Social entrepreneurs are highly effective in connecting multiple sectors and bridging siloed systems (Drayton, Brown, & Hillhouse, 2006; Harting, Kunst, Kwan, & Stronks, 2010). Such an approach is directly relevant to mental health equity, which is determined by many factors and suffers in most contexts due to fragmented and poorly coordinated service systems. Social entrepreneurs also generate community-based solutions to problems, an approach that is relevant if not necessary to effectively address mental illness in many ethnocultural contexts.

While SE is a framework would seem useful in articulating models through which mental health equity can be addressed, investigation into its applicability to health is very limited. One exploratory study that examined the work of rural health care providers in Tanzania from an SE perspective highlighted factors such as the credibility of the providers and their ability to bridge different sectors (Farmer & Kilpatrick, 2009). Another study in Holland examined the use of health brokers for marginalized groups and likewise emphasized their role in building social capital, also noting the importance of systemic entrepreneurship—embedding SE principles in service systems (Harting, Kunst, Kwan, & Stronks, 2011). Overall, and as was the case in a recent systematic review (Short, Moss, & Lumpkin, 2009), research into social entrepreneurship in health is minimal and we were unable to find a single example that focused specifically on mental health.

Study Aims

The aim of this study is to examine the meaning of social entrepreneurship in the context of mental health services for persons experiencing mental health inequity and to examine which SE components are present in services that have proven to be effective and sustainable. The goal of this line of inquiry is twofold:

1. to develop a SE roadmap for mental health equity, providing a template for those seeking to develop effective services in this area; and
2. to identify models of entrepreneurship so that we might enhance the ability of decision-makers to recognize and cultivate such individuals and services.

Using the search framework of Ashoka (www.ashoka.org; Bornstein, 2007), we identified organizations that embody SE principles in addressing mental health equity in Toronto and employed a multiple case study design to articulate the key components that underlie their effectiveness. The services studied focused on Aboriginal, immigrant, refugee, homeless, and LGBTQ populations.

METHODS

Context

This project focused on services targeting Aboriginal people, homeless, lesbian, gay, bisexual, transgender, and queer persons (LGBTQ), immigrants, and refugee groups, as each of these groups face pervasive inequity in many domains including mental health. In this search we concentrated on services operating in Toronto, Ontario. The population of Toronto is 5.5 million and it is one of the most diverse cities in the world, with half of this population having been born outside of Canada (City of Toronto, 2011).

Participating Organizations

The first step of this project was to use a purposeful sampling strategy to identify service providers who could be considered among the most effective social entrepreneurs working to promote equity in mental health. The search process was modelled after that of Ashoka (Bornstein, 2007). A search committee was assembled of 9 recognized leaders in service provision in one or more of the sectors of interest. These committee members had extensive experience in service delivery and management and also had an extensive knowledge of and contact with Toronto providers in each sector. They were oriented to the key criteria characterizing social entrepreneurs and given the task of using their knowledge base and networks to identify services that aligned with these core criteria.

A total of 46 services were recommended by the committee. Each of these organizations were contacted, the nature of the project described to them, and they were asked to submit a brief written description outlining (i) the types of services offered, (ii) how their work is innovative, (iii) challenges faced and how they have been overcome, (iv) how they engage the communities served, (v) the impact of their work, and (vi) their vision for the future of their work. They were advised that they could be helped to produce the description of their work. Twenty-one of the services contacted expressed an interest in participating and provided us with the written description.

The committee reviewed the descriptions provided by the organizations with the goal of determining services that would go on to be interviewed. A consensus process was used, reviewing the key components of SE as they applied to each of the organizations, making use of both the written descriptions and the committee's knowledge about the organizations. Through this process 3 organizations in each sector were chosen to participate in interviews to gather further details about their work.

The directors of the organizations selected for interviews were interviewed by two people involved in the project—one member of the research team and one member of the committee with expertise in the relevant service sector. These interviews revolved largely around obtaining story of their organization: how it emerged and developed, challenges and successes that occurred in their development, and the model through which they did their work. Through these interviews we sought elaboration on the key domains of social entrepreneurship and we also sought to determine if they were able to articulate the process of development clearly. Since a primary goal of this project was to describe models of social entrepreneurship in mental health equity, if those details could not be derived we would be much less able to identify key components. The selection process was then based on a 9 question rating scale.

In our final meeting with the committee, the selection of one representative organization in each sector was made. Organizations were chosen that were (i) highly representative of the key concepts of social entrepreneurism, and (ii) able to articulate their development in detail. The selected organizations included:

1. A centre providing an array of services to survivors of torture and war.
2. A group of people with lived experience of mental illness who use their personal stories and experiences to successfully influence housing policy.
3. A service grounded in Indigenous values and self-determination that offers extensive and wide-ranging programs to Indigenous families.
4. A coalition of 15 health and social service agencies working in partnership with the goal of coordinating services and influencing public policy concerning accessibility and appropriate care for marginalized and vulnerable populations.
5. A multi-service program with a focus on lower-income, street-involved, homeless, sex-working and marginalized members of trans communities.

Case Studies

Case studies were conducted with each of the organizations identified in the selection process in a multiple case study analysis (Stake, 2006). This approach was chosen as it provides an effective framework for integrating a set of case studies in an *instrumental* design, one in which a case or cases are used to provide insight into a broader issue. Since the focus of the project was on the developmental trajectory of the organizations and their model of service delivery, the analysis was situated within a narrative/developmental framework. The sources of information were semi-structured interviews with senior management and direct service staff and a review of documentation (e.g., reports, websites, policies, mission/values statements). The investigation did not extend to interviews with clients. In each organization the service leader or leaders were interviewed, in most cases on multiple occasions over 2 to 3 hours; past leaders were sought out for interviews, and direct service staff (range from 2 to 10 direct service staff per organization) participated in individual and group interviews. Investigators also attended meetings and events held by the organization, taking ethnographic field notes. The project was reviewed and approved by an institutional ethics review board.

In each case, audio recorded interviews, ethnographic observation, and document analysis focused on obtaining the following: (1) A detailed history tracking the trajectories and turning points in services offered, service structures/models, goals and values, leveraging support, and relationships with stakeholders and supporters. (2) Identifying instances of adversity and how they were overcome, as well as instances of achievement and how they were attained. (3) Inquiry into the roles and activities of key people within the organization and external partners. (4) Examination of their relationships with other services and place within the larger service system. (5) Discussion of the impacts of their work. (6) Inquiry into their vision for the future of their organization.

Data Analysis

Data analysis proceeded in three stages, using the rigorous content analysis procedure articulated by Charmaz (1995) in the context of grounded theory, though the analysis in this study did not extend to theory generation. First, for each of the organizations all of the materials were analyzed for recurrent themes through a content analysis triangulated by source of information (interview respondent and written materials). Through this content analysis a detailed organizational narrative was developed, with key themes and processes highlighted with quotes, field note entries, and extracts from documents. These narratives were further revised as a second investigator examined the coding structure and in some instances requested further information and clarification. In the second step, the reports were given to the members of the organizations who were interviewed in a member checking process that led to further revision and expansion of the content in some areas. In the third step, all of the reports were examined through content analysis to identify common themes running across all of the organizations, with attention paid to patterns of variability that emerged in some themes/areas of inquiry. This integrated analysis was in turn reviewed by all of the investigators, with feedback given to ensure reliable linkages with the individual case study data; feedback was also sought from the directors of each of the participating organizations.

RESULTS

Overview

Five core themes emerged in the analysis:

1. how the service started, including the types of people involved and the problems they sought to address;
2. a very active period of clarifying values and mission, conceptualizing an approach, and engaging community and partners;
3. applying a highly innovative approach;
4. maintaining focus, keeping current, and exceeding expectations; and
5. acting more as a service working from within a community than a service for a community.

While the five organizations varied widely in the problems that they addressed, there was a remarkable degree of similarity in the components that were described as crucial to their effectiveness and success, both in their organizational structure and their specific activities. These components are as follows.

When the Right People Meet a Specific Problem

Each of the case studies revealed that these organizations began in response to a very specific problem, which may have led to the development of a clear purpose as is described in the subsequent section. Specific problems included the closing of a hospital, the murders of two trans sex-trade workers, large numbers of Aboriginal children being placed in white families, poor housing quality for persons with severe mental illness, and the challenges South American torture victims faced in the immigration process.

There were also a number of shared characteristics across the founders of these organizations. All had a very personal investment. This was not seen as a job so much as a mission that held a deep personal meaning. In all cases the founders invested large amounts of time and resources on a volunteer basis and there was an active involvement, if not membership, in the communities served.

> Almost everybody in that room could name a relative with a negative experience of child welfare. (Interviewee speaking about the founding of the Aboriginal service)

All of the founders of these services had experience in service delivery and they all had an extensive network of helpful contacts. These were individuals with access to large amounts of social capital—collective social and political resources. The founders of all of these organizations knew how to work with political systems, were angry and passionate while still being able to build a broad base of supporters, and were both patient and extremely persistent—in some cases maintaining focus through years of setbacks.

Getting Aligned, Oriented to an Approach, and Connected

All of the organizations commented on the importance of a social justice framework as the foundation of all of their activities. Most saw themselves as advocates, if not activists, working to address social inequity. All worked to explicitly develop a clear focus or mission, seeking out board members and staff who shared their investment and aligned with the agreed upon mission.

> We responded with ... a burning concern with social justice, political action, and the impatience and frustration against a confused world of passive bystanders. (Interviewee from the service for victims of torture)

A key component of this effort to clarify their purpose and gain consensus/agreement was a close consultation with their communities. Through both formal research and informal contact all of these organizations constantly consult and involve their communities. In many ways, these organizations operate from within the community, through volunteers, former clients coming back and working as staff, and an active involvement of members of the communities in decision making. This ranged from staff in essence being the community to services that acted at the systems level, with each member being a leader of a service within a community of services.

> The key to our impact is that it is by community for community. (Interviewee from the service that works with trans clients)

> Along with the strong community-based and social justice foundations, they had a holistic approach to their work. None saw their work as being focused on the mental illness of a person; they all work at individual, family, social, cultural, and political levels in an integrated manner.

> What we want to do is help them to build their own community, and slowly move to coalition building ... so it is a circle from the individual to the group, from the group to the community, and from the community to civic responsibility and advocacy. (Interviewee from the service for victims of torture)

They also had a strong orientation towards action. In each case they all are "doers," preferring to attempt something that might fail rather than continue to just talk about it.

The time for studies is over. There have been numerous studies of Native people already. (At a planning meeting in 1985 for the service for Aboriginal populations)

Another element shared and emphasized by these organizations is the degree to which they sought out strategic partnerships. Within the organizations, this meant a careful consideration of the composition of staffing and boards, looking to bring on people with expertise in service delivery, connections with decision-makers, legal experts, and skilled grant writers. What was most remarkable was the extent to which they all actively if not aggressively pursued partnerships outside of their organizations. They all worked to develop close relationships with policy-makers, academics, leaders of other service organizations, and community leaders. They also all actively sought to have a maximum amount of visibility in the community. Holding events open to the public, getting media attention, and consistently working to raise awareness about the problem being addressed.

What the [service] has very successfully done is they have built a strong cadre of supporters, whether its advisors or coordinators or sponsors ... they continually work to maintain those relationships. (Interviewee from the advocacy organization that influences housing policy)

The Innovative Approach

The proposal of highly innovative approaches to the problem being considered was another commonality between the five organizations. Having assembled extremely strong groups, developed strategic partnerships, and assessed the needs of their communities, the solutions that they proposed were in each case unique. The service for victims of torture was one of two such services in the world when it was developed. The Aboriginal service is still the only urban Aboriginal-run child protection service in Canada. In each case these organizations offered a solution grounded in the needs of the community that was a fresh approach to the problem and that was a compelling and convincing alternative.

Keeping Focused, Keeping Current, and Exceeding Expectations

Once established, each of these organizations put in place processes to regularly revisit and maintain its original focus/mission, whether it was embedded in the structure of meetings or reiterated through key advisory groups and retreats. Also critical, however, was the longevity of a core person or group. All of the organizations described the importance of having people involved, whether staff or partners, for a long period of time to provide stability and a memory of the "original marching orders." Not only was this critical in keeping focus, but this organizational memory and longevity also helped to deepen informal and formal connections with partners. Having such established relationships greatly increases efficiency.

It's about collaboration. It's about how those interpersonal relationships at those very high levels allow for things to be dealt with really quickly: It allows for someone to just pick up the phone, and call a director, so there can be a coordinated network for care. (Interviewee from the service coalition)

While all of these organizations successfully maintained a stable focus in their mission, in their activities and engagement with the communities they serve they are highly reflexive and organic. In each case, they continued to deepen existing relationships with partners, cultivate relationships with new partners and communities, and remain sensitive to the ebb and flow of the communities they serve. This ability to be sensitive to the needs of the community is greatly enhanced by the blurring of boundaries between service providers and those served.

Through advisory boards, extensive networks of volunteers from the community, former clients coming back as staff, and highly active outreach activities, these organizations are embedded more than connected. For instance, the centre that treats victims of torture was developed for South American refugees but has embraced each new wave of refugees and their unique needs, whether they came from Eastern Europe or Somalia. In each case, whether they be new services, new projects, or new methods of working, these organizations carefully do their research, collaborate, develop an effective practice, and rapidly implement it. For services working within larger organizations, such flexibility and ability to rapidly implement services was described as being greatly aided by there being a "buffer." This buffer between the SE service and the larger organization allowed for a degree of flexibility that would be lost in the context of the bureaucratic processes present in the latter.

Another critical ingredient shared by these five organizations is their effectiveness and efficiency. In each case they radically outperform what is expected of them by partners, funders, and the public. The centre that treats victims of torture—with a small staff and budget—serves 1,500 clients annually from over 100 countries. The trans community service delivered training on trans issues to 3,000 providers on a budget for 300.

More a Community than a Service for a Community

The final point that unites these organizations, and one less tangible than some of the other uniting factors, is the manner in which their shared passion and focus, their embeddedness in the community and reflexivity, and their ability to welcome new partners creates a vital community in and of itself. All of the organizations cultivate a sense of family, of shared and united purpose, of safety, and of a valued identity.

Our uniqueness is a result of creating the sense of the lost village of survivors left behind and we have created a safe haven. (Interviewee from the service for victims of torture)

DISCUSSION

This study aimed to articulate, using a social entrepreneurship (SE) framework, the characteristics shared by service organizations that are highly effective in their ability to address mental health inequity for marginalized groups. This, to our knowledge, is the first research application of an SE approach in mental health.

The organizations' creativity, relentless effort to create social value, continuous engagement despite adversity and limited resources, integration with the community, and social capital were readily evident. The work of the organizations chosen was also reflected in aspects of entrepreneurial orientation that receive more commentary in the business literature than the SE literature (Rauch, Wiklund, Lumpkin, & Frese, 2009). These include aggressiveness and a willingness to take risks by venturing into new and uncertain domains of service delivery. While not necessarily framed in the light of "competitive aggressiveness" (Rauch, Wiklund, Lumpkin, & Frese, 2009, p. 763), these services were indeed aggressive in their advocacy and awareness-raising activities (e.g., taking the province of Ontario to court on discrimination charges) as well as in their outputs.

A major finding of this study is the highly strategic and coherent approach to their work. A complex and nuanced set of characteristics emerged that, while fundamentally grounded in the communities in which they work, also reads like a guide to effective management. Their efficiency and effectiveness would seem to be driven by three core attributes.

First, the personal investment and involvement of the leaders and staff in the communities that they are serving. This leads them to: (i) readily recognize what is needed by the communities they serve; (ii) recognize the importance of being flexible to those needs and implement changes; (iii) use highly leveraged approaches in which interventions can have the largest possible impact on many determinants of health, thus increasing efficiency; and (iv) foster an intense and personally invested focus and shared passion about the problems at hand, since these are their own problems, leading to an action orientation and an emphasis upon rapid implementation. All of these characteristics, aside from personal involvement being highlighted as the key motivator, are also closely associated with the success of these organizations as they are in business (Rauch, Wiklund, Lumpkin, & Frese, 2009) and organizations in general (Barrett, Balloun, & Weinstein, 2005).

Second, the work is driven by a social justice framework. All of the organizations focus on specific problems and work actively to adhere to and maintain their core values through policy, organization structure, and the longevity of leaders. While adherence to a clear and simple primary goal is also a characteristic of successful businesses (Heath & Heath, 2007), it is not surprising that these organizations need to be extremely active in their efforts to avoid "drift," given the complexity of the problems being addressed, the need to work closely with and be responsive to a range of funders with at times disparate agendas, and factors such as low pay and extremely high work levels. The latter point would seem to be addressed both by personal investment and the family-like relationships cultivated by staff and leadership.

The third and final major attribute can be described as social capital. While fundamentally grounded in a "by the community for the community" framework, all of these organizations are extremely active in their efforts to make meaningful and lasting connections with other providers, policy-makers, researchers, and the public. They focused on building shared interest and investment in their cause and creating large amounts of social capital around their work. This ability to create bridges between stakeholders has likewise been commented on by the few other studies examining SE and health (Farmer & Kilpatrick, 2009; Harting, Kunts, Kwan, & Stronks, 2011; Myers & Nelson, 2011), and social capital has been found in the business literature to reduce transaction costs, facilitate information flow, and foster creativity, just as it did in the present study (Arregle, Hitt, Sirmon, & Very, 2007).

GLOSSARY

The Big Society: A movement in the United Kingdom that involves a shift in the responsibility for social problems from the public sector to small groups, charities, and businesses at a community level (Scott, 2011).

Marginalized groups: Those that are systematically denied access to the rights, resources, and opportunities afforded to others (Hall, 1999).

Mental health equity: The absence of avoidable differences in mental health among groups of people regardless of social, economic, demographic, or geographic difference (WHO, 2016).

Social entrepreneurs: "People with new ideas to address major problems who are relentless in the pursuit of their visions, ... [and] who will not give up until they have spread their ideas as far as they possibly can" (Bornstein, 2007, p. 1).

DISCUSSION QUESTIONS

1. What are the characteristics of leaders of successful organizations that address mental health equity?
2. Can you name three characteristics of interventions of social entrepreneurs in the area of mental health equity?
3. What is the relationship between service recipients and providers in successful organizations in this area?

REFERENCES

Aisenberg, E. (2008). Evidence base practice in mental health care to ethnic minority communities: Has its practice fallen short of its evidence? *Social Work, 53*, 297–306.

Arregle, J., Hitt, M., Sirmon, D., & Very, P. (2007). The development of organizational social capital: Attributes of family firms. *Journal of Management Studies, 44*, 73–95.

Barrett, H., Balloun, J., & Weinstein, A. (2005). Success factors for organizational performance: Comparing business services, health care, and education. *SAM Advanced Management Journal, 70*, 16–27.

Bhui, K., Warfa, N., Edonya, P., McKenzie, K., & Bhugra, D. (2007). Cultural competence in mental health care: A review of evaluations. *BMC Health Research, 7*, 15.

Bornstein, D. (2007). *How to change the world: Social entrepreneurs and the power of new ideas.* New York: Oxford University Press.

Cabinet Office (2010). *Building the big society.* Retrieved from https://www.gov.uk/government/publications/building-the-big-society

Cantor-Graae, E., & Selton, J. (2005). Schizophrenia and migration: A meta-analysis and review. *American Journal of Psychiatry, 162*, 12–24.

Charmaz, K. (1995). Grounded theory, In J. A. Smith, R. Harre & L. V. Langenhove (eds.), *Rethinking methods in psychology* (pp. 27–49). Thousand Oaks, CA: Sage.

City of Toronto. (2011). *Toronto's racial diversity.* Retrieved from http://www.toronto.ca/toronto_facts/diversity.htm

Cochran, S., & Mays, V. (2009). Burden of psychiatric morbidity among lesbian, gay and bisexual individuals in the California quality of life survey. *Journal of Abnormal Psychology, 118*, 647–658.

Department of Health UK. (2005). *Delivering race equality in mental health care: An action plan for reform inside and outside services and the Government's response to the independent inquiry into the death of David Bennett.* Retrieved frrom http://www.dh.gov.uk/en/Publicationsandstatistics/Publications/PublicationsPolicyAndGuidance/DH_4100773

Department of Health UK. (2009). *Delivering race equality a review.* Retrieved from http://www.nmhdu.org.uk/our-work/mhep/delivering-race-equality/delivering-race-equality-in-mental-health-a-review

Drake, R., Goldman, H., Leff, S., Lehman, A., Dixon, L., Mueser, K., & Torrey, W. (2001). Implementing evidence-based practices in routine mental health service settings. *Psychiatric Services, 52*, 179–182.

Drayton, B., Brown, C., Hillhouse, K. (2006). Integrating social entrepreneurs into the "Health for All" framework. *Bulletin of the World Health Organization, 84*, 591.

Farmer, J., & Kilpatrick, S. (2009). Are rural health professionals also social entrepreneurs? *Social Science & Medicine, 69*, 1651–1658.

Germak, A., & Singh, K. (2010). Social entrepreneurship: Changing the way social workers do business. *Administration in Social Work, 34*, 79–95.

Hall, J. M. (1999). Marginalization revisited: Critical, postmodern, and liberation perspectives. *Advances in Nursing Science, 22*, 88–102.

Harting, J., Kunst, A., Kwan, A., & Stronks, K. (2011). A 'health broker' role as a catalyst of change to promote health: An experiment in deprived Dutch neighbourhoods. *Health Promotion International, 26*, 65–81.

Heath, C., & Heath, D. (2007). *Made to stick: Why some ideas survive and others die.* New York: Random House.

Kirmayer, L. J., Brass, G. M., Holton, T. L., Paul, K., Simpson, C., & Tait, C. L. (2007). *Suicide among Aboriginal peoples in Canada.* Ottawa: Aboriginal Healing Foundation.

Mental Health Commission of Canada. (2012). *Changing direction, changing lives: The mental health strategy for Canada.* Calgary: Mental Health Commission of Canada.

Myers, P., & Nelson, T. (2011). Considering social capital in context of social entrepreneurship. In A. Fayolle & H. Matley (eds.), *Handbook of research on social entrepreneurship.* Cheltenham, UK: Edward Elgar.

Paredo, A., & McLean, M. (2006). Social entrepreneurship: A critical review of the concept. *Journal of World Business, 41,* 56–65.

Rauch, A., Wiklund, J., Lumpkin, T., Frese, M. (2009). Entrepreneurial orientation and business performance: An assessment of past research and suggestions for the future. *Entrepreneurship Theory and Practice, 33,* 761–787.

Roy, E., Haley, N., Leclerc, P., Sochanski, B., Boudreau, J., Boivin, J. (2004). Mortality in a cohort of street youth in Montreal. *Journal of the American Medical Association, 292,* 569–574.

Savaya, R., Packer, P., Stange, D., & Namir, O. (2008). Social entrepreneurship: Capacity building among workers in public human service agencies. *Administration in Social Work, 32,* 65–86.

Scott, M. (2011). Reflections on 'The Big Society.' *Community Development Journal, 46,* 132–137.

Shaw, E., & Carter, S. (2007). Social entrepreneurship: Theoretical antecedents and empirical analysis of entrepreneurial processes and outcomes. *Journal of Small Business and Enterprise Development, 14,* 418–434.

Short, J., Moss, T., & Lumpkin, G. (2009). Research in social entrepreneurship: Past contributions and future opportunities. *Strategic Entrepreneurship Journal, 3,* 161–194.

Stake, R. (2006). *Multiple case study analysis.* New York: Guilford.

Standing Senate Committee on Social Affairs, Science and Technology. (2006). *Out of the shadows at last: Transforming mental health, mental illness and addiction services in Canada.* Retrieved from http://www.parl.gc.ca/Content/SEN/Committee/391/soci/rep/rep02may06-e.htm

Wei-Skillern, J. (2010). Networks as a type of social entrepreneurship to advance public health. *Preventing Chronic Disease, 7,* 1–5.

World Health Organization. (2016). *Equity.* Retrieved from http://www.who.int/healthsystems/topics/equity/en

CHAPTER 20

Youth Futures: A Program and Its Evaluation

Vivien Runnels and Caroline Andrew

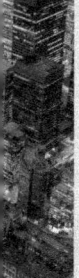

TAKE-HOME MESSAGE

- Evaluation of the Youth Futures program allowed for a number of learning opportunities and benefits, including the expansion of the partnership and rationalization of the program's structure, and consideration of how different forms of engagement—community, parental, and political—can be used effectively to enhance the program's impacts.

BACKGROUND

This chapter describes an evaluation of a program called Youth Futures (Avenir Jeunesse in French). The aim of the program is to encourage participation in post-secondary education. The working theory is that participation in post-secondary education leads to better employment and income which, in turn, affects health and social outcomes for individuals and their families.

The evaluation was carried out in 2011–2012 and sought to determine if Youth Futures was being implemented as planned. If it was, the theoretical likelihood that Youth Futures benefits those who participated in it is increased. An implementation or process evaluation is not intended to measure outcomes or the end results of an intervention (this is possible using different research designs), but it is an important means of researching and assessing an intervention that can be conducted in the early stages of its development and implementation. The chapter concludes with some selected reflections on Youth Futures and its evaluation. Readers are encouraged to refer to the PHIRN Working Paper (Runnels, 2012) and, in particular, to read the narrative reconstruction of a participant's experience of Youth Futures to gain some perspective on a youth's experience of the program.

WHY YOUTH FUTURES WAS CREATED

Social and health outcomes are significantly shaped by social, educational, and economic determinants of health (WHO, 2008). Disadvantaged high school students may not be in a position to consider or benefit from many of life's opportunities that their more advantaged peers can use to their recourse, such as exposure to post-secondary education. As a consequence, they may not engage with post-secondary education, which has been shown to increase life chances, including improved employment, higher salaries, and enhanced health outcomes. Exposure to post-secondary education while in high school may be critical for influencing decisions to pursue post-secondary education (Hoffman, Vargas, & Santos, 2008).

Youth Futures was developed in Ottawa to encourage high school students who experience disadvantage to access and participate in post-secondary education. The program's broad vision is to break the cycle of disadvantage and poverty through access to post-secondary education, transforming the lives and influencing the health of young people and their families over time, making Canada a more equitable society. An intensive and comprehensive bilingual intervention, Youth Futures is organized and administered at no cost to participants through a partnership among the City of Ottawa, the University of Ottawa, Ottawa Community Housing, and several other organizations. The participants in the program are francophone and anglophone young women and men aged 16–21 who are from low-income backgrounds and may be the first in their families to attain post-secondary education.

WHY AN EVALUATION OF THE PROGRAM?

An evaluation can help to ensure that a program:

- is reaching its intended audience (population);
- is being implemented in the manner in which it was planned (process);
- has its combination of components working effectively to meet its goals (content); and
- is satisfactory to participants and other stakeholders (satisfaction).

The Youth Futures partners determined that an evaluation designed to address questions about population, process, content, and satisfaction was necessary. It would also provide all Youth Futures stakeholders with information to help make educated decisions about the program in the present and the future.

The first steps involved setting up and carrying out the evaluation, including striking an evaluation committee and appointing an evaluator; developing a program vision, mission statement, and program logic model; and producing a set of questions to guide the evaluation (see Box 20.1).

Box 20.1: Youth Futures/Avenir Jeunesse Implementation Evaluation Questions

---

Recruitment, selection, and population:
Is the intervention reaching the intended population? Did the selected students match the targeted population for the course? What are the barriers and facilitators for participation in the Youth Futures program? What improvements could be made to the recruitment and selection process?

Program process:
What is the program process? Were any problems encountered? Is Youth Futures being implemented in the way it was planned? How could the process be improved?

Program content:
Does the content (program components) match what it has set out to accomplish? Does the content match the participants' interests? Were any problems encountered with the content? Is the content in keeping with the mission, vision, and values of Youth Futures?

Program satisfaction:
How satisfied are the participants and the stakeholders with the program? What is the perceived impact of the program?

In addition to a brief review of the literature on the background of the intervention itself, two methods were selected to answer the evaluation questions: a review of the Youth Futures documentation (both hard copies and electronic documentation) and key informant interviews. Documentation included research papers and notes, governance records, program implementation notes, previously collected participants' survey responses, and website content. Key informant interviews were conducted with as many individuals as possible who could be contacted who had contributed to the governance of the Youth Futures partnership and the coordination and implementation of the program. Those interviewed were guaranteed anonymity, and their participation in an interview was held confidential by the interviewer. The evaluation's methods were granted ethical approval by two research ethics boards: the University of Ottawa and Saint Paul University. Interviews were transcribed, coded, and synthesized. The results of the document review and interviews were presented in the PHIRN Working Paper with a number of recommendations.

TARGETING THE "RIGHT" POPULATION

Youth Futures sought to recruit the "right" population by targeting its promotion and recruitment efforts at selected areas and locations in Ottawa. Promotion and recruitment of Youth Futures was undertaken largely by City of Ottawa staff and outreach workers and Ottawa Community Housing staff (a key partner in the program), and accomplished largely through neighbourhood, community (e.g., community houses, community health and resource centres), and school presentations. Dissemination of information was also carried out through distribution of flyers and personal contacts. Word of mouth was noted as a particularly important means of knowledge dissemination for certain ethnic/cultural groups. Administrators of social programs also provided information to families. The evaluation recommended that Youth Futures partners should institute a sex/gender analysis of program participants, and attempt to examine barriers to participation in the program that may overly impact one group over another, to ensure equity in participation.

Stakeholders agreed that Youth Futures does reach and recruit the intended population, but there was also acknowledgement of missing groups within the broadly described population. One group that was sought but did not participate at all (at the time) was Aboriginal youth. Francophone youth participated but to a lesser extent than anglophone youth. One respondent thought "a group that is generally missing [is] multi-generational mainstream Canadian youth living in social housing." The specialized knowledge and personal touch that outreach staff brought to community work was recognized as having an encouraging effect, particularly for immigrant youth.

PROGRAM PROCESS AND CONTENT

> Youth Futures is a quite intense program. It's not just intense for the youth—it's intense for the staff ... you live and breathe it. (Interview participant)

After submitting a written application that allowed a first filtering-out of candidates who did not meet the target population, youth were assessed for their fit to the program. If they were a match, they were offered a place. On acceptance, participants took part in an orientation session. They then received intensive leadership and employment training (the Advanced Leadership Program), which included what it means to be employable, job interview skills and practice, resumé writing, and other skills for the workplace. There were also opportunities to volunteer in local communities.

> I think the leadership program is a fantastic idea, and it's addressing an inequity ... we're giving kids who might not normally have access ... we know from the literature ... that kids who are poor or a minority don't have as much access. They get the drug treatment programs, they get the "you'd better behave" programs, the programs for youth-at-risk. They don't get the piano lessons, the sports, the leadership training, so I think that's addressing a real inequity. (Interview participant)

The next part of the process was the introduction to the post-secondary sector, which covers many aspects of post-secondary attendance including lectures in different subject areas by university professors, workshops on subjects such as budgeting and financing, and how to fill out applications offered by the University of Ottawa's Student Academic Success Service (SASS) and Financial Aid and Financial Awards Services. The summer phase entailed formal job interviews and six weeks of paid employment with public and private sector employers. The whole process incorporated mentoring and support provided by university students. At the end of the program, the process was completed with celebration of participants' achievements. The celebration was attended by Youth Futures participants, leadership training and coordinating staff, members of the Coordinators' Table and the governing Champions' Table, post-secondary staff and professors, as well as VIPs, mentors, parents, family members, and friends.

During all phases of Youth Futures, participants were assigned to mentors, paid University of Ottawa students who provided individual support to participants. The types of support they provided include moral and practical support, such as ensuring that participants got to the right location at the right time for a job interview. For some respondents, mentoring was the key thread or glue that allowed continuity and support, and for some individuals who presented challenges, it was the means by which they retained their place in the program.

How the process and program components linked with each other, and whether they fulfilled the process as planned, was assessed for sufficiency of program resources, staffing (including the mentors), governance, and coordination. Participation in the meetings of coordinators came to be seen as critically important and an indication of the partners' participation and engagement with Youth Futures. Coordinators' own supervisors and other stakeholders attended these meetings voluntarily. Several recommendations were made as a result of the evaluation. One such recommendation concerned the curriculum for leadership training. According to some key informants, the content made certain assumptions about the participants, their understanding of the program, and the experiences they brought to the program. Typically participants of leadership programs have had some personal experience of summer recreational camps and programs, but Youth Futures participants had rarely had this experience. They therefore had no views on what to expect from the leadership training program, their performance and participation in it, or what the eventual outcomes might be. Taking these issues into consideration, and redesigning the curriculum and presentation of its contents, meant that participants could benefit more from the leadership and skills training component. However, it also reinforced the need of Youth Futures participants to undergo this type of training in order to acquire work and to succeed in a job. As one respondent noted, "I think it's almost impossible to go without that training otherwise we will have perpetual exclusion."

> There are cultural aspects of behaviour that whoever is running the program may not be well aware of and ... there might be conditions that immigrant youth themselves or the participants in general are dealing with in their lives living in low income neighbourhoods. [These conditions] are not well communicated or communicable to program managers or individuals ... things like not having

a bus ticket and taking a long time to arrive at the meeting and these kinds of difficulties. If there's no accommodation of these challenges, if there's no real understanding, they [the youth] will continue to be marginalized ... it requires care and not giving up on the youth, but trying to understand.... (Interview participant)

Crucial to these linkages between process and content was the role of the overall co-ordinator who coordinated all the parts of the program, while others coordinated specific components. This design resulted in a distributed model of coordination, in which the load is shared and individuals with expertise in their own area fully contribute. Having an overall coordinator produced a process that appeared to work smoothly, encouraged regular communication and knowledge sharing, but ensured that no one partner had overall ownership of the program.

PROGRAM SATISFACTION

Here we were with a kid from a low income community who had never had an opportunity to participate in anything meaningful.... This [youth] was hesitant [to participate in Youth Futures] initially but didn't want to disobey ... so this [youth] did come and participate and the first couple of weeks were a little rough but the [youth] stuck with it.... After the program, ... the youth now started to think about university or post-secondary as an option. All of a sudden that becomes part of the youth's mind. [The youth was] granted a special student status at [a post-secondary institution] ... I remember one of the most powerful things [the youth] said was, "When I received ... my student card, I stared at that card for over an hour because I could not believe that I was in [a post-secondary institution]."
Some totally blossomed and that was amazing to see.... And their self-esteem, they just went from quiet, timid, shy people who wouldn't look you in the eye, to really confident ... some of them just really changed, which is the amazing thing in the program. (Interview participant)

One of the major findings from the interviews was that the coordinators derived great satisfaction from their own participation in the program. They were able to observe tangible changes in individual youth participants through opening up opportunities that the youth would otherwise have never accessed. Many stories of success were reported by the respondents following themes of growing awareness of the opportunity of post-secondary education and its meanings for the future.

This was an awesome program ... it was a lot of work and kind of emotional at times. It's a program that really, really changes about 10% of the youth's lives, profoundly changes them, takes them from a student ... who doesn't think they're going anywhere, doesn't see any chance of postsecondary education, who doesn't really think they'll make anything of themselves, to someone who's positive, like their whole life does a 360. So for that 10% I think it's totally worth it. (Interview participant)

THE VALUE OF EVALUATION FOR YOUTH FUTURES

As a result of this evaluation, the Youth Futures partnership has learned that evaluation brings many opportunities to learn, and several benefits to be gained. Even though it might compete with important and necessary actions such as implementing this annual program or strengthening partnerships, evaluation has helped to provide a written explicit framework to the program, whereas what existed before was somewhat implicit. The evaluation provided data for the direction of the program and feedback on its values and operation; an assessment of different facets of program; help in making improvements to the program; information for program stakeholders, members of the public, and funders; and systematically collected evidence for the development of future research and evaluation proposals. The evaluation also contributed to the expansion of the partnership and rationalization of the program's structure, enabled the partnership to direct attention to its own development, and considered how different forms of engagement—community, parental, and political—can be used effectively to enhance the program's influence.

GLOSSARY

Intervention: "A combination of program elements or strategies designed to produce behavior changes or improve health status among individuals or an entire population. Interventions may include educational programs, new or stronger policies, improvements in the environment, or a health promotion campaign.... Interventions may be implemented in different settings including communities, worksites, schools, health care organizations, faith-based organizations or in the home" (Missouri Department of Health and Senior Services, 2017).

Post-secondary education: Any education beyond high school. In Canada, this may include "apprenticeship or trades certificate or diploma (including 'centres de formation professionnelle'); college, CEGEP or other non-university certificate or diploma; university certificate or diploma below bachelor level; or a university degree (bachelor's degree; university certificate or diploma above bachelor level; degree in medicine, dentistry, veterinary medicine or optometry; master's degree; earned doctorate)" (Statistics Canada, 2010). Also referred to as higher education.

DISCUSSION QUESTIONS

1. What could be some of the reasons why Aboriginal youth (and to some extent francophones) did not participate in this program? What barriers might have limited accessibility to this segment of the population?
2. What is the relationship between access to employment for youth and health?

REFERENCES

Hoffman, N, Vargas, J., & Santos, J. (2008). Blending high school and college: Rethinking the transition. *New Directions for Higher Education*, 144, 15–25.

Missouri Department of Health and Senior Services. (2017). What is an intervention? Retrieved from http://health.mo.gov/data/InterventionMICA/index_4.html

Runnels, V. (2012). Youth Futures/L'Avenir Jeunesse: A process evaluation. Ottawa: Population Health Improvement Research Network. Retrieved from http://rrasp-phirn.ca/images/stories/docs/workingpaperseries/Download_2340_KB.pdf

Statistics Canada. (2010). Definition of postsecondary education. Retrieved from http://www.statcan.gc.ca/pub/81-004-x/2010001/def/posteducation-educpost-eng.htm

WHO. (2008). Closing the gap in a generation: Health equity through action on the social determinants of health. Commission on Social Determinants of Health final report. Retrieved from http://apps.who.int/iris/bitstream/10665/43943/1/9789241563703_eng.pdf

CHAPTER 21

Designing and Implementing Rights-Based Provincial/Territorial Strategies to Address Homelessness and Poverty

Bruce Porter

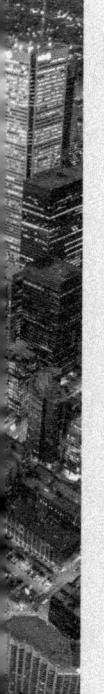

TAKE-HOME MESSAGE

- A number of provinces have implemented anti-poverty and housing strategies affirming commitments to improve particular program outcomes and evidence-based assessments of progress in alleviating poverty and homelessness. However, provincial/territorial strategies have continued to treat access to housing and an adequate standard of living as aspirational goals rather than enforceable human rights and as such are outdated and inconsistent with provincial/territorial obligations under international human rights law.
- The effect of recognizing rights to housing and an adequate standard of living as legal rights in provincial/territorial strategies would not be to transfer decision making to courts but rather to infuse all decision-making and policy design with human rights norms, aligned with the obligation under international human rights to take all reasonable measures to eliminate poverty and homelessness.
- Provinces and territories should establish social rights commissions to monitor the implementation of strategies, to assess compliance with rights to housing and an adequate standard of living, and to receive complaints. Alternatively, or in addition, the mandate of the provincial/territorial human rights commissions and tribunals could be expanded to include these rights.

INTRODUCTION

The modern conception of social rights (such as the right to housing, food, and an adequate standard of living) understands these as rights that, like civil and political rights, can be claimed and enforced and must be subject to effective remedies. This understanding provides a new paradigm for the design and implementation of housing and anti-poverty strategies that would breathe life into and enhance the effectiveness of existing poverty reduction and homelessness-reduction strategies.

Rather than simply affirming commitments to improve particular program outcomes and enhanced evidence-based assessment, provincial/territorial housing and anti-poverty strategies should be reframed as commitments to implementing fundamental human rights to an adequate standard of living, adequate food, and adequate housing. Reconstructing these strategies around international human rights and constitutional values would ensure that the strategies engage with the broad spectrum of law, policy, and program administration that is involved. Aspirational commitments and targets that are too often divorced from actual decision-making would be transformed into enforceable human rights obligations that would inform decisions and policies in all relevant government activities. Under the rights-based model, accountability mechanisms would be linked to the ability of individuals and groups to claim and enforce social rights when decisions are made that affect their ability to live with dignity and security.

Affirming social rights as legal obligations does not require an excessive reliance on courts. As legally binding human rights norms have become accepted in other areas, such as those regarding disability or sexual orientation, they have only rarely relied on judicial enforcement. Courts have clarified the meaning of the legal rights, but the social transformation and policy reform necessary to give effect to these rights has occurred without extensive judicial intervention. Recognizing legally-binding social rights will similarly depend on courts only in rare cases, in order to clarify the meaning and application of these rights in particular circumstances. The courts' role will remain that of interpreting and applying rights, not designing or implementing social policy. Recognizing the right to adequate housing and an adequate standard of living as legally enforceable rights in each province and territory would, however, change the framework of values and rights that guides decision-makers and hence inform the design and administration of policies and programs. It would challenge the systemic social exclusion that lies behind homelessness and poverty in Canada by implementing decision making that is informed by and consistent with fundamental human rights that are already binding on decision-makers but are too often ignored.

While the proposed social rights–based approach requires a significant paradigm shift from current housing and poverty reduction strategies, this can be accomplished without major legislative change or significant institutional reform. As will be explained below, provincial/territorial statutory bodies and administrative decision-makers already have obligations to exercise their authority in a way that safeguards, wherever reasonably possible, the right to an adequate standard of living, adequate food, and adequate housing. Provincial/territorial governments need only affirm and promote their existing obligations under international human rights and domestic constitutional law. Rather than legislatively ignoring and, when challenged in court, contesting social rights to housing and an adequate standard of living as has been done in the past, provinces and territories would instead recognize and affirm their social rights commitments by framing anti-poverty and housing strategies within existing human rights frameworks.

Using Ontario's anti-poverty and housing strategies as an example, this paper will consider what is lacking from a human rights standpoint in provincial/territorial strategies and contemplate the benefits of a rights-based approach based on international and constitutional norms. It will explore whether a new rights-based framework for housing and anti-poverty strategies could be implemented in Ontario and other provinces and territories without major institutional or legislative changes, and consider what roles existing institutions and agencies might play.

ONTARIO'S HOUSING AND ANTI-POVERTY STRATEGIES: THE MISSING RIGHTS

An unprecedented 400,000 people now rely on Ontario food banks and approximately 900,000 households experience food insecurity (Food Banks Canada, 2012; Tarasuk, Mitchell, & Dachner, 2013). The number of homeless families seeking emergency shelter in Toronto has sharply increased and a record number of households are now on the waiting list for subsidized housing (Housing Connection, 2014; Toronto.ca, n.d.). Behind these numbers are hundreds of thousands of personal experiences of the dire mental and physical health consequences of homelessness and poverty, including broken families, violence, and prematurely ended lives.

United Nations committees have expressed grave concern about the extent of these kinds of violations of social rights in as affluent a country as Canada. Ontario and other provinces and territories have responded to these concerns by reporting on their housing and anti-poverty strategies primarily in terms of improved outcome-focused service delivery and provision of support, with little evidence of any end in sight to serious and widespread human rights violations. Such responses to UN committees overseeing government compliance with international human rights do not effectively address the concern and shock that homelessness and poverty have been allowed to reach such critical proportions in one of the most affluent countries to appear before the UN Committee on Economic, Social and Cultural Rights (CESCR, 1998, 2006). There is a significant asymmetry between the CESCR's concerns about a systemic human rights crisis and the presentation of strategies for improvements in program and service delivery, as well as modest (and continually deferred) targets such as Ontario's target of reducing child poverty by 25 percent.

There is certainly nothing wrong with governments making efforts to ensure improved outcomes from housing or income support programs, or commitment to making progress on addressing child poverty based on agreed measures and indicators. However, the absence of any reference to the human rights at stake in strategies to address violations of the right to adequate housing and to an adequate standard of living is significant. Strategies for effective public management are no substitute for commitments to protect and ensure human rights to dignity, security, life, and health.

There is no reference to the right to an adequate standard of living or to any other human rights—either domestic or international—in Ontario's 2008 *Breaking the Cycle: A Poverty Reduction Strategy* (Government of Ontario, 2008), the Poverty Reduction Act

(Legislative Assembly of Ontario, 2009), or the recent *Realizing Our Potential: Ontario's Poverty Reduction Strategy: 2014–2019* (Government of Ontario, 2014). Ontario's Long-Term Affordable Housing Strategy (Ministry of Municipal Affairs and Housing, 2010) makes no reference to Ontario's obligations to ensure the right to adequate housing under the International Covenant on Economic, Social and Cultural Rights (ICESCR), making only passing reference to the right to equal treatment without discrimination. The Strong Communities through Affordable Housing Act (Legislative Assembly of Ontario, 2011c) makes no reference at all to human rights.

Existing strategies do affirm a number of principles that resonate with human rights values. The Poverty Reduction Act commits to such principles as the full participation of groups facing discrimination; respect for individual dignity, diversity, and recognition of unique needs of particular groups; participation of stakeholders in program design; and cooperation among various levels of government (Legislative Assembly of Ontario, 2009). Ontario's long-term affordable housing strategy similarly affirms that housing programs must be based on strong partnerships among all levels of government, housing providers, and those in need of housing, inclusive of groups facing discrimination and providing necessary support services (Ministry of Municipal Affairs and Housing, 2010). All Ontario municipalities have been required to develop local housing and homelessness plans to address issues defined as provincial interests. Plans must provide measures to prevent homelessness, including eviction prevention and the provision of supports appropriate to clients' needs; adopt a "housing first" philosophy; and facilitate transitioning people from the street and shelters to safe, adequate, and stable housing (Ministry of Municipal Affairs and Housing, 2011). The new Poverty Reduction Strategy (2014–2019) makes a firmer commitment to "end homelessness" in Ontario, though goals, timelines, and evidence-based indicators of progress have yet to be developed (Government of Ontario, 2014).

Unfortunately, the "principles" of the anti-poverty strategy and "provincial interests" in the homelessness strategies do not reference any human rights obligations under international human rights or domestic law. Even the obligation to provide supports necessary for people with disabilities and to address the needs of groups facing discrimination, which are existing legal obligations under human rights legislation and the Canadian Charter of Rights and Freedoms, are affirmed only as "principles." There is no acknowledgement that these are human rights, and no reference to mechanisms by which they can be claimed and enforced.

The emphasis in the existing strategies on the need for evidence-based, measurable goals and on community consultation and collaboration is compatible with the rights-based approaches to housing and anti-poverty strategies recommended to Canadian governments by United Nations bodies (United Nations Office of the High Commissioner for Human Rights, 2006). In all provincial/territorial strategies, however, indicators and targets remain aspirational, with no meaningful accountability mechanisms in place to ensure that decisions that run contrary to these commitments can be reviewed or that necessary policies and program changes will be implemented to attain the stated targets.

ASPIRATIONAL TARGETS OR HUMAN RIGHTS OBLIGATIONS?

The distinction between governmental aspirations and human rights obligations is critical to assessing whether anti-poverty and housing strategies comply with international human rights law. This distinction has been central to UN human rights bodies' concerns about the status of social rights in Canadian provinces. In all of its periodic reviews of Canada dating back to 1993, the CESCR has stressed that the right to adequate housing, food, and an adequate standard of living must not be reduced to mere policy objectives (CESCR, 1998). The CESCR has recommended that Covenant rights "be enforceable within provinces and territories through legislation or policy measures, and that independent and appropriate monitoring and adjudication mechanisms be established" (2006, p. 6).

Ontario's Poverty Reduction Strategy has been criticized for lacking "teeth." Critics have noted that little attention has been paid to equality issues for socially marginalized groups, and that the strategy lacks independent monitoring of progress in meeting targets (Registered Nurses' Association of Ontario, 2009). Similar concerns have been expressed about the lack of a rights-based framework in the Long-Term Affordable Housing Strategy (Legislative Assembly of Ontario, 2011a, 2011b). The missing ingredients in the housing strategy were most clearly laid out by Miloon Kothari, the UN Special Rapporteur on Adequate Housing, who conducted a mission to Canada in 2008. In his 2009 report, his central recommendation was to create a national rights-based housing strategy engaging both provincial and federal governments (United Nations Human Rights Council, 2009). Ontario's Long Term Affordable Housing Strategy was subsequently introduced without any reference to the right to adequate housing. Kothari wrote to the Honourable Rick Bartolucci, Minister of Municipal Affairs and Housing, urging the government to consider amendments to include an improved human rights framework that would:

- include firm goals and timetables for the elimination of homelessness;
- provide for independent monitoring and review of progress and for consideration of complaints of violations of the right to adequate housing;
- prioritize the needs of groups most vulnerable to homelessness and discrimination; and
- ensure meaningful follow-up to concerns and recommendations from UN human rights bodies (M. Kothari, personal communication, April 6, 2011).

Similar recommendations have been made by many other experts and organizations in Canada in relation to housing and anti-poverty strategies. A House of Commons Standing Committee, after holding extensive hearings, concluded that poverty reduction strategies must not "only be guided by moral principles, but must be set within a human rights framework, specifically the recognition that governments have a duty to enforce socio-economic and civil rights" (Standing Committee on Human Resources, Skills and Social Development and the Status of Persons with Disabilities, 2010). The Ontario

Human Rights Commission has recommended that Ontario pass legislation affirming a legal right to adequate housing and adopting a provincial housing strategy (Ontario Human Rights Commission, 2008).

A federal private member's bill, Bill C-400, received support from all opposition parties but was defeated by the majority Conservative members. Bill C-400 included the following requirements (Parliament of Canada, 2012):

- Engagement with all levels of government, Aboriginal communities, and civil society
- Focus on marginalized groups particularly vulnerable to homelessness
- Private sector as well as governmental engagement
- Financial supports for those who cannot otherwise afford housing
- Clear targets and timelines to eliminate homelessness
- Monitoring of progress by an independent agency to ensure ongoing accountability
- Mechanisms to ensure that affected individuals and groups can identify violations of the right to housing and get needed responses and actions

These components are consistent with the requirements of international human rights norms (Porter, 2014).

WHY DO PROVINCES AND TERRITORIES NEED A RIGHTS-BASED APPROACH?

While rights-based approaches have been widely recommended, it is sometimes unclear to policy-makers and legislators what the added value would be of implementing a new framework based on human rights. In order to answer that question, it is important for the proponents of human rights–based solutions to explain how homelessness and poverty are in fact human rights problems that require rights-based solutions. Rights-based approaches emerge from improved understandings of the human rights dimensions of the problem housing and anti-poverty strategies seek to address.

Social rights approaches understand hunger or homelessness as resulting at least in part from "entitlement system failures" (Sen, 1988). When access to food and housing are not given the status of fundamental rights within a broader system of entitlements, these rights are not prioritized over other interests and to not properly inform decision-making. Homelessness, hunger, and poverty do not flow from a scarcity of food or affordable housing per se, but from entitlement system failures tied to a broad range of policy choices, legislation, and program administration decisions in which access to adequate housing and food have not been considered as fundamental human rights.

A vast array of laws, regulations, decisions, and policies create a legislative and policy framework in each province and territory that, among other things, has left certain individuals and groups homeless or otherwise living in poverty. When these decisions are made without consideration of their link to the protection of fundamental human rights of vulnerable groups, then violations of rights will invariably occur. Access to adequate housing among vulnerable groups, for example, is affected by a myriad of decisions, including the determination of the shelter component of social assistance; benefits accorded to part-time workers; minimum wage; budgets for subsidized housing and rent supplements; and rent regulation or conditions under which a tenancy may be terminated. Adopting a rights-based approach to housing strategies means engaging with decision making and program design in these and other areas that affect access to housing. In order to do this, the right to adequate housing must be accorded the status of primacy—informing and guiding all decision making. In other words, it must be accorded the same legal status as other human rights, such as rights to freedom from discrimination. Decisions that result in homelessness or hunger must come to be viewed in the same light as decisions that blatantly discriminate on prohibited grounds or violate other legal rights. Rather than framing strategic obligations solely as governmental aspirations or political commitments, a human rights approach therefore starts by engaging directly with the decision-making processes through which these commitments must be realized, tying rights to firm legal obligations of governments and ensuring that rights-holders have access to hearings and effective remedies where necessary.

The right to adequate housing is not to be confused with a claim to housing as a direct entitlement from government. One does not have an entitlement to be provided housing but rather an entitlement to a *system* that ensures this right by entrenching it within the normative framework for decision-making in a range of policies and programs. Social rights must therefore be embedded within housing and anti-poverty strategies as fundamental rights that will inform all relevant policies and decisions. It is this all-encompassing human rights framework that transforms a system of entitlements that denies vulnerable groups access to adequate housing, adequate food, and an adequate standard of living into one that remedies these exclusions and progressively realizes substantive social rights.

STATUTORY INTERPRETATION, REASONABLENESS, AND ADMINISTRATIVE DISCRETION

Fortunately, there is an existing legal framework in Canada for the requirement that decisions in a range of policy and program areas must comply with the right to adequate housing and to an adequate standard of living. The Supreme Court of Canada has affirmed that all legislation should be interpreted and applied consistently with international human rights law (Jackman & Porter, 2012). In the seminal case of *Baker v. Canada (Minister of Citizenship and Immigration)*, L'Heureux-Dubé found for the majority of the Court that the values reflected in international human rights should inform how statutes are interpreted (Supreme Court of Canada, 1999). She cited Ruth Sullivan's *Driedger on the Construction of Statutes* in support of this interpretive principle:

[T]he legislature is presumed to respect the values and principles enshrined in international law, both customary and conventional. These constitute a part of the legal context in which legislation is enacted and read. In so far as possible, therefore, interpretations that reflect these values and principles are preferred. (Supreme Court of Canada, 1999)

The application of this interpretive principle to administrative decision making by administrative or governmental officials exercising conferred authority is critical to implementing international human rights in Canada. Conferred decision making must be exercised reasonably, in accordance with international human rights values, including the right to adequate housing and to an adequate standard of living. The Supreme Court has also established that the Canadian Charter of Rights and Freedoms should be presumed to provide human rights protections that accord with Canada's international human rights obligations (Supreme Court of Canada, 1989). Reasonable decisions must be consistent with the Canadian Charter, including Charter values such as dignity, equality, and security. All decision-makers thus have an obligation to consider and apply a human rights framework that embraces both constitutional and international human rights values (Supreme Court of Canada, 2012). The Supreme Court has also developed a new and more robust rights-informed standard of reasonableness in the administrative law context. This provides a critical framework for ensuring that decision making across a range of policies, programs, and administrative bodies is consistent with the realization of rights to housing and an adequate standard of living. In adopting a rights-based approach based on this framework, provincial/territorial housing and anti-poverty strategies would simply implement and enforce obligations that are already binding but have been largely ignored.

RECOMMENDATIONS

There are a number of relatively simple ways in which a rights-based framework can be created for anti-poverty and housing strategies in each province and territory in Canada, based on existing laws and relying primarily on existing institutional structures.

Recommendation 1

Each province and territory should affirm that it recognizes the right to an adequate standard of living, including the rights to adequate food and adequate housing as per article 11 of the ICESCR. Governments should also recognize that measures to reduce and eventually eliminate poverty are required to protect the rights to life, liberty, and security of the person, and the right to equality in sections 7 and 15 of the Charter. Provincial/territorial attorneys general should take the position publicly and before the courts that the Charter can and should be interpreted so as to provide effective remedies to violations of these rights caused by poverty or homelessness.

Recommendation 2

Legislation should be adopted that implements housing and anti-poverty strategies and which state that all provincial or territorial statutes are to be interpreted consistently with Canadian governments' obligations under international human rights law to progressively realize the right to an adequate standard of living and the right to adequate housing. Where municipalities are delegated roles in implementing housing and anti-poverty strategies, all municipalities should be required to recognize the right to adequate housing as a framework for local decision making.

Recommendation 3

Every province and territory in Canada should affirm in legislation that all decision-makers operating under provincial statutes should consider the rights to an adequate standard of living and to adequate housing as fundamental values to be applied when exercising decision-making authority. Direction should be given to courts, delegated decision-makers, municipalities, and private actors that ratified international human rights to adequate housing, food, and an adequate standard of living must be fully respected as fundamental rights and as components of Canadian Charter rights. These initiatives would clarify and promote compliance with existing international and constitutional obligations.

Recommendation 4

Each province and territory should establish by legislation an independent Social Rights Commission with the authority to monitor compliance regarding the rights to an adequate standard of living and adequate housing, and assess progress in implementing social rights. The commission should be authorized to institute a complaints procedure through which it may receive complaints of social rights violations and, where it is in the public interest, hold hearings and issue recommendations as to appropriate remedies. A committee of the legislature should be responsible for receiving and ensuring follow-up to recommendations made by the Social Rights Commission.

CONCLUSION

The central change necessary to transform current provincial/territorial anti-poverty and housing strategies into rights-based strategies is to make the rights to an adequate standard of living and to adequate housing legally binding on all relevant decision-makers.

Additional modest institutional reforms should provide for external monitoring and a complaints procedure. Such procedures would create a quasi-judicial space for constructive dialogue between rights-claimants, democratic institutions, and policy-makers, and avoid excessive reliance on courts. A Social Rights Commission, as recommended, would ensure a specialized expertise in relation to social rights. If a provincial or territorial government wishes to avoid creating a new institution, an alternative possibility would be to invest provincial/territorial human rights commissions with the authority to provide external monitoring and allow human rights tribunals to hear complaints of social rights violations. As noted above, the judicial enforceability of social rights will serve primarily to clarify obligations and ensure that the new status of these rights ripples out to other decision-makers.

A social rights paradigm will become truly transformative when the executive branch of government consistently exercises conferred decision-making authority in compliance with its obligations to protect the rights to housing and an adequate standard of living. Whether it is an executive decision to set the shelter component of social assistance at a rate that is known to be unmanageable in today's rental market, or a residential tenancy board member's decision to evict a family into homelessness when they owe only a month's rent, the important change that must occur is for such decisions to come to be considered unreasonable and unacceptable. A new legal standard of reasonableness consistent with international human rights would also become a moral one, creating a new consensus about what constitutes acceptable policy.

Since Canada ratified the International Covenant on Economic, Social and Cultural Rights (ICESCR) in 1976, we have become used to food banks, homeless families, and other violations of social rights that would not have been imagined when Canada ratified the Covenant. The perspective of international human rights is critically important to challenging current widespread complacency. It provides some reflective distance that enables us to see the absurdity and injustice of aspects of our society to which we have become accustomed. Canada and its provinces and territories are perfectly situated to become world leaders in fully protecting and ensuring the right to adequate food, housing, and a life of dignity for all. It is time to retrieve and reaffirm the fundamental human rights values that define us by reimagining provincial/territorial housing and anti-poverty strategies within the framework of fundamental human rights.

GLOSSARY

Accountability mechanisms for human rights: Procedures through which governments' actions, decisions, or policies can be assessed against human rights obligations and corrective measures implemented. Such mechanisms range from court hearings and enforcement of remedies to violations of rights to informal monitoring and recommendations by independent panels or ombudspersons.

Committee on Economic, Social and Cultural Rights (CESCR): A United Nations human rights treaty body, made up of 18 independent experts, which monitors state compliance with the ICESCR.

International Covenant on Economic, Social and Cultural Rights (ICESCR): A human rights treaty adopted by the United Nations General Assembly that came into force in January 1976 and was ratified by Canada in May 1976. The ICESCR and the International Covenant on Civil and Political Rights are the two international human rights treaties that codified the Universal Declaration of Human Rights (UDHR).

Socioeconomic rights (social and economic rights, social rights): The category of rights contained in the ICESCR, including the rights to health, education, work (including just and favourable conditions of work), social security, and an adequate standard of living, including adequate food, clothing, and housing. In addition to being components of the right to an adequate standard of living, rights to adequate housing, food, water, and sanitation have subsequently been recognized as self-standing socio-economic rights.

DISCUSSION QUESTIONS

1. What might be some of the government's concerns about recognizing rights to housing and to an adequate standard of living as enforceable human rights? How would you address these concerns?
2. Can you think of examples demonstrating how recognizing particular human rights as legally enforceable has transformed a range of policies and programs and become embedded in the way decisions are made? Is it realistic to think the same process could occur in relation to the rights to housing and an adequate standard of living? What kinds of decisions might be affected?
3. Do you think the mandate of human rights commissions and human rights tribunals should be extended to include social rights, or is it better to maintain the focus on discrimination?

REFERENCES

CESCR. (1998). *Consideration of reports submitted by states parties under articles 16 and 17 of the covenant: Concluding observations of the Committee on Economic, Social and Cultural Rights: Canada.* Retrieved from http://www.refworld.org/docid/3f6cb5d37.html

CESCR. (2006). *Consideration of reports submitted by states parties under articles 16 and 17 of the covenant: Concluding observations of the Committee on Economic, Social and Cultural Rights: Canada.* Retrieved from http://www.refworld.org/docid/45377fa30.html

Food Banks Canada. (2012). *Hunger count 2012.* Toronto: Food Banks Canada.

Government of Ontario. (2008). *Breaking the cycle: Ontario's poverty reduction strategy.* Retrieved from https://dr6j45jk9xcmk.cloudfront.net/documents/3367/breaking-the-cycle.pdf

Government of Ontario. (2014). *Realizing our potential: Ontario's poverty reduction strategy: 2014–2019.* Retrieved from https://www.ontario.ca/page/realizing-our-potential-ontarios-poverty-reduction-strategy-2014-2019-all

Housing Connections. (2014). *Quarterly activity report: 2nd quarter 2014.* Retrieved from http://www.housingconnections.ca/information/reports.asp

Jackman, M., & Porter, B. (2012). *Constitutional framework for rights-based strategies to address homelessness and poverty as social determinants of health.* Ottawa: PHIRN.

Legislative Assembly of Ontario. *Poverty reduction act.* (2009). Retrieved from http://www.ontla. on.ca/web/bills/bills_detail.do?locale=en&BillID=2147

Legislative Assembly of Ontario. (2011a). *Official report of debates (Hansard).* http://www.ontla. on.ca/house-proceedings/transcripts/files_pdf/24-MAR-2011_L097.pdf

Legislative Assembly of Ontario. (2011b). *Official report of debates (Hansard).* Retrieved from http://www.ontla.on.ca/house-proceedings/transcripts/files_pdf/31-MAR-2011_L101.pdf

Legislative Assembly of Ontario. (2011c). *Strong communities through affordable housing act.* Retrieved from http://www.ontla.on.ca/web/bills/bills_detail.do?locale=en&BillID=2440

Ministry of Municipal Affairs and Housing. (2010). *Building foundations: Building futures: Ontario's long-term affordable housing strategy.* Retrieved from http://www.mah.gov.on.ca/ AssetFactory.aspx?did=8590

Ministry of Municipal Affairs and Housing. (2011). *Ontario housing policy statement.* Retrieved from http://www.mah.gov.on.ca/AssetFactory.aspx?did=9262

Ontario Human Rights Commission. (2008). *Right at home: Report on the consultation on human rights and rental housing in Ontario.* Retrieved from http://www.ohrc.on.ca/en/right-home-report-consultation-human-rights-and-rental-housing-ontario

Parliament of Canada. (2012). *Bill C-400: An act to ensure secure, adequate, accessible and affordable housing for Canadians.* Retrieved from http://www.parl.ca/DocumentViewer/ en/41-1/bill/C-400/first-reading

Porter, B. (2014). International rights in anti-poverty and housing strategies: Making the connection. In M. Jackman & B. Porter (eds.), *Advancing social rights in Canada* (pp. 33–64). Toronto: Irwin Law.

Registered Nurses' Association of Ontario. (2009). *Bill 152: Poverty reduction act, 2009.* Retrieved from http://rnao.ca/policy/submissions/bill-152-poverty-reduction-act

Sen, A. (1988). Property and Hunger. *Economics and Philosophy, 4*(1), 57–68.

Standing Committee on Human Resources, Skills and Social Development and the Status of Persons with Disabilities. (2010). *Federal poverty reduction plan: Working in partnership towards reducing poverty in Canada.* Retrieved from http://ywcacanada.ca/data/research_ docs/00000177.pdf

Supreme Court of Canada. (1989). *Slaight Communications Inc. v. Davidson.* Retrieved from https:// scc-csc.lexum.com/scc-csc/scc-csc/en/item/450/index.do

Supreme Court of Canada. (1999). *Baker v. Canada (Minister of Citizenship and Immigration).* Retrieved from http://scc-csc.lexum.com/scc-csc/scc-csc/en/item/1717/index.do

Supreme Court of Canada. (2012). *Doré v. Barreau du Québec.* Retrieved from https://scc-csc. lexum.com/scc-csc/scc-csc/en/item/7998/index.do

Tarasuk, V., Mitchell, A., & Dachner, N. (2013). *Household food insecurity in Canada, 2011.* Retrieved from http://nutritionalsciences.lamp.utoronto.ca

Toronto.ca. (n.d.). *Quick facts about homelessness and social housing in Toronto.* Retrieved from http://www1.toronto.ca/wps/portal/contentonly?vgnextoid=f59ed4b4920c0410VgnVCM1 0000071d60f89RCRD&vgnextchannel=c0aeab2cedfb0410VgnVCM10000071d60f89RCRD

United Nations Human Rights Council. (2009). *Report of the special rapporteur on adequate housing as a component of the right to an adequate standard of living, and on the right to non-discrimination in this context, Miloon Kothari: Addendum: Mission to Canada.* Retrieved from http://www.refworld.org/docid/49b7af2c2.html

United Nations Office of the High Commissioner for Human Rights. (2006). *Principles and guidelines for a human rights approach to poverty reduction strategies.* Geneva: OHCHR.

CHAPTER 22

International Human Rights in Anti-Poverty and Housing Strategies: Making the Connection

Bruce Porter

TAKE-HOME MESSAGE

- Widespread poverty and homelessness in an affluent country such as Canada are not simply social "problems"; they are human rights violations that require urgent action and rights-based solutions.
- Human rights are not just goals to be realized; they also provide a framework for achieving these goals through enhanced participation of stakeholders, respect for dignity, effective monitoring and accountability of governments, and access to justice for effective remedies to human rights violations.
- United Nations human rights bodies have expressed growing concern about the extent of poverty and homelessness in Canada and have urged the adoption of coordinated housing and anti-poverty strategies based on human rights.

INTRODUCTION

Calls for a rights-based approach to addressing poverty and homelessness have recently become commonplace, particularly within the United Nations (UN) human rights system. Since the mid-1990s, UN human rights bodies have urged Canadian governments to address the crisis of increasing poverty and homelessness within a human rights framework that recognizes the rights to adequate housing and an adequate standard of living as guaranteed in international human rights law ratified by Canada. These recommendations have been echoed by parliamentary committees, civil society organizations, and human rights, legal, and policy experts (Jackman & Porter, 2012a).

What is meant by a rights-based approach, however, is not always clear. Is the point of affirming social rights in the context of housing and anti-poverty strategies simply to create a moral imperative on governments to improve housing and income support programs? Does a rights-based strategy rely on allocating a central role to courts? Does it affect the design and content of housing and anti-poverty strategies or merely describe their goal?

In earlier years, socioeconomic rights such as the right to housing and an adequate standard of living were relegated to a "second generation" of human rights, considered aspirational goals of government policy rather than enforceable rights. Socioeconomic rights are now understood within the UN as equal in status to civil and political rights, claimable by rights-holders and subject to adjudication and effective remedies. The modern conception of social rights calls for a new understanding of the interplay between human rights and socioeconomic policy, which could frame a more effective approach to anti-poverty and housing strategies. Social rights claims are now seen as a critical means to challenge and address the structural disadvantage, social exclusion, and political powerlessness that lies behind the troubling phenomenon of homelessness and poverty in the midst of affluence.

Rights-based approaches address poverty and homelessness as denials not only of basic needs, but also of equal citizenship, dignity, and rights. The new social rights paradigm expands human rights practice beyond individualized denials of rights and brings broader strategic aspects of policy and program development into the field. Under the new framework, whether homelessness is caused by an individual act of discrimination by a housing provider or by a failure of governments to implement reasonable programs and strategies to ensure access to adequate housing, those whose rights are affected must have access to effective remedies. Under the new paradigm, however, effective remedies are not restricted to judicial remedies. Adjudication and remedy of rights claims is no longer relegated to a separate legal sphere but is instead incorporated into program and policy design. The new paradigm obliges governments to facilitate the design of strategies and programs to realize social rights within well-defined time frames, goals, and targets; to recognize the central role of rights claimants; and to strengthen accountability through complaints procedures, monitoring, and evaluation.

The International "Common Understanding" of Rights-Based Approaches

During the 1990s, the United Nations Committee on Economic, Social and Cultural Rights (CESCR), charged with monitoring compliance with the International Covenant on Economic Social and Cultural Rights (ICESCR), wrestled with growing poverty and widening inequality in both developed and developing countries in the context of periodic reviews of state parties to the Covenant. The Committee identified a critical need for a better understanding of the role of human rights in poverty reduction strategies and, in 2001, asked the UN Office of the High Commissioner for Human Rights (OHCHR) to develop guidelines for integrating human rights into poverty reduction strategies. In 2002 the OHCHR published *Draft Guidelines: A Human Rights Approach to Poverty Reduction*

Strategies (OHCHR, 2002). In 2003 the UN development agencies adopted a "common understanding of a rights-based approach," outlined in *The Human Rights-Based Approach to Development Cooperation: Towards a Common Understanding Among the UN Agencies* (known as the Common Understanding; United Nations Development Group, 2003).

The Common Understanding identified four key ingredients of rights-based programming:

1. Identifying the central human rights claims of rights-holders and the corresponding duties of "duty-bearers," and identifying the structural causes of the non-realization of rights.
2. Assessing the capacity of rights-holders to claim their rights and of duty-bearers to fulfill their obligations, and develop strategies to build these capacities.
3. Monitoring and evaluating both outcomes and processes, guided by human rights standards and principles.
4. Ensuring that programming is informed by the recommendations of international human rights bodies and mechanisms.

The Common Understanding called for interdependent social policy, human rights principles, and legal entitlements (United Nations Development Group, 2003). It required that strategies and programs ensure meaningful engagement with, and participation of, those living in poverty as rights-claimants, with access to effective remedies (United Nations Development Group, 2003). Rights-based programming, the UN agencies affirmed, recognizes stakeholders as key actors and participation as both a means and a goal—empowering marginalized and disadvantaged groups, promoting local initiatives, adopting measureable goals and targets, developing "strategic partnerships," and supporting "accountability to all stakeholders" (United Nations Development Group, 2003).

The 2006 publication *Principles and Guidelines for a Human Rights Approach to Poverty Reduction Strategies* affirmed that "the adoption of a poverty reduction strategy is not just desirable but obligatory for States which have ratified international human rights instruments" (OHCHR, 2006, pp. 4–4). It recommended that poverty reduction strategies include four categories of accountability mechanisms: judicial, quasi-judicial, administrative, and political (OHCHR, 2006). No singular mechanism is sufficient for effective accountability and remedies. Poverty reduction strategies must recognize the role of human rights institutions and adjudication processes and "build on, and strengthen links to, those institutions and processes that enable people who are excluded to hold policymakers to account" (OHCHR & WHO, 2008, p. 8).

The shift from needs-based to rights-based approaches is linked both to a more unified conception of human rights that includes social rights and to a fundamental reconceptualization of poverty and homelessness. No longer seen solely as economic deprivation, poverty and homelessness are now understood as deprivations of rights and capacity—symptomatic of failures not just of social and economic programs and policies, but also of legal and administrative regimes, justice systems, human rights institutions, and other participatory mechanisms through which governments can be held accountable and rights-holders can become active citizens. Among other sources, the new approach has drawn inspiration from the work of Nobel Prize–winning economist Amartya Sen. In his early groundbreaking research, Sen showed that poverty and famine were not generally caused by a scarcity of goods or discrete failures of programs. They involved broader "entitlement system failures" that largely arose from a devaluing of the basic rights claims of the most vulnerable members of society (Sen, 1988). This led to Sen's later understanding of poverty as a deprivation of capabilities that is tied, but not reducible, to low income levels (Sen, 1992, 2000). Eliminating poverty and homelessness is about more than addressing economic needs. It requires re-valuing the rights claims of those living in poverty; empowering them as rights-holders; identifying the entitlement system failures that lie behind poverty and homelessness; challenging systemic barriers to equality that confront marginalized and disadvantaged groups; redressing failures of governmental accountability; and remedying the discrimination, and social exclusion, experienced by people living in poverty. In short, poverty and homelessness are human rights problems that demand rights-based solutions.

INTERNATIONAL HUMAN RIGHTS NORMS RELEVANT TO ANTI-POVERTY AND HOUSING STRATEGIES IN CANADA

The Right to Effective Remedies for Rights Violations

Although international human rights are not directly enforceable in Canada except through domestic law, they provide the normative framework for the rights-based approach that has emerged internationally. International human rights are an important source of both substantive and procedural rights protections for people living in poverty or denied adequate housing in Canada. As noted by the Senate Subcommittee on Cities in its seminal report, *In from the Margins: A Call to Action on Poverty, Housing and Homelessness*, international human rights are a persuasive source for interpreting the Charter and other domestic laws and are implemented through domestic legislation (Subcommittee on Cities of the Standing Senate Committee on Social Affairs, Science and Technology, 2009). Moreover, international human rights violations may be remedied by way of periodic review procedures before UN treaty bodies; the Universal Periodic Review (UPR) before the UN Human Rights Council; optional complaints procedures before human rights treaty bodies; or fact-finding missions and recommendations from "mandate holders" such as the UN Special Rapporteur on Adequate Housing. Those affected by poverty and homelessness in Canada have increasingly turned to these international human rights procedures to advance claims that are not being heard by Canadian courts.

International procedures alone, however, are insufficient without domestic remedies for human rights violations. An overriding obligation under international law, and one implicit in the principle of the rule of law, is to provide effective domestic remedies for violations of human rights (CESCR, 1998b). Where judicial remedies are not available, alternative, effective remedies for violations must be implemented, outside of courts (CESCR, 1998b). For example, human rights commissions have broad authority to review legislation, hold inquires, and develop policy statements, and thus can play a remedial role. Many other administrative bodies involved in housing or income assistance could likewise provide new opportunities for rights claimants to obtain a fair hearing and secure effective remedies.

Beyond judicial review, a rights-based approach also requires the implementation of other accessible, affordable, and timely procedures to ensure effective remedies. Judicial and quasi-judicial mechanisms should be integrated with effective informal and administrative procedures for claiming and enforcing social rights under legislated housing and poverty reduction strategies.

There are multiple forums in which rights to housing and an adequate standard of living can be claimed, defined, and applied, and many ways in which rights can and should affect policies and programs, short of court orders. The Supreme Court of Canada (1992) has yet to decide to what degree programs to remedy poverty or homelessness are constitutionally mandated, but it has affirmed that such measures are constitutionally "encouraged" by Charter values. Rights-based strategies for eliminating poverty and homelessness serve to reclaim rights that have not been adequately protected by courts, providing access to new types of adjudication and remedies.

Progressive Realization and the Obligation to Implement Strategies

Under both domestic and international law, key components of economic and social rights are subject to progressive realization. Obligations are assessed relative to a state party's available resources and the stage of development of its institutions and programs (OHCHR, 1966). Article 2(1) of the ICESCR requires a state party "to take steps ... to the maximum of its available resources, with a view to achieving progressively the full realization of the rights recognized in the present Covenant by all appropriate means, including particularly the adoption of legislative measures" (OHCHR, 1966). The CESCR has consistently emphasized that even if the full implementation of Covenant rights cannot be achieved immediately, there is still an overriding obligation to "adopt a detailed plan of action for the progressive implementation" of each of the rights contained in the Covenant (CESCR, 1989, para. 4). The steps taken "should be deliberate, concrete and targeted as clearly as possible towards meeting the obligations recognized in the Covenant" (CESCR, 1990, para. 2). "Moreover, the obligations to monitor the extent of the realization, or more especially of the non-realization, of economic, social and cultural rights, and to devise strategies and programs for their promotion, are not in any way eliminated as a result of resource constraints" (CESCR, 1990, para. 11). In General Comment No. 4 on the right to adequate housing the CESCR (1991) noted that compliance with the right to adequate housing "will almost invariably require the adoption of a national housing strategy." Legal remedies must be available to groups facing evictions, inadequate housing conditions, or discrimination in access to housing (CESCR, 1991).

The Reasonableness Standard

The Optional Protocol to the ICESCR prescribes a standard of "reasonableness" in assessing steps taken to achieve progressive realization of ICESCR rights, requiring compliance with the substantive guarantees in Part II of the ICESCR while recognizing "that the State Party may adopt a range of possible policy measures for the implementation of the rights" (OHCHR, 2008).

The wording used in the Optional Protocol was taken from the now famous Grootboom decision (Constitutional Court of South Africa, 2000) on the right to adequate housing in South Africa, in which the South African Constitutional Court first developed its reasonableness standard for reviewing compliance with constitutional economic and social rights (Porter, 2009).

In general comments and in concluding observations on periodic reviews of state parties, the CESCR has further clarified the requirements of policies and strategies for compliance with Article 2(1) of the ICESCR. Comprehensive and purposive legislative measures are almost always required (CESCR, 1990), and strategies must be informed by an equality framework that prioritizes the needs of disadvantaged groups and protects against discrimination (CESCR, 2009b; United Nations Commission on Human Rights, 1987). Strategies must specifically address issues of systemic discrimination and remedy historic discrimination, and should include "efforts to overcome negative stereotyped images" (CESCR, 2009b, para. 41). They should rely on effective "coordination between the national ministries, regional and local authorities" (CESCR, 2003, para. 51). Human rights institutions may scrutinize existing laws, identify appropriate goals and benchmarks, provide research and education, monitor compliance, and examine complaints (CESCR, 1998c). Monitoring should include assessment of budgetary measures (CESCR, 1990), based on information such as the percentage of the budget allocated to specific rights compared to states with similar levels of development (CESCR, 2009a; Griffey, 2011; Ssenyonjo, 2011).

As Sandra Liebenberg and Geo Quinot (2011) have argued in relation to the reasonableness standard in South African jurisprudence, the requirement of reasonableness itself demands a rights-conscious strategy, commensurate with the special status of "rights" compared to other policy objectives:

> It is not enough that the objectives which the State sets itself fall within the broad range of what are regarded as 'legitimate' State objectives. These objectives must be consistent with the normative purposes of the rights. This implies a rights-conscious social policy, planning and budgeting process. (p. 649)

The Supreme Court of Canada has developed a standard of reasonableness that is compatible with South African and international standards. In the Eldridge case, in which people with hearing impairments challenged the British Columbia government's decision not to fund interpreter services for the deaf and hard of hearing in hospitals and other health services, the Court found that the duty to provide program or services to accommodate needs of disadvantaged groups is a component of the guarantee of equality in section 15 and of "reasonable limits" under section 1 of the Charter (Supreme Court of Canada, 1997). In the Baker case the Court affirmed that reasonable decision making in domestic law must conform with the Charter and international human rights values (Supreme Court of Canada, 1999). More recently in *Doré v. Barreau du Québec* the Court adopted a new "robust" administrative law test of reasonableness that applies Charter values in administrative decisions so as to provide essentially the same level of protection of Charter rights as a full Charter review and section 1 analysis (Supreme Court of Canada, 2012). Where decisions impact on the rights to life and security of the person, discretion must also be exercised in conformity with principles of fundamental justice (Supreme Court of Canada, 2011), which include international human rights norms (Supreme Court of Canada, 2002). Drawing on this jurisprudence, there is support for the application of both domestic and international standards of reasonableness as legal requirements of strategies and programs to address poverty and homelessness in Canada (Jackman & Porter, 2012b).

Recommendations for Housing and Anti-Poverty Strategies in Canada

Concerns among international human rights bodies about the growing crisis of poverty and homelessness in Canada have reached unprecedented levels in recent years. The centrepiece of the CESCR's recommendations regarding poverty and homelessness in Canada has been a strategy for the reduction of homelessness and poverty that integrates economic, social, and cultural rights (CESCR, 1998a). The CESCR has emphasized that a Canadian strategy should include "measurable goals and timetables, consultation and collaboration with affected communities, complaints procedures, and transparent accountability mechanisms, in keeping with Covenant standards" (CESCR, 2006, para. 62).

The CESCR's recommendations were reinforced during the 2007 mission to Canada of the UN Special Rapporteur on Adequate Housing, Miloon Kothari. A key recommendation in Kothari's report was for "a comprehensive and coordinated national housing policy based on indivisibility of human rights and the protection of the most vulnerable" (UNHRC, 2009a, para. 90). Kothari reiterated the CESCR's recommendations that the strategy include measurable goals and timetables, complaints procedures, and transparent accountability mechanisms (UNHRC, 2009a). He recommended that federal and provincial governments cooperate to "commit stable and long-term funding to a comprehensive national housing strategy" (UNHRC, 2009a, para. 92) and that the "right to adequate housing be recognized in federal and provincial legislation as an inherent part of the Canadian legal system" (UNHRC, 2009a, para. 88).

The UN Human Rights Council's two reviews of Canada under the new Universal Periodic Review (UPR) procedure have also highlighted the need for anti-poverty and housing strategies based on human rights. Among the recommendations in Canada's 2009 UPR were that Canada develop "a national strategy to eliminate poverty" and "consider taking on board the recommendation of the Special Rapporteur on adequate housing, specifically to extend and enhance the national homelessness programme" (UNHRC, 2009b, p. 20). Recommendations for strategies to address homelessness and poverty were made again in Canada's 2013 UPR, supplemented by further recommendations for strategies to ensure food security and the rights to water and sanitation (UNHRC, 2013).

A range of domestic authorities have also called for national rights-based housing and anti-poverty strategies in Canada. In its report *In from the Margins* (Subcommittee on Cities of the Standing Senate Committee on Social Affairs, Science and Technology, 2009), the Senate Subcommittee on Cities noted that feedback from numerous experts and civil society representatives emphasized the need for rights-based approaches and called for a national housing and homelessness strategy (Subcommittee on Cities of the Standing Senate Committee on Social Affairs, Science and Technology, 2009). The report cited then UN High Commissioner on Human Rights Louise Arbour's statement that poverty "describes a complex of interrelated and mutually reinforcing deprivations, which impact on people's ability to claim and access their civil, cultural, economic, political and social rights. In a fundamental way, therefore, the denial of human rights forms part of the very definition of what it is to be poor" (Subcommittee on Cities of the Standing Senate Committee on Social Affairs, Science and Technology, 2009, p. 71). The subcommittee recommended that the federal government "explicitly cite international obligations ratified by Canada in any new federal legislation or legislative amendments relevant to poverty, housing and homelessness" (Subcommittee on Cities of the Standing Senate Committee on Social Affairs, Science and Technology, 2009, p. 16).

In 2010 the House of Commons Standing Committee on Human Resources, Skills and Social Development and the Status of Persons with Disabilities (HUMA Committee) held hearings and issued a report on a federal poverty reduction plan. The committee reported that:

> The Committee was told that we also need a shift in perspective if we are to significantly reduce poverty in Canada. Poverty reduction measures must not be seen only as charity work or only be guided by moral principles, but must be set within a human rights framework, specifically the recognition that governments have a duty to enforce socio-economic and civil rights. Adopting a human rights framework also limits the stigmatization of people living in poverty. The Committee fully endorses such a framework in this report. (HUMA Committee, 2010, p. 2)

The HUMA Committee (2010) noted the importance of Canada's international obligations under the Universal Declaration of Human Rights (UDHR) and in ratified human rights treaties to ensure an adequate standard of living, including adequate housing. It recommended the federal government "endorse the United Nations Declaration on the Rights of Indigenous Peoples and implement the standards set out in this document" (HUMA Committee, 2010, p. 2). The Committee also emphasized the importance of ensuring that measures to reduce poverty among people with disabilities are linked to human rights protections, including the Convention on the Rights of Persons with Disabilities (CRPD) (HUMA Committee, 2010). The HUMA Committee recommended a federal poverty reduction action plan that incorporates a human rights framework and provides for engagement with provincial and territorial governments, Aboriginal governments and organizations, the public and private sector, and people living in poverty (HUMA Committee, 2010).

CONCLUSION: EMERGING SITES FOR SOCIAL RIGHTS PRACTICE IN CANADA

Provincial governments have taken important steps in implementing housing and anti-poverty strategies. However, the strategies to date have remained largely within the older paradigm of social rights as moral aspirations. They have failed to consider the need for revitalized human rights institutions and rights-claiming mechanisms as promoted by the UN (Greason, 2014).

The model of rights-based approaches to poverty and homelessness that has evolved within international human rights is highly relevant to the ongoing crisis of poverty and homelessness in Canada and to the design of strategies to address it. Sen's early insight that famine and hunger are linked to entitlement system failures rather than resource scarcity certainly applies to homelessness and poverty in Canada. Economic deprivation amidst affluence must be understood as a socially constructed systemic failure of law, policy, and decision making, deriving from the devaluing of the rights of those who have been stigmatized and marginalized. Social program cuts and budgetary decisions have occurred within this broader context. As Marie-Eve Sylvestre and Céline Bellot (2014) observed,

> As programmatic responses that addressed the causes of homelessness such as social housing, investment in health care, or employment policies have been reduced or eliminated, governments have adopted unprecedented measures based on the stigma of homelessness as a perceived moral failure and designed to make homeless people disappear from the public sphere, rendering these social and economic changes invisible. (p. 168)

It is no accident that historically unprecedented social program cuts in Canada have been accompanied by withdrawal of funding and support for any rights-based advocacy on behalf of the groups most affected. The attack on programs and the attack on rights are inextricably linked (Porter, 2007).

What will rights-based strategies look like in Canada? They will start from the understanding of social rights as claimable rights that has emerged internationally. Goals and timelines for reducing and eliminating homelessness will not simply be targets for governments to aim toward, but legal entitlements to decision making that is consistent with meeting the targets. Human rights norms will be included in a range of programs and legislation, reforming the mandate of administrative bodies such as human rights commissions, landlord and tenant groups, social benefits, and labour tribunals to ensure that their decisions are consistent with the rights to housing and an adequate standard of living. Courts will be required to engage more constructively with the obligations of governments to implement effective strategies and to progressively realize social rights. All of these changes will begin to ensure that the myriad of entitlement system failures that create and perpetuate poverty and homelessness are brought within a human rights lens and made subject to effective remedies.

It is time that governments in Canada responded to the chorus of recommendations, from the UN, parliamentary bodies, experts, and community grassroots movements, to incorporate Canada's international human rights obligations into housing and anti-poverty strategies. Rights-based strategies for the elimination of poverty and homelessness may serve as the next critical frontier through which these rights—too long ignored—can be reclaimed.

GLOSSARY

Concluding observations: Assessments of the implementation of human rights treaties by a state. They are issued by the respective treaty bodies after their examination of the state reports.

General Comments: A treaty body's interpretation of the content of particular human rights provisions or clarifications of the obligations of states.

Periodic reviews: Reviews conducted by United Nations human rights treaty monitoring bodies to assess state compliance with each human rights treaty that they have ratified. States that have ratified a human rights treaty are required to submit periodic reports approximately every five years and to send a delegation to appear before a treaty monitoring body, such as the UN Committee on Economic, Social and Cultural Rights.

Socioeconomic rights (social and economic rights or social rights): The category of rights contained in the ICESCR, including the rights to health, education, work (including just and favourable conditions of work), social security, and an adequate standard of living (including adequate food, clothing, and housing). Rights to adequate housing, food, water, and sanitation have subsequently been recognized as self-standing rights.

Structural disadvantage or inequality: A pattern or system of unequal relations in roles, power, participation, functions, rights, and opportunities affecting particular social groups, such as women, people with disabilities, or people living in poverty.

DISCUSSION QUESTIONS

1. How would a rights-based strategy to address homelessness and poverty in Canada differ from current approaches? Do you think it would be more effective?
2. Should courts consider homelessness or hunger in Canada as violations of human rights in the same way that they have found bans on same-sex marriage or preventing medically assisted death to be violations of human rights? Why or why not?
3. What are some of the most common discriminatory stereotypes about people who are homeless or living in poverty, and how might these be overcome?

REFERENCES

CESCR. (1989). *General comment 1: Report by states parties.* Retrieved from http://www.refworld.org/docid/4538838b2.html

CESCR. (1990). *General comment 3: The nature of states parties' obligations (art. 2, para. 1 of the covenant).* Retrieved from http://refworld.org/docid/4538838e10.html

CESCR. (1991). *General comment 4: The right to adequate housing (art. 11(1) of the covenant).* Retrieved from http://www.refworld.org/docid/47a7079a1.html

CESCR. (1998a). *Consideration of reports submitted by states parties under articles 16 and 17 of the covenant: Concluding observations of the Committee on Economic, Social and Cultural Rights: Canada.* Retrieved from http://www.refworld.org/docid/4af181b00.html

CESCR. (1998b). *General comment 9: The domestic application of the covenant.* Retrieved from http://www.refworld.org/docid/47a7079d6.html

CESCR. (1998c). *General comment 10: The role of national human rights institutions in the protection of economic, social and cultural rights.* Retrieved from http://www.refworld.org/docid/47a7079c0.html

CESCR. (2003). *General comment 15: The right to water. (art 11 & 12).* Retrieved from http://www.refworld.org/docid/4538838d11.html

CESCR. (2006). *Consideration of reports submitted by states parties under articles 16 and 17 of the covenant: Concluding observations of the Committee on Economic, Social and Cultural Rights: Canada.* Retrieved from http://www.refworld.org/publisher,CESCR,,CAN,45377fa30,0.html

CESCR. (2009a). *Consideration of reports submitted by states parties under articles 16 and 17 of the covenant: Concluding observations of the Committee on Economic, Social and Cultural Rights: Democratic Republic of Congo.* Retrieved from http://www.refworld.org/docid/4ef9fee12.html

CESCR. (2009b). General comment 20: Non-discrimination in economic, social and cultural rights (art. 2 para. 2, of the International Covenant on Economic, Social and Cultural Rights). Retrieved from http://www.refworld.org/docid/4a60961f2.html

Constitutional Court of South Africa. (2000). *Government of the Republic of South Africa and Others v. Grootboom and Others.* Retrieved from http://www.saflii.org/za/cases/ZACC/2000/19.html

Greason, V. (2014). Poverty as a human rights violation (except in government anti-poverty strategies). In M. Jackman & B. Porter (eds.), *Advancing social rights in Canada* (pp. 55–86). Toronto: Irwin Law.

Griffey, B. (2011). The 'Reasonableness' Test: Assessing violations of state obligations under the optional protocol to the International Covenant on Economic, Social and Cultural Rights. *Human Rights Law Review, 11,* 275–327.

HUMA Committee (House of Commons, Standing Committee on Human Resources, Skills and Social Development and the Status of Persons with Disabilities). (2010). *Federal poverty reduction plan: Working in partnership towards reducing poverty in Canada.* Retrieved from http://www.parl.gc.ca/HousePublications/Publication.aspx?DocId=4770921&File=9

Jackman, M., & Porter, B. (2012a). *International human rights, health and strategies to address homelessness and poverty in Ontario: Making the connection.* Ottawa: PHIRN. Retrieved from http://rrasp-phirn.ca/images/stories/docs/workingpaperseries/wps_feb2012_report.pdf

Jackman, M., & Porter, B. (2012b). *Rights-based strategies to address poverty and homelessness in Ontario: The constitutional framework.* Ottawa: PHIRN. Retrieved from http://socialrightscura.ca/documents/publications/BP-MJ-PHIRN-Making-the-Connection.pdf

OHCHR. (1966). *International Covenant on Economic, Social and Cultural Rights.* Geneva: OHCHR.

OHCHR. (2002). *Draft guidelines: A human rights approach to poverty reduction strategies.* Geneva: OHCHR.

OHCHR. (2006). *Principles and guidelines for a human rights approach to poverty reduction strategies.* Geneva: OHCHR.

OHCHR. (2008). *Optional protocol to the International Covenant on Economic, Social and Cultural Rights.* Geneva: OHCHR.

OHCHR & WHO. (2008). *Human rights, health and poverty reduction strategies.* Geneva: OHCHR & WHO.

Porter, B. (2007). Claiming adjudicative space: Social rights, equality and citizenship. In M. Young, S. B. Boyd, G. Brodsky, & S. Day (eds.), Poverty: Rights, social citizenship, and legal activism (pp. 77–95). Vancouver: University of British Columbia Press.

Porter, B. (2009). The Reasonableness Of Article 8(4) – Adjudicating claims from the margins. *Nordisk Tidsskrift For Menneskerettigheter, 27*(1), 39–53.

Quinot, G., & Liebenberg, S. (2011). Narrowing the band: Reasonableness review in administrative justice and socio-economic rights jurisprudence in South Africa. *Stellenbosch Law Review 22*(3), 639–663.

Sen, A. (1988). Property and hunger. *Economics and Philosophy, 4*(1), 57–68.

Sen, A. (1992). *Inequality reexamined.* New York: Russell Sage Foundation.

Sen, A. (2000). *Development as freedom.* New York: Anchor Books.

Ssenyonjo, M. (2011). Reflections on state obligations with respect to economic, social and cultural rights in international human rights law. *International Journal of Human Rights, 15,* 969–1012.

Subcommittee on Cities of the Standing Senate Committee on Social Affairs, Science and Technology. (2009). *In from the margins: A call to action on poverty, housing and homelessness.* Retrieved from http://www.parl.gc.ca/Content/SEN/Committee/402/citi/rep/rep02dec09-e.pdf

Supreme Court of Canada. (1992). *Schachter v. Canada.* Retrieved from http://scc-csc.lexum.com/scc-csc/scc-csc/en/item/903/index.do

Supreme Court of Canada. (1997). *Eldridge v. British Columbia (Attorney General)*. Retrieved from http://scc-csc.lexum.com/scc-csc/scc-csc/en/item/1552/index.do

Supreme Court of Canada. (1999). *Baker v. Canada (Minister of Citizenship and Immigration)*. Retrieved from http://scc csc.lexum.com/scc-csc/scc-csc/en/item/1717/index.do

Supreme Court of Canada. (2002). *Suresh v. Canada (Minister of Citizenship and Immigration)*. Retrieved from https://scc-csc.lexum.com/scc-csc/scc-csc/en/item/1937/index.do

Supreme Court of Canada (2011). *Canada (Attorney General) v. PHS Community Services Society.* Retrieved from http://scc-csc.lexum.com/scc-csc/scc-csc/en/item/7960/index.do

Supreme Court of Canada. (2012). *Doré v. Barreau du Québec.* Retrieved from https://scc-csc.lexum.com/scc-csc/scc-csc/en/item/7998/index.do

Sylvestre, M. (2011). *Affidavit for Tanudjaja v. Canada (Ont Sup Ct File no CV-10-403688)*. Retrieved from http://www.acto.ca/assets/files/cases/Afd.%20of%20M%20E%20SYLVESTRE,%20Associate%20professor%20of%20Law%20&%20Director%20of%20the%20Ph.d%20Program%20in%20Law,%20University%20of%20Ottawa%20-%20FINAL.pdf

Sylvestre, M., & Bellot, C. (2014). Challenging discriminatory and punitive responses to homelessness in Canada. In M. Jackman & B. Porter (eds.), *Advancing social rights in Canada* (pp. 107–127). Toronto: Irwin Law.

United Nations Commission on Human Rights. (1987). *Note verbale dated 86/12/05 from the permanent mission of the Netherlands to the United Nations Office at Geneva addressed to the Centre for Human Rights.* Retrieved from http://www.refworld.org/docid/48abd5790.html

United Nations Development Group. (2003). *The human rights based approach to development cooperation: Towards a common understanding among the UN agencies.* Retrieved from http://hrbaportal.org/the-human-rights-based-approach-to-development-cooperation-towards-a-common-understanding-among-un-agencies

UNHRC. (2009a). *Report of the Special Rapporteur on Adequate Housing as a Component of the Right to an Adequate Standard of Living, and on the Right to Non-discrimination in this Context, Miloon Kothari: Addendum: Mission to Canada.* UNHRC. Retrieved from http://www.refworld.org/docid/49b7af2c2.html

UNHRC. (2009b). Report of the working group on the universal periodic review: Canada. Retrieved from http://www.refworld.org/docid/49f964ec2.html

UNHRC. (2013). *Draft report of the working group on the universal periodic review: Canada.* Retrieved from http://www.international.gc.ca/genev/mission/UN_Per_Rev_Sec_Rep_Canada_2013-Deux_Rap_Ex_Pol_NU_Canada_2013.aspx?lang=eng

CHAPTER 23

Taxing Private Health Insurance to Fund Programs for the Poor in Ontario

Jamie Moeller and Carlos Quiñonez

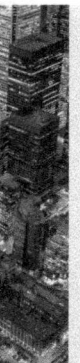

TAKE-HOME MESSAGE

- Taxing private health insurance to fund programs for the poor enjoys considerably less support from the general public in Ontario than policies that reallocate existing resources to disease prevention or health-creating services, such as basic education or housing.
- Socioeconomic differences exist among those who favour this policy, and peoples' personal and political values and preferences significantly guide their policy preferences.

INTRODUCTION

In Canada, services provided within hospitals, or by physicians in private practices, are largely free at the point of access. Other health care services—notably dental care, pharmaceutical care, and vision care—are primarily financed through private insurance coverage or out-of-pocket payments by patients. During the development of Canada's publicly funded health care system, these services were excluded for a variety of reasons, namely legislative priorities, professional resistance, sociocultural values, and political or economic constraints (Boothe, 2013; Quiñonez, 2013).

As demand for these health care services remained strong in the absence of public financing, the model of private financing for these services that exists today began to emerge. With the growth in unionization during the decade following the passing of the 1966 Medical Care Act, employment-based (private) health insurance that generally includes variable coverage of prescription drugs, vision care, and dental care became a common non-wage benefit offered through employee-employer contracts (Quiñonez & Grootendorst, 2013). To encourage increased growth of these private health insurance plans, federal and provincial governments in Canada maintained and expanded policies that exempted non-wage benefits from taxation as income (Hurley & Guindon, 2008). These tax exemptions, or subsidies, partly drove the growth of workplace health insurance plans in Canada during that time, and are still in effect today in Ontario and much of the country (Quiñonez & Grootendorst, 2013). More recently though, the premiums paid for employment-based health insurance have become subject to a provincial tax of 2 to 4 percent, still far below the marginal income tax rate (Hurley & Guindon, 2008).

These tax exemptions are problematic for two reasons. First, the distribution of these subsidies is highly inequitable. Because private health insurance and other non-wage benefits are more commonly associated with higher-paying jobs, the benefits disproportionately favour those in higher socioeconomic positions (Smythe, 2001). Second, a 2002 figure estimated the forgone tax revenue for Canadian governments to be over $3 billion (Royal Commission of Health Care in Canada, 2002). A more recent estimate suggests the value of this tax exemption is $2.6 billion for the federal government alone (Department of Finance, 2008; Hurley & Guindon, 2008). Not only could this revenue be used to be fund health care programs and services for the poor and the uninsured, but the poor and other economically-disadvantaged groups pay additional taxes (income taxes, gasoline taxes, and sales taxes) in order to make up for the revenue governments forgo, thus arguably exacerbating existing inequities (Leake, 2006).

For these reasons, there have been invitations by some for governments to reform the current policy by taxing employment-based health care insurance premiums as income (Leake, 2006; Royal Commission of Health Care in Canada, 2002; Smythe, 2001). In 1993, Quebec became the first province to implement this policy. Despite evidence demonstrating that the reforms in Quebec have had only a mild impact on the provision of private health insurance to employees by employers (Finkelstein, 2002; Stabile, 2001), Quebec remains the only Canadian province to have enacted this policy.

Certainly, professional groups where this type of financing is relevant overwhelmingly oppose such a policy (Quiñonez, Figueiredo, & Locker, 2009), and government officials in Ontario are likely wary of being seen by voters as raising taxes in the current political climate. However, it is not clear if Ontario residents would support this initiative if the revenue were used to provide care for the poor. Given that these reforms would assuage the inequitable distribution of benefits among different socioeconomic groups in Ontario—particularly if the tax revenues are used to finance programs for the poor—it may be useful for government officials, policy-makers, and public health planners to be informed about the saliency of this proposal among the general public in Ontario.

To be sure, earmarking of government revenues for specific spending purposes has been proposed for several public initiatives in recent years by governments in Canada (Federation of Canadian Municipalities, 2015; Miedema, 2012). In particular, earmarking remains popular for allocating revenues that are generated by activities closely linked to the favoured spending category, such as sin taxes on cigarettes used to fund health care services for cigarette users (World Health Organization, 2012). However, government revenues are fungible—that is, earmarked revenues can be, and often are, diverted from their intended purpose if they are less than the funds received from general revenue financing (Dye & Mcguire, 1992; Evans & Zhang, 2007; Garrett, 2001; Phuong, 2015; World Health Organization, 2012); it is unclear whether revenue generated from taxing private health insurance would be used exclusively to expand existing health programs or introduce new health programs that are targeted at the poor.

Nevertheless, this study aims to expand the research on the dynamics of public opinion and government spending on health care in Ontario by examining public support for taxing private health insurance in order to finance public programs for the poor. The objectives of this study are to: (1) determine the proportion of respondents that support taxing private health insurance if the funds raised are used to fund programs for the poor; (2) identify the personal values, political preferences, socioeconomic characteristics, and demographic profiles of respondents who are most likely to support this proposal; and (3) to compare the level of public support for this policy with the level of support for other initiatives targeted at improving the health of the poor.

METHODS

Data Source

The data used for this analysis was gathered from 2,006 Ontarians aged 18 years and over in 2010 through a telephone interview survey using random digit dialing. The market-based research firm contracted to conduct the survey used a random sampling of landline telephone numbers in Ontario, and was required to meet quotas in terms of sex, age, and location. No personal identifiers were collected, and surveys were conducted only in English. The study was approved by the University of Toronto's Office of Research Ethics (Protocol Reference No. 25583). Sample data were weighted by age and sex according to 2006 Canadian Census data, and all data analyses were completed using Statistical Package for the Social Sciences (SPSS) Version 22.0 for Windows.

Variables and Data Analysis

This analysis focuses on measuring the level of support for taxing private health insurance among participants by using the following survey question:

> Right now in Ontario, people are not taxed on their private health and dental insurance. This is not the case in other provinces. Do you think the government should tax these private health benefits to fund programs for the poor?

Participants could respond, "yes," "no," or "don't know/no response." Participants were also provided with two other potential solutions targeted at improving the health of the

Table 23.1: Percentage of Respondents Who Support the Proposed Solutions to Narrow Health Differences between the Rich and the Poor

	Question/Statement	Message
1	Assuming limited financial resources to pay for new services, would you support transferring money from health care treatment resources to disease-prevention services like health education campaigns?	Opinions about possible solutions to address inequalities in health between the rich and the poor
2	Assuming limited financial resources to pay for new services, would you support transferring money from health care treatment resources to health-creating services like basic education and affordable housing?	
3	Right now in Ontario, people are not taxed on their private health and dental insurance. This is not the case in other provinces. Do you think the government should tax these private health benefits to fund programs for the poor?	
4	In Ontario, all people are equally healthy and can expect to live for more or less the same amount of time.	Awareness of income-related health inequalities between the rich and the poor
5	In Ontario, people who are rich are much healthier than those who are poor.	
6	In Ontario, people who are poor are less likely to live into their 80s than people who are rich.	
7	Over the last few years, people who are rich have become healthier while people who are poor have become less healthy.	
8	People should take responsibility for their own health and not expect the government to do it for them.	Opinions about the importance of narrowing differences in health between the rich and the poor
9	It is important for governments to find ways of narrowing differences in health between the rich and the poor.	
10	Government should work to close the health gap between the rich and the poor even if it means raising taxes.	
11	Government should work to close the health gap between the rich and the poor even if it means shifting resources away from the better off to the less well-off.	

poor, both of which focused on reallocating existing resources within the Canadian health care system for programs targeted at the poor.

Responses to these three potential solutions are not mutually exclusive—respondents were not required to support any of the options, and were allowed to support more than one option. As well, respondents were asked to agree or disagree with statements related to their perceived awareness of income-related health inequalities in Ontario, attitudes about fairness and equity, and opinions about the importance of narrowing differences in health between the rich and poor (Table 23.1). For all statements, participants were presented with the response options of strongly agreeing, agreeing, disagreeing, strongly disagreeing, or neither agreeing nor disagreeing.

Demographic characteristics were also collected, including: sex (male, female), age (18–34 years, 35–54 years, and 55+ years), location (urban, rural), employment status (employed, unemployed), educational attainment (high school diploma or less, college education, or university degree), visible minority status, political voting intention (Progressive Conservative, Liberal, New Democratic Party), total annual household income (less than $20,000, $20,000–39,999, $40,000–59,999, $60,000–79,999, $80,000–99,999, and more than $100,000), and private health insurance (yes, no). Of note, we considered respondents' affirmation of dental insurance coverage a proxy for private health insurance coverage, given that private dental insurance coverage in Canada is the health benefit most often provided to individuals through private health insurance plans (Hurley & Guindon, 2008).

For the analysis, we first computed the percentage of respondents who supported each of the three policies proposed to improve the health of the poor. Next, we used binary logistic regression to determine the socioeconomic and demographic characteristics of those respondents who thought the government should tax private health insurance to fund programs for the poor. Finally, binary logistic regression was used to identify the personal values and government policy preferences of those respondents who support taxing private health insurance to fund programs for the poor.

RESULTS

The response rate and demographic profile of participants are described in another publication (Shankardass, Lofters, Kirst, & Quiñonez, 2012). Briefly, the survey had a response rate of 5.5 percent after excluding for numbers that were not in service, fax machines, busy signals, answering machines, no answer, language barriers, and ill or incapable participants. Roughly 52 percent of participants were female, and 73 percent of participants reported living in an urban area (defined as a geographic area with an urban core of more than 100,000 residents). Roughly 70 percent of participants reported an annual household income greater than $40,000, and just over 25 percent of participants reported a high school diploma or less as the highest attained education.

Among the three proposed policy proposals to improve the health of the poor, taxing private health insurance in order to fund programs for the poor received the lowest support from respondents (31%). In contrast, policies that reallocated existing resources to disease-prevention services like health education campaigns (58%) or to health-creating services like basic education and affordable housing (54%) enjoyed considerably more support from respondents (Figure 23.1).

Bivariately, support for taxing private health insurance in order to fund programs for the poor appeared to be linked to socioeconomic variables as indicated by household income, age, educational attainment, and dental insurance coverage. Specifically, respondents from the lowest-income households were three times as likely as those from the highest-income households to support taxing private health insurance to fund

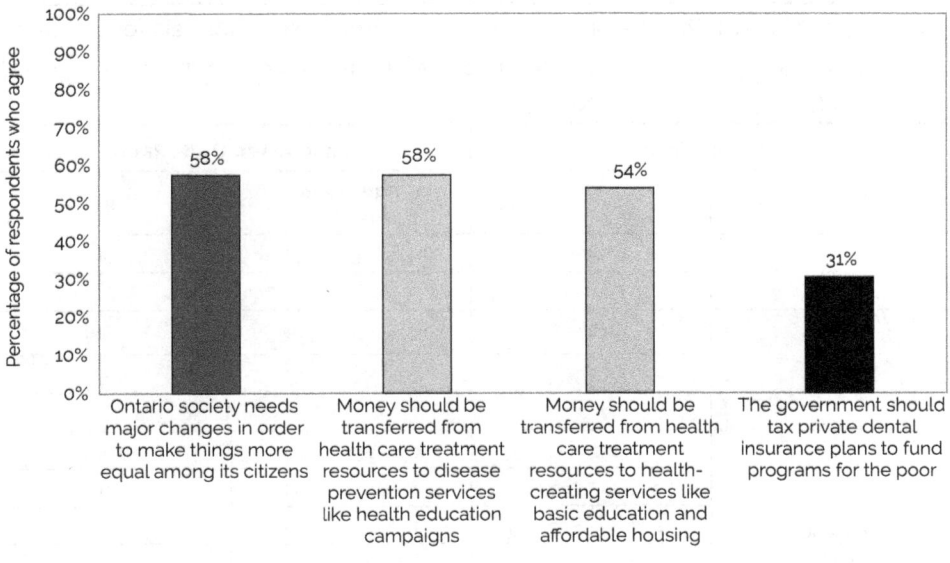

Figure 23.1: Eleven Statements and Questions Presented to Survey Respondents

programs for the poor, and those with dental insurance were about half as likely as those without it to support this policy. As well, the youngest respondents were twice as likely as the oldest to support this initiative, as were those respondents who identified as visible minorities compared to non-visible minority respondents.

In addition, support for taxing private health insurance to fund programs for the poor was considerably more likely among those respondents who were aware of health differences between the rich and poor and among those who favoured government intervention to address income-related health inequalities between the rich and poor, as well as among those who agreed that Ontario needs major changes to make things more equal among its citizens. This likelihood increased among those respondents who favoured redistribution of wealth and higher taxes to address inequalities between the rich and the poor. Those respondents who intended to vote for political parties more traditionally aligned with conservative values were less likely to favour this policy. Specifically, those who considered health to be a personal responsibility, and those who intended to vote for the Progressive Conservative Party of Ontario (relative to the traditionally more left-leaning New Democratic Party) were about half as likely to support taxing private health insurance.

DISCUSSION

In this study, we found that more than half of respondents in Ontario, Canada's most populated province, supported policies that reallocated existing resources to disease-prevention services like health education campaigns (58 percent) or to health-creating

Table 23.2: Model 1: Results of Bivariate Logistic Regression Analysis for the Odds of Support Taxing Health Care Insurance Premiums as Income in Order to Fund Programs for the Poor (Yes = 1; No = 0)

Characteristic		Unadjusted Odds Ratio*	
		Odds Ratio (95% CI)	P
Sex	Male	1.10 [0.91 – 1.33]	0.344
	Female	Reference	
Age	18–34	1.86 [1.46 – 2.38]	<0.001
	35–54	0.89 [0.70 – 1.13]	0.350
	55+	Reference	
Household income	<$20,000	2.76 [1.91 – 3.98]	<0.001
	$20,000 – $39,999	1.84 [1.34 – 2.54]	<0.001
	$40,000 – $59,999	1.32 [0.95 – 1.84]	0.102
	$60,000 – $79,999	1.12 [0.79 – 1.59	0.521
	$80,000 – $99,999	1.15 [0.79 – 1.68]	0.460
	$100,000+	Reference	
Educational attainment	Post-secondary	0.75 [0.60 – 0.93]	0.008
	High school or less	Reference	
Dental insurance coverage	Dental insurance	0.55 [0.45 – 0.68]	<0.001
	No dental insurance	Reference	
Residence status	Urban	1.18 [0.95 – 1.47]	0.138
	Rural	Reference	
Employment status	Employed	0.83 [0.56 – 1.22]	0.332
	Unemployed	Reference	
Visible minority status	Visible minority	1.67 [1.29 – 2.15]	<0.001
	Non-visible minority	Reference	

* Model 1 entered all variables independently.

services like basic education and affordable housing (54 percent), whereas taxing private health insurance in order to fund programs for the poor enjoyed considerably less support from respondents (31 percent). These results generally reflect respondents' opinions to addressing health inequalities in general. For example, a significant majority of Ontarians agree that it is important for governments to find ways to narrow differences in health between the rich and poor; however, support drops if this is conditional on the redistribution of wealth, or on paying for programs with higher taxes (Kirst et al., 2015).

Further analysis revealed important socioeconomic differences among those favouring taxing private health insurance in Ontario, namely support from disadvantaged

Table 23.3: Model 2: Results of Bivariate Logistic Regression Analysis for the Odds of Support Taxing Health Care Insurance Premiums as Income in Order to Fund Programs for the Poor (Yes = 1; No = 0)

Statement		Unadjusted OR*	
		Odds Ratio (95% CI)	P
Opinions about the importance of addressing health inequalities between the rich and the poor	Ontario needs major changes in order to make things more equal among its citizens.	1.98 [1.61 – 2.44]	<0.001
	People should take responsibility for their own health and not expect the government to do it for them.	0.71 [0.57 – 0.89]	<0.001
	It is important for governments to find ways of narrowing differences in health between the rich and the poor.	2.28 [1.61 – 3.25]	<0.001
	Government should work to close the health gap between the rich and the poor even if it means shifting resources away from the better off to the less well off.	2.88 [2.21 – 3.75]	<0.001
	Government should work to close the health gap between the rich and the poor even if it means raising taxes.	2.94 [2.37 – 3.65]	<0.001
Attitudes about fairness	Everyone in Ontario should have the same opportunity to live a long and healthy lifestyle.	1.09 [0.52 – 2.30]	0.822
	Everyone in Ontario does have the same opportunity to live a long and healthy lifestyle.	0.72 [0.59 – 0.87]	<0.001
Awareness of income-related health inequalities	In Ontario, all people are equally healthy and can expect to live for more or less the same amount of time.	0.90 [0.73 – 1.12]	0.349
	In Ontario, people who are rich are much healthier than those who are poor.	1.34 [1.01 – 1.63]	0.023
	In Ontario, people who are poor are less likely to live into their 80s than people who are rich.	1.36 [1.10 – 1.68]	0.007
	Over the last few years, people who are rich have become healthier while people who are poor have become less healthy.	1.24 [1.01 – 1.52]	0.031
Political affiliation	Progressive Conservative	0.50 [0.35 – 0.70]	<0.001
	Liberal	0.85 [0.60 – 1.19]	0.212
	New Democratic	Reference	

*Model 2 entered all variables independently.

adults: those with low income, with no private health insurance, and with low education. Certainly, these findings support previous studies, which demonstrate that there is a moderate level of demand for expanded and more accessible health services among these marginalized groups in Canada (Ramji & Quiñonez, 2012a, 2012b; Wlezien, 1995). Alternatively, it may simply highlight differences in lived experiences between the rich and poor, in which those from lower-income households better understand the benefits the poor would derive from increased resources devoted to the socially and economically marginalized (Kraus, Piff, & Keltner, 2009).

In addition, those with more individualistic worldviews and conservative politics were considerably less likely to support taxing private health insurance than those who favoured government intervention to address social ills. These findings may be a reflection of the socioeconomic divisions outlined above. Indeed, those with greater wealth tend to exhibit a greater degree of psychological entitlement, reduced levels of empathy, and a greater value placed on personal independence (Kraus et al., 2012; Piff, 2013). In contrast, those from lower socioeconomic classes endorse contextual explanations of economic trends, and are generally more concerned with the needs of others (Piff et al., 2010).

Respondents who reported more awareness of income-related health inequalities were more likely to favour taxing private health insurance than those who were unaware that the poor suffer disproportionately worse health than the rich. In addition, those who agree that Ontario needs major changes to make things more equal among its citizens were more likely to support taxing private health insurance to fund programs for the poor. These results may indicate that those who wish to see changes to the current policy of exempting private health insurance premiums from income taxation would benefit most by raising public awareness about the health differences observed between the rich and poor in Ontario.

It should be stressed that support by respondents for this policy proposal was conditional on the idea that the funds raised through these taxes would and/or could be used for programs targeted at the poor. However, revenues are fungible and there exists little evidence to suggest that earmarking—allocating specific taxes to finance narrowly defined government programs—would result in increased financial support for any support program (Anesi, 2006; McCleary, 1991). Given that there is evidence that Canadians tend to view taxes much more favourably if the revenue is allocated to support like-minded programs (Gratzer, 2012), it is unclear whether public support for this policy would remain as observed in this study without guarantees of government oversight to account for revenue generated through this tax.

On the other hand, governments in Canada today face the difficult task of addressing the needs of those most marginalized in society in the context of finite government resources. Our findings must therefore be considered within the larger context of increasing economic and social inequality in Ontario (Brzozowski, Gervais, Klein, & Suzuki, 2010; Reitz & Banerjee, 2009). In particular, this study demonstrates that there is an appetite among Ontarians to narrow differences in health between the rich and poor. Although taxing private health insurance in order to fund programs for the poor enjoys less support than other policies presented to respondents, recent evidence suggests that Ontarians underestimate the extent of the wealth gap that exists in Canada, and may be even more receptive to measures that produce a more equitable distribution of wealth if this knowledge is increased (Broadbent Institute, 2014). In this context, a policy that attenuates the inequities produced by these tax exemptions, while also offering governments the potential to raise a considerable amount of revenue in order to expand new or existing programs to improve the health of the poor, may receive more public support than is found in this study.

It is important to note the limitations of this study. First, we considered dental insurance coverage to be a proxy for private health insurance coverage among the survey's respondents. The survey did not differentiate between public insurance, employer-sponsored insurance, or privately-purchased insurance plans. However, recent estimates show that dental insurance is the most commonly provided health benefit through private health insurance plans (Hurley & Guindon, 2008), and an estimated 90 percent of those with dental insurance coverage have private insurance plans (Statistics Canada, 2012), suggesting that its use as a proxy for private health insurance is reliable, though imperfect. Second, telephone surveys exclude households without conventional landlines, and thus raise concerns about the representativeness of the sample population (Ramji & Quiñonez, 2012a). However, the sample was weighted by age, sex, and location according to 2006 Census data to yield a representative sample of Ontario. Finally, participants may display social desirability bias, in which they answer questions in a manner that will be viewed favourably by others, and not necessarily in a manner reflective of their true opinions. However, the telephone survey was anonymous, limiting participants' tendency to conform to what they view as socially desirable.

CONCLUSION

Taxing private health insurance to fund programs for the poor enjoys the least amount of public support among the three policies presented to participants in this study. There are significant socioeconomic differences among those who favour this policy, and peoples' personal and political values and preferences significantly guide their policy preferences. Ultimately, these results may be used by policy leaders to gauge public support or resistance for a variety of policy options to improve the health of the poor, but also to facilitate broader discussions about equity in health care for some of the most marginalized groups in Ontario.

GLOSSARY

1966 Medical Care Act: In response to the 1964 Royal Commission on Health Services' recommendation for a national plan covering all medical costs for all Canadians, this legislation was passed to provide universal public coverage of hospital and doctors' services to all Canadians (Health Canada, 2012).

Earmarking: The practice of assigning revenue, generally through statute or constitutional clause, from specific taxes or groups of taxes to specific government activities or areas of activity (McCleary, 1991).

Economic inequality: The uneven distribution of income, wealth, or consumption between individuals within a given population; also discussed as income inequality, wealth inequality, or the wealth gap (Stiglitz, 2012).

Employer-sponsored insurance: A form of private health insurance that is financed through private non-income-related payments (premiums) made to an insuring entity by the employer on behalf of the employee. The insurance entity then provides payment or reimbursement for health services according to the terms and conditions of a contract (Colombo & Tapay, 2014).

Fungibility: The potential for earmarked funds to be diverted from their initial purpose (Garrett, 2001).

Privately purchased insurance: A form of private health insurance that is financed entirely by an individual through after-tax income made to an insuring entity. A unique contract outlines the terms and conditions for payment or reimbursement of health services (Colombo & Tapay, 2014).

Public health insurance: Government-financed health services that are financed through government revenues. In Canada, select individuals are eligible for health services not delivered by physicians or in a hospital setting, such as dental care, vision care, and pharmaceutical drugs (Ramsay, 2002).

Public opinion: The aggregate of public attitudes or beliefs about government or politics (Bianco & Canon, 2013).

Social inequality: The uneven distribution of resources between members of a given population, producing unequal rewards and opportunities for individuals dependent upon social positions within a group or society (Sernau, 2013).

DISCUSSION QUESTIONS

1. What might this study's findings suggest about the limits of different levels of government to address inequities and inequalities in Ontario?

2. How might governments and community organizations use the findings from this study to address social, economic, and health inequalities in Ontario, or Canada more broadly?

3. The authors offer several possible explanations for the demographic and socioeconomic differences observed among those who support and those who do not support taxing private health insurance premiums to fund programs for the poor. How might governments in Ontario use these results in a broader policy context to narrow inequalities between the rich and the poor?

REFERENCES

Anesi, V. (2006). Earmarked taxation and political competition. *Journal of Public Economics, 90*, 679–701.

Bianco, W. T., & Canon, D. T. (2013). *American politics today* (3rd ed.). New York: WW Norton.

Boothe, K. (2013). Ideas and the limits on program expansion: The failure of nationwide pharmacare in Canada Since 1944. *Canadian Journal of Political Science, 46*, 419–53.

Broadbent Institute. (2014). *The wealth gap: Perceptions and misconceptions in Canada*. Ottawa: Broadbent Institute Retrieved from http://www.broadbentinstitute.ca/the_wealth_gap

Brzozowski, M., Gervais, M., Klein, P., & Suzuki, M. (2010). Consumption, income, and wealth inequality in Canada. *Review of Economic Dynamics, 13*, 52–75.

Colombo, F., & Tapay, N. (2014). *Private health insurance in OECD countries: The benefits and costs for individuals and health systems*. Paris: OECD. Retrieved from http://www.oecd-ilibrary.org/social-issues-migration-health/private-health-insurance-in-oecd-countries_527211067757

Department of Finance. (2008). *Tax expenditures and evaluations 2007*. Ottawa: Government of Canada.

Dye, R. F., & Mcguire, T. J. (1992). The effect of earmarked revenues on the level and composition of expenditures. *Public Finance Review, 20*, 543–556.

Evans, W. N., & Zhang, P. (2007). The impact of earmarked lottery revenue on K–12 educational expenditures. *Education Finance and Policy, 2*, 40–73.

Federation of Canadian Municipalities. (2015). *Policy statement: Municipal infrastructure and transportation policy*. Ottawa: Federation of Canadian Municipalities.

Finkelstein, A. (2002). The Effect of tax subsidies to employer-provided supplementary health insurance: Evidence from Canada. *Journal of Public Economics, 84*, 305–339.

Garrett, T. A. (2001). Earmarked lottery revenues for education: A new test of fungibility. *Journal of Education Finance, 26*, 219–238.

Gratzer, D. (2012). Are soda taxes a cure for obesity? Montreal: Montreal Economic Insitute. Retrieved from http://www.iedm.org/files/note1212_en.pdf

Health Canada. (2012). *Canada's health care system*. Ottawa: Government of Canada. Retrieved from http://www.hc-sc.gc.ca/hcs-sss/pubs/system-regime/2011-hcs-sss/index-eng.php

Hurley, J., & Guindon, G. E. (2008). *Private health insurance in Canada*. Hamilton: Center for Health Economics and Policy Analysis.

Kirst, M., Shankardass, K., Singhal, S., Lofters, A., Muntaner, C., & Quiñonez, C. (2015). *Addressing health inequities in Ontario, Canada: What solutions do the public support?* Manuscript submitted for publication.

Kraus, M. W., Piff, P. K., & Keltner, D. (2009). Social class, sense of control, and social explanation. *Journal of Personality and Social Psychology, 97*, 992–1004.

Kraus, M. W., Piff, P. K., Mendoza-Denton, R., Rheinschmidt, M. L., & Keltner, D. (2012). Social class, solipsism, and contextualism: How the rich are different from the poor. *Psychological Review, 119*, 546–572.

Leake, J. L. (2006). Why do we need an oral health care policy in Canada? *Journal of the Canadian Dental Association, 72*(40), 317a–317j.

McCleary, W. (1991). The earmarking of government revenue: A review of some world bank experience. The *World Bank Research Observer, 6*, 81–104.

Miedema, D. (2012). *Government — gambling's biggest addict.* Ottawa: Parliament of Canada.

Phuong, N.-H. (2015). Volatile earmarked revenues and state highway expenditures in the United States. *Transportation, 42*, 237–256.

Piff, P. K. (2013). Wealth and the inflated self: Class, entitlement, and narcissism. *Personality and Social Psychology Bulletin, 40*, 34–43.

Piff, P. K., Kraus, M. W., Côté, S., Cheng, B. H., & Keltner, D. (2010). Having less, giving more: The influence of social class on prosocial behavior. *Journal of Personality and Social Psychology, 99*, 771–784.

Quiñonez, C. (2013). *Why was dental care excluded from Canadian medicare?* Toronto: Network for Canadian Oral Health Research.

Quiñonez, C., & Grootendorst, P. (2013). Equity in dental care among Canadian households. *International Journal for Equity in Health, 10*, 14–23.

Quiñonez, C. R., Figueiredo, R., & Locker, D. (2009). Canadian dentists' opinions on publicly financed dental care. *Journal of Public Health Dentistry, 69*, 64–73.

Ramji, S., & Quiñonez, C. (2012a). Government spending on dental care: Is it a public priority? *Journal of Public Health Dentistry, 72*, 246–251.

Ramji, S., & Quiñonez, C. (2012b). Public preferences for government spending in Canada. *International Journal for Equity in Health, 11*, 64–74.

Ramsay, C. (2002). *A framework for determining the extent of public financing of programs and services.* Discussion Paper No. 16. Ottawa: Commission on the Future of Health Care in Canada.

Reitz, J. G., & Banerjee, R. (2009). Racial inequality and social integration. In J. G. Reitz, R. Breton, K. K. Dion, K. L. Dion (eds.), *Multiculturalism and social cohesion: Potentials and challenges of diversity* (pp. 123–155). New York: Springer.

Royal Commission of Health Care in Canada. (2002). *Building on values: The future of health care in Canada.* Ottawa: Health Canada.

Sernau, S. (2013). *Social inequality in a global age* (4th ed.). Thousand Oaks, CA: Sage.

Shankardass, K., Lofters, A., Kirst, M., & Quiñonez, C. (2012). Public awareness of income-related health inequalities in Ontario, Canada. *International Journal for Equity in Health, 11*, 26–36.

Smythe, J. G. (2001). *Tax subsidization of employer-provided health care insurance in Canada: Incidence analysis.* Edmonton: University of Alberta.

Stabile, M. (2001). Private insurance subsidies and public health care markets: Evidence from Canada. *Canadian Journal of Economics, 34*, 921–942.

Statistics Canada. (2012). *Canadian community health survey - annual component.* CHASS Statistics Database. Ottawa: Statistics Canada.

Stiglitz, J. (2012). *The price of inequality.* New York: WW Norton.

Wlezien, C. (1995). The Public as thermostat: Dynamics of preferences for spending. *American Journal of Political Science, 39,* 981–1000.

World Health Organization. (2012). *Tobacco taxation and innovative health-care financing.* New Delhi: World Health Organization.

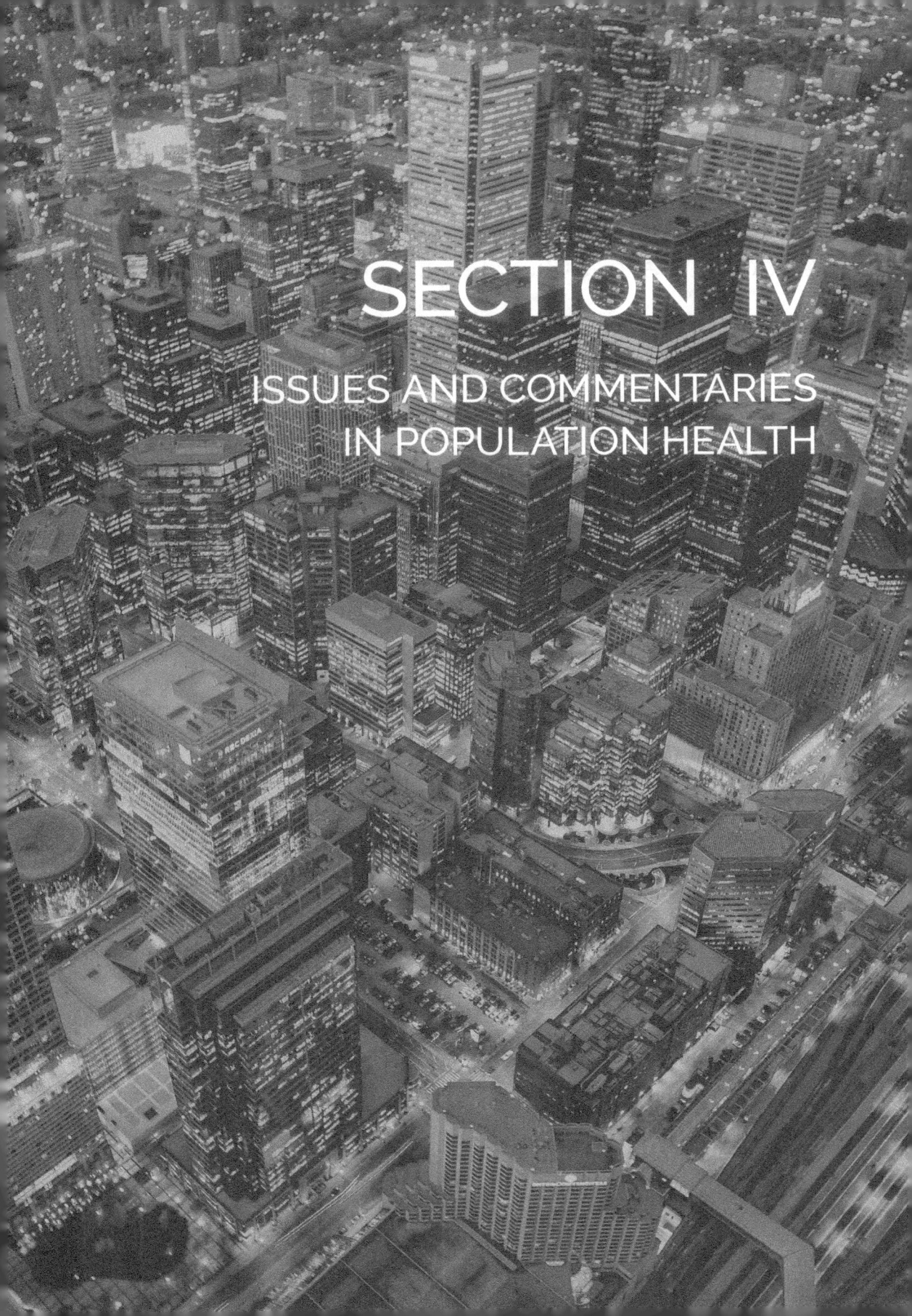

SECTION IV

ISSUES AND COMMENTARIES IN POPULATION HEALTH

CHAPTER 24

Social Determinants of Health: Bad News and Good on the Inequality Front

Ted Schrecker

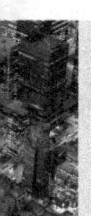

TAKE-HOME MESSAGE

- Increased income inequality is closely connected to population health inequalities; the wider the gaps, the lower the levels of health and well-being.

The Commission on Social Determinants of Health was emphatic about the role of "the inequitable distribution of power, money and resources" in sustaining socioeconomic gradients in health. Remarkably, over the past few years economic inequality has moved to centre stage in the academic world (see Box 24.1) and in policy circles that have not historically been much concerned with inequality, or with health. Addressing the 2014 annual joint meeting of the World Bank and the International Monetary Fund, the Fund's managing director Christine Lagarde (2014) described the growth in inequality worldwide as "staggering." A 2015 report from the Organisation for Economic Co-operation and Development (OECD), the club of high-income (and some middle-income) governments, noted that inequality has reached "historical highs" in some countries, driven partly by rising income shares at the top of the income distribution (OECD, 2015). Canadian economists noted in 2012 that 14 percent of total income in Canada flowed to the top 1 percent of the income distribution, up from about 8 percent in the late 1970s. "Such an uneven distribution of income has not been seen since the dark days of the Great Depression" (Fortin et al., 2012, p. 127). The OECD report pointed to another, equally disturbing pattern: "In recent decades, as much as 40% of the population at the lower end of the distribution has benefited little from economic growth in many countries" (2015, p. 21), with the incomes of some actually falling in inflation-adjusted terms.

Many influences contribute to the rise in inequality. Structural economic change, in particular the collapse of manufacturing employment and the rise of low-wage, often precarious service sector employment is one. But this trend itself is more pronounced in

Box 24.1: Recent Academic Treatments of Economic Inequality

Atkinson, Anthony B. (2015). *Inequality: What can be done?* Cambridge, MA: Harvard University Press.

Bourguignon, François* (2015). *The globalization of inequality.* Princeton: Princeton University Press.

Clark, Tom, & Heath, Anthony (2014). *Hard times: The divisive toll of the economic slump.* New Haven: Yale University Press.

Piketty, Thomas (2014). *Capital in the twenty-first century.* Cambridge, MA: Belknap Press of Harvard University Press.

Stiglitz, Joseph E.*† (2015). *The great divide.* London: Penguin Random House.

* Former chief economist, World Bank
† Nobel laureate in Economics

some countries than others. An extensive comparative study of labour markets (Gautié & Schmitt, 2010) found that in the mid-2000s low-wage work, defined with reference to the median wage, was three times as common in the US as in Denmark, and twice as common as in France. Movement toward the US norm was clearly evident over the 1980–2005 period in some countries, like the UK, but not in others. A recent study of a larger number of countries identified labour market characteristics, such as minimum wages and the level of unionization (in decline across much of the high-income world) as contributors to inequality (Jaumotte & Buitron, 2015). Labour market institutions are affected by public policy—think, for example, about the attack on unions by the Thatcher government and its successors in the UK—but they are only part of the picture. The extent to which taxes and transfers of all kinds reduce inequalities in market income is substantial, and varies widely among countries. This can be seen in Figure 24.1, which shows a threefold variation in the extent to which tax and transfer policies in selected OECD countries shrink the number of people who would live in poverty if they had to rely on their market incomes. (The figure actually understates the differences, because it does not take into account the value of in-kind transfers like publicly financed health care, quality public education, or support for public transportation.) Part of the increase in Canadian economic inequality is related to rising market incomes at the top of the distribution, but an important part of the explanation is the retreat from redistribution that began at both national and provincial levels in the 1990s (Heisz, 2007; Fortin et al., 2012). An earlier OECD report (2011) observed that this retreat was widespread in OECD countries, although the extent of the retreat varied considerably.

The good news is that the connection between inequality and policy is now more widely understood. The iconoclastic Canadian health economist Robert Evans argues that rising inequality and the growing share of national income flowing to the top 1 percent of the income distribution "are to a considerable extent a consequence of conscious, deliberate

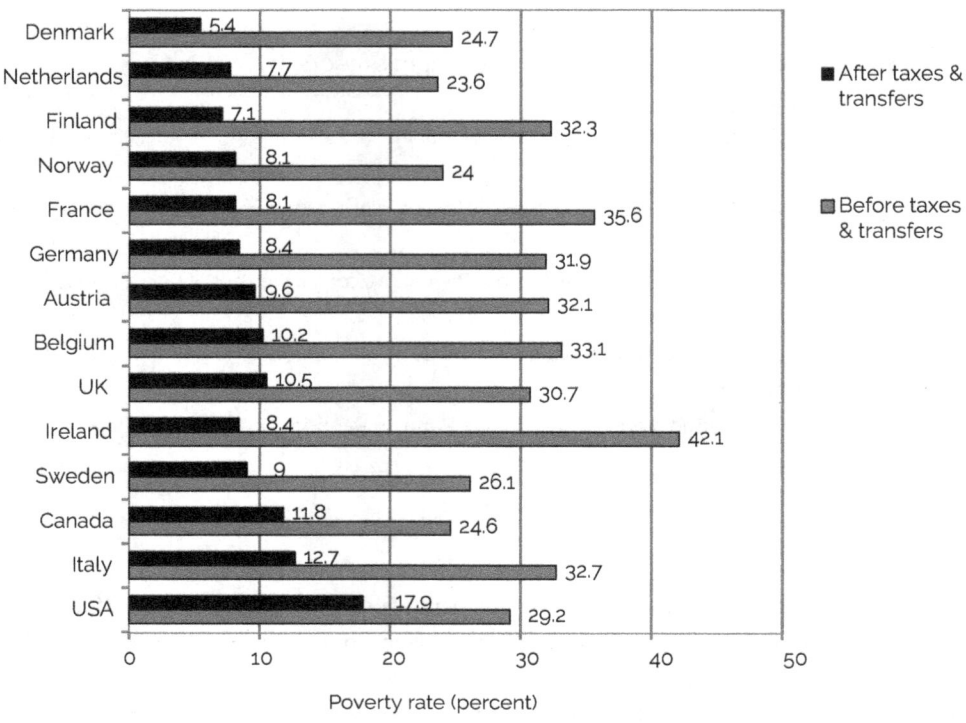

Figure 24.1: Poverty Rates Before and After Taxes and Transfers, Selected OECD
Countries, 2012

Source: OECD, n.d.

agency by more or less organized and coherent interest groups" (2012, p. 17). And Thomas
Piketty, the French economist whose book on inequality turned into a surprise bestseller,
has emphasized that "inequality does not follow a deterministic process.... There are powerful forces pushing alternately in the direction of rising or shrinking inequality. Which
one dominates depends on the institutions and policies that societies choose to adopt"
(Piketty & Saez, 2014, pp. 842–843).

Population health researchers must be concerned with rising inequality for several reasons. First is the directly debilitating effects of poverty—although many of these
are amenable to policy intervention given the necessary political will. Second, socioeconomic gradients in health usually exist across the entire income spectrum. Intuitively,
we would expect these gradients to be steeper when economic gradients are also steeper,
other things being equal, although this is a difficult proposition to test because of the differential impact of policies that do not directly affect income distribution. Third, income
inequality is only part of the story: wealth inequality, which is more difficult to measure,
is greater than income inequality, and insecure and precarious jobs (which have their own
health implications, including higher exposure to on-the-job hazards) are concentrated at

the bottom of the income scale. Fourth, it is argued—notably by Wilkinson and Pickett (2010)—that higher levels of economic inequality within a society lead to overall lower levels of health and well-being. Although the mechanisms of action remain unclear, a review of the evidence five years after the appearance of Wilkinson and Pickett's *The Spirit Level* concluded that the evidence base is now considerably stronger than at the time of its publication (Pickett & Wilkinson, 2015).

A final reason has received less attention, and it involves a phenomenon that former US Cabinet secretary Robert Reich (1991) called the "secession of the successful." Past a certain high level of income and wealth, people need less from government, and different things. As one Arizona resident interviewed for an article on politics in that state put it: "People who have swimming pools don't need state parks. If you buy your books at Borders you don't need libraries. If your kids are in private school, you don't need K–12. The people here, or at least those who vote, don't see the need for government" (Silverstein, 2010). We could add that people who can afford to drive or fly everywhere don't need public transportation; people with secure incomes gain little from public financing of social or subsidized housing; people who can afford private insurance may resist paying taxes to keep a public health insurance system afloat for the less healthy and less wealthy; and so on. Evans wonders, "If we are back to a pre-war income distribution, how much of our post-war social policies can survive?" (2006, p. 24). As mainstream politicians appear determined to ignore this question, it becomes more important than ever.

GLOSSARY

Economic structural change: A shift or change in the basic ways a market or economy functions or operates.

Redistribution: Redistribution of income and redistribution of wealth are respectively the transfer of income and of wealth (including physical property) from some individuals to others by means of a social mechanism such as taxation, charity, welfare, public services, land reform, monetary policies, confiscation, divorce, or tort law. The term typically refers to redistribution on an economy-wide basis rather than between selected individuals, and it almost always refers to redistribution from those who have more to those who have less.

DISCUSSION QUESTION

1. To what extent can redistributive social and economic policies address health inequalities?

REFERENCES

Evans, R. G. (2006). From world war to class war: The rebound of the rich. *Healthcare Policy, 2*(1), 14–24.

Evans, R. G. (2012). A casualty in the class war: Canada's medicare. *Healthcare Policy, 7*(3), 14–22.

Fortin, N. M., Green, D. A., Lemieux, T., Milligan, K., & Riddell, W. C. (2012). Canadian inequality: Recent development and policy options. *Canadian Public Policy, 38*, 121–145.

Gautié, J., & Schmitt, J. (eds.) (2010). *Low-wage work in the wealthy world.* New York: Russell Sage Foundation.

Heisz, A. (2007). *Income inequality and redistribution in Canada: 1976 to 2004.* Analytical Studies Branch Research Paper Series No. 298. Ottawa: Statistics Canada. Retrieved from: http://www.statcan.gc.ca/pub/11f0019m/11f0019m2007298-eng.pdf

Jaumotte, F., & Buitron, C. O. (2015). *Inequality and labor market institutions.* IMF Staff Discussion Note SDN/15/14. Washington, DC: International Monetary Fund. Retrieved from: http://www.imf.org/external/pubs/ft/sdn/2015/sdn1514.pdf

Lagarde, C. (2014). *The IMF at 70: Making the right choices—yesterday, today and tomorrow.* Speech to IMF/World Bank Annual Meeetings, Washington, DC. Retrieved from http://www.imf.org/external/np/speeches/2014/101014.htm

OECD. (n.d.). *OECD Stat: Income distribution and poverty.* Retrieved from http://stats.oecd.org/Index.aspx?DataSetCode=IDD

OECD. (2011). *Divided we stand: Why inequality keeps rising.* Paris: OECD.

OECD. (2015). *In it together: Why less inequality benefits all.* Paris: OECD.

Pickett, K. E., & Wilkinson, R. G. (2015). Income inequality and health: A causal review. *Social Science & Medicine, 128*, 316–326.

Piketty, T., & Saez, E. (2014). Inequality in the long run. *Science, 344*, 838–843.

Reich, R. (1991, January 20). Secession of the successful. *New York Times Magazine,* 16–17, 42–45.

Silverstein, K. (2010, July). Tea party in the Sonora: For the future of G.O.P. governance, look to Arizona. *Harper's,* 35–42. Retrieved from http://harpers.org/archive/2010/07/tea-party-in-the-sonora

Wilkinson, R., & Pickett, K. (2010). *The spirit level: Why equality is better for everyone.* London: Penguin.

CHAPTER 25

Healthy, Equitable, and Sustainable Transportation: A New Frontier for Action on Health Equity?

Ted Schrecker

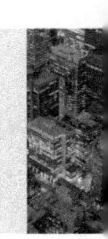

TAKE-HOME MESSAGE

- Transportation is an important area for action to reduce health inequity; public policy (in addition to the health sector) can influence social determinants of health.

In December 1995, Cynthia Wiggins was hit by a truck while crossing several lanes of traffic in suburban Buffalo, New York; shortly afterward, she died from her injuries. The 17-year-old African-American woman had to cross the arterial road to her job in the posh Walden Galleria mall because the bus that brought her from downtown was not allowed on mall property. The local public transportation authority had for years tried, unsuccessfully, to get permission to stop in the mall's parking lot. In 1999, a lawsuit charging the mall's owners with racial discrimination was settled for $2.55 million (to benefit Ms. Wiggins's son) without admission of liability (Chen, 1999).

Ms. Wiggins's death is an especially dramatic example of the connections between transportation policy and social exclusion: specifically, support for a form of spatial apartheid in the United States long after *de jure* forms of racial segregation were limited in law. Although some such extremes are distinctive to the United States, an important and neglected 2009 Canadian study of mobility and social exclusion in Hamilton, Toronto, and Montreal concluded that "the evidence uncovered in terms of mobility and accessibility patterns is suggestive of social exclusionary processes that may prevent various vulnerable groups," specifically low-income people, seniors, and single-parent households, "from accessing the places required for their daily needs" (Páez et al., 2009, p. xiii). Since social exclusion functions as a determinant of (ill) health (Popay et al., 2008), the role of transportation in social exclusion should automatically be of concern to the public health community.

More immediate reasons also exist for concern. One involves the health consequences of transport-related (mainly automotive) air pollution. In 2013 the

International Agency for Research on Cancer (IARC), a historically cautious agency of the World Health Organization, classified outdoor air pollution, to which automobiles are a major contributor, as a Group 1 carcinogen (Loomis et al., 2013)—the category with the strongest evidence of cancer causation in human beings—although the monograph supporting this decision only appeared in 2016 (IARC Working Group, 2016). A second issue is the relationship between metropolitan form and injuries and deaths from road accidents. Ewing, Schieber, and Zeeger (2003) developed a "sprawl index" for metropolitan counties in the United States, matched this against "all-mode" traffic fatality statistics, and concluded that "sprawl is a significant risk factor for traffic fatalities, especially for pedestrians" (p. 1544). In the 10 counties with the most compact urban form, fatality rates were roughly one-fifth those in the most sprawling counties. However, hazardous environments for pedestrians are common even in cities that are relatively compact by North American standards.

A third reason for concern involves the relationship among transport policy, the built environment, and overweight and obesity. The idea of obesogenic environments has gained widespread acceptance (Townshend & Lake, 2009), and represents an essential challenge to the emphasis on "lifestyles" or "healthy choices" that characterizes many health-promotion efforts. Isolating the specific contribution of transport to obesogenic environments can be difficult, but some evidence suggests a direct link. For example, a 2004 study using a sprawl index (not the same one used by Ewing and colleagues) and self-reports of body mass index (BMI) found that each 1-point increase in the sprawl index (on a scale of 100; values for large US metropolitan areas ranged from 6 to 100) was associated with a 0.5 percent increase in the risk of obesity, after individual-level variables were controlled for (Lopez, 2004). Almost by definition, urban sprawl implies a high reliance on automobiles for transportation (Newman & Kenworthy, 2011), with economic, social, and health consequences. A hard-hitting fact sheet on urban sprawl and health produced by Alberta Health Services (2009) is especially useful.

Equity must be a special concern: as with other social determinants of health, socioeconomic gradients are common. A 2011 report from the UK's Sustainable Development Commission (since disbanded) documented the role of car-centred transport systems in reinforcing social exclusion, finding that among the poorest fifth of households, fewer than half had a car, with the figures even lower among those relying on benefits; the study also found a variety of direct effects on health inequalities (Kay, 2011), including that road traffic deaths and injuries were found to be much more frequent in deprived areas and among lower-income households. A socioeconomic gradient probably exists in exposure to auto-related air pollution, although the issue is complicated by the limitations of using residential location as a proxy for exposure, since most adults don't spend most of their time at home; it is probably more important to consider pollution from automobiles as just one contributor to environmental injustice (*American Journal of Public Health*, 2011) and an ingredient in complex metropolitan "riskscapes" that generate health inequity (Morello-Frosch & Shenassa, 2006)

As in many other areas where public policy outside the health sector influences social determinants of health, the evidence base for policy responses to reduce health inequity is substantial, although heterogeneous. (The discomfort of many epidemiologists with that heterogeneity is another story; see Schrecker & Taler, Chapter 9, this volume.) A WHO evidence review identified transportation as an important area for action to reduce health inequity (Albrecht et al., 2011). A review by Canada's National Collaborating Centre for Healthy Public Policy (Bellefleur & Gagnon, 2011) offers a detailed list of both small- and large-scale "traffic calming" measures. Kenworthy (2006) has listed "ten key transport and planning decisions for sustainable city development," including de-emphasis of freeway and road construction; planning for employment and housing growth in the city centre and sub-centres; and a planning process that allows for meaningful debate about future choices and directions rather than just planning roads to match computer projections of future demand for car travel (see also Milne, 2012). A growing number of British local governments have adopted 20-mph speed limits in residential areas based on evidence that these substantially reduce road traffic injuries (Cairns et al., 2015). Apart from the pricing of gasoline, which is taxed far less heavily in North America than in Europe, a good start in tax policy might be to cut back on subsidies for company cars; Canada provides only a small subsidy, but Germany underwrites the operation of the average company car to the tune of almost €2,500 per year (OECD, 2014). Other measures include congestion charges (which have resulted in a dramatic reduction in traffic volumes in central London) and toll roads—the list goes on.

So far as I know, the acronym HEST (healthy, equitable, and sustainable transportation) is my own invention, although the idea is not new. Without necessarily going as far as Douglas, Watkins, Gorman, and Higgins (2011), who wonder whether "cars are the new tobacco," it seems clear that reducing health inequity in car-dominated societies will require some fundamental rethinking of priorities, starting with a recognition that organizing settlement patterns around the presumption of universal automobility in fact represents a recipe for cementing social exclusion and spatial segregation. HEST also offers a fine illustration of how health equity is best advanced by thinking in terms of synergies with other areas of social and economic justice.

GLOSSARY

Obesogenic environment: An environment (the surroundings, opportunities, or conditions of life) that promotes weight gain or is not conducive to weight loss (Swinburn, Egger, & Raza, 1999).

DISCUSSION QUESTIONS

1. Aside from mobility/transportation, can you think of other factors that can contribute to social exclusion and their impacts on health and health equity?

2. This chapter demonstrates that it would be ideal for the public health community to work together with other public sectors. Discuss.

REFERENCES

Alberta Health Services (2009). *Urban sprawl and health.* Edmonton: Alberta Health Services. Retrieved from http://www.albertahealthservices.ca/poph/hi-poph-hpp-info-urban-sprawl.pdf

Albrecht, D., Zamora, G., Banister, D., Valentine, N., & Dora, C. (2011). *Transport (road transport): Shared interests in sustainable outcomes.* Social Determinants of Health Sectoral Briefing Series No. 3. Geneva: World Health Organization. Retrieved from http://www.actionsdh.org/site/DefaultSite/filesystem/documents/OMS-EET_SectorBriefing-Transport-20111013v14.pdf

American Journal of Public Health (2011). Towards environmental justice and health equity. Special Issue. *American Journal of Public Health, 101.* Retrieved from http://ajph.aphapublications.org/toc/ajph/101/S1

Bellefleur, O., & Gagnon, F. (2011). Urban traffic calming and health: A literature review. Quebec City: National Collaborating Centre for Healthy Public Policy. Retrieved from http://www.ncchpp.ca/docs/ReviewLiteratureTrafficCalming_En.pdf

Cairns, J., Warren, J., Garthwaite, K., Greig, G., & Bambra, C. (2015). Go slow: An umbrella review of the effects of 20 mph zones and limits on health and health inequalities. *Journal of Public Health, 37*(3), 515–520.

Chen, D. W. (1999, November 18). Suit accusing shopping mall of racism over bus policy settled. *New York Times.*

Douglas, M. J., Watkins, S. J., Gorman, D. R., & Higgins, M. (2011). Are cars the new tobacco? *Journal of Public Health, 33,* 160–169.

Ewing, R., Schieber, R. A., & Zegeer, C. V. (2003). Urban sprawl as a risk factor in motor vehicle occupant and pedestrian fatalities. *American Journal of Public Health, 93,* 1541–1545.

IARC Working Group on the Evaluation of Carcinogenic Risks to Humans (2016). *Outdoor Air Pollution,* IARC Monograph 109. Lyon: International Agency for Research on Cancer.

Kay, D. (2011). *Fairness in a car-dependent society.* London, UK: Sustainable Development Commission. Retrieved from http://www.sd-commission.org.uk/data/files/publications/fairness_car_dependant.pdf

Kenworthy, J. R. (2006). The eco-city: Ten key transport and planning dimensions for sustainable city development. *Environment and Urbanization, 18,* 67–85.

Loomis, D., Grosse, Y., Lauby-Secretan, B., El Ghissassi, F., Bouvard, V., Benbrahim-Tallaa, L., Guha, N., Baan, R., Mattock, H., & Straif, K. (2013). The carcinogenicity of outdoor air pollution. *The Lancet Oncology, 14*(13), 1262–1263.

Lopez, R. (2004). Urban sprawl and risk for being overweight or obese. *American Journal of Public Health, 94,* 1574–1579.

Milne, E. M. G. (2012). A public health perspective on transport policy priorities. *Journal of Transport Geography, 21*, 62–69.

Morello-Frosch, R., & Shenassa, E. D. (2006). The environmental "riskscape" and social inequality: Implications for explaining maternal and child health disparities. *Environmental Health Perspectives, 114*, 1150–1153. Retrieved from http://www.ncbi.nlm.nih.gov/pmc/articles/PMC1551987/pdf/ehp0114-001150.pdf

Newman, P., & Kenworthy, J. (2011). 'Peak Car Use': Understanding the demise of automobile dependence. *World Transport, Policy & Practice, 17*, 31–42. Retrieved from http://www.eco-logica.co.uk/pdf/wtpp17.2.pdf

OECD (Organisation for Economic Co-operation and Development) (2014, September 30). Under-taxing drivers is bad for environment and health, OECD says. *OECD*. Retrieved from http://www.oecd.org/newsroom/under-taxing-drivers-is-bad-for-environment-and-health.htm

Páez, A., Mercado, R. G., Farber, S., Morency, C., & Roorda, M. (2009). *Mobility and social exclusion in Canadian communities: An empirical investigation of opportunity access and deprivation from the perspective of vulnerable groups*. Ottawa: Policy Research Directorate, Human Resources and Social Development Canada.

Popay, J., Escorel, S., Hernández, M., Johnston, H., Mathieson, J., & Rispel, L. (2008). *Understanding and tackling social exclusion: Final report to the WHO Commission on Social Determinants of Health from the Social Exclusion Knowledge Network*. Lancaster: Lancaster University. Retrieved from http://www.who.int/social_determinants/knowledge_networks/final_reports/sekn_final%20report_042008.pdf

Swinburn, B., Egger, G., & Raza, F. (1999). Dissecting obesogenic environments: The development and application of a framework for identifying and prioritizing environmental interventions for obesity. *Preventive Medicine 29*, 563–570.

Townshend, T., & Lake, A. A. (2009). Obesogenic urban form: Theory, policy and practice. *Health & Place, 15*, 909–916.

CHAPTER 26

So You Think You Have Free Health Care?

Sarah Giles

TAKE-HOME MESSAGE

- A robust formulary of a range of medications is needed in order for physicians to provide the best care. Drugs that are effective, safe, and minimally addictive should be on formularies for those who need help accessing medications.
- Poverty, a social determinant of health, can prevent patients from receiving the care they need to become well.
- Health care providers must acknowledge poverty as a social determinant of health and work with governments to decrease poverty and improve the population's health.

Many doctors do not openly discuss the social determinants of health. It's the dirty little secret of Canadian medicine: income makes a huge difference to your health. In the land of "free" health care, living in poverty is still going to have the biggest effect on a patient's health. At the 2012 Canadian Medical Association (CMA) annual meeting in Yellowknife, doctors finally seemed to acknowledge the fact that poverty equals poor health. Why has it taken so long for doctors to acknowledge the problem? A cynic might say that it is because the vast majority of doctors come from privileged backgrounds, have an income in the top 5 percent of Canadians, and generally don't care about or understand the poor. A more forgiving person might argue that, coming from such privileged backgrounds and having little to no formal teaching on the subject, many doctors are unaware of the devastating impact of poverty on their patients. And, in fairness, some doctors do not get much exposure to the poor.

A wise physician once told me, "If you don't know your patient's financial situation, you don't know your patient." Truer words have never been uttered. Yesterday I saw a wheezing little boy in clinic. He is a known asthmatic who had not taken his puffers in three months. It would have been easy to dismiss the mother as lazy and "non-compliant."

Instead, the aunt (who recently gained custody of the little boy) explained to me that she was now looking after four children and could not afford the insurance co-pay on these potentially life-saving medications. She didn't qualify for income support and she had insurance, but she still couldn't afford the medications. So much for a comprehensive social safety net.

Patients with low socioeconomic status face a number of challenges within our system. For the homeless, the first challenge is getting a health card. You need a fixed address to get one, and then the organizational skills to hold on to it and renew it every few years. Small wonder that the homeless go to the ER more than almost any other population—it's the only place they can be seen without a health card.

Let's say that you are on income support or disability. Your health should be good, right? You likely have housing, your meds are covered, and you can even access some allied health resources. But can you afford to eat? Studies show that, in fact, in Ontario you can't afford to eat a healthy diet on income support. And, even if you could, you likely live in an area where there are lots of expensive "convenience" stores but very few places to buy fresh produce or healthy foods with a short shelf-life. It's much easier to buy unhealthy food than anything with nutritional value. So, you put on some weight and develop diabetes. Your meds are covered but, since your family doctor isn't part of one of those fancy health teams that you get in rich neighbourhoods, you can't access a dietitian because your community health centre hasn't been able to fill the position. All of the other dietitians charge $70 per hour to tell you what you already know—eat better (more expensive and inaccessible) food.

Now let's pretend that you have developed crippling insomnia. You can't sleep. You got fired from your last job for falling asleep during the day because you couldn't sleep at night. You are now on income support, but that's going to run out soon. You are sure you could get back into the workforce if you could just sleep six hours per night. You have tried trazodone and amitriptyline—the infamously ineffective sleep aids—but they didn't work. Your doctor now gives you an option: try zopiclone, a sleep aid that works and has some addictive properties and a low street value, or try clonazepam, a highly addictive benzodiazepine that requires higher and higher doses as your body becomes habituated to it—and a drug with considerable street value. The choice is obvious: you want zopiclone. Unfortunately, the provincial formulary will only cover the highly addictive medication with a street value. Zopiclone will cost you at least a dollar a day—a dollar you don't have.

Nobody ever claimed that life was fair. It is intuitively obvious that the more money you have, the more access you have to goods and services. But should money make such a difference that it can determine how healthy you will be or how long you will live? If we, as Canadians, want to continue to be proud of our "universal" health care, we need to make some changes.

Provincial and non-insured health benefits (NIHB) formularies are set by a bunch of experts sitting in a room. The formulary, to those of us in practice, seems to be arbitrary. There is no publically available explanation as to why one drug is covered and another is not. Recent drug shortages have made life even more difficult, as drugs that I would commonly use as a substitute are often not on formulary. (For instance, amitriptyline is covered but I couldn't get any; gabapentin is not covered for anything other than seizures, so I have nothing to give my patients with neuropathic pain.) I'm not sure why we need 10 drugs in one category covered when we could have three instead, buy in bulk, and use those savings to incorporate other drugs into the formulary.

Provincial and NIHB formularies need to help doctors decrease addictions to opioids and benzodiazepines. They could do this by covering medications that are currently believed to be less addictive. For instance, I can prescribe OxyNEO (the new version of Oxycontin) until the cows come home, but prescribing a long-acting fentanyl patch or long-acting codeine requires special forms. Doctors can prescribe massive doses of narcotics but need a special license to prescribe the meds required to help people break their addictions (Suboxone and methadone). Certain nonsteroidal anti-inflammatory drugs (NSAIDs) require special permission, but massive doses of benzodiazepines don't raise flags in the system. Private insurance fills these gaps for many patients but creates a two-tiered system.

When poor people get injured, their lack of access to outpatient allied health services (such as physiotherapy) and non-addictive medications decreases their chances of returning to the workforce. If outpatient allied health services were easily available to patients, they would be able to get off of income support faster and be less likely to remain in chronic pain.

Imagine if the thousands of people off work for mental health reasons were able to easily access free psychological help? In Ottawa, the going rate for a psychologist is $160/hr. I know of very few people who can afford this. If they could afford it, many people could remain in the workforce or stay off of the streets. Instead, we rely on NGOs to provide care that should really be universally available.

In short, I'm tired of seeing such discrepancies in the availability of care and medication, and in the overall health status between the poor and the rich. I am glad that the CMA is finally taking note of the problem—but how are we going to address it? Having the Harper government pull the social safety net out from under those who are most vulnerable is not going to help matters. Is it only a matter of time before I recommend that patients find a way to get sent to jail so that they can get the medication, rehab, and care they require? There has got to be a better way.

GLOSSARY

Formulary: A list of approved medications from which physicians can prescribe for a given population.
Social determinants of health: The conditions in which people are born, grow, work, live, and age, and the wider set of forces and systems shaping the conditions of daily life.

DISCUSSION QUESTIONS

1. How can students in health care professions learn about the impact of poverty on their patients and clients?
2. Should health care practitioners routinely screen their patients for poverty?
3. How would you begin to advocate for formulary changes?

CHAPTER 27

Our Big Fat Complicated Population Health Problem: Even Tougher than You Thought?

Ted Schrecker

TAKE-HOME MESSAGE
- Overweight and obesity are a substantial public health problem.
- Tackling overweight and obesity represents an important opportunity to reduce health inequities, and is an example of the need for action involving policy fields outside health and health systems.

Overweight and obesity contribute directly to a variety of adverse health outcomes. At least in high-income countries, these conditions also exhibit a pronounced socioeconomic gradient. For example, an article co-authored by the director of health assessment and epidemiology for Los Angeles County's Department of Public Health found "a striking fourfold difference in childhood obesity prevalence between the communities with the highest and lowest levels of EH [economic hardship]" in the sprawling county (Shih, Dumke, Goran, & Simon, 2013, p. 5). Reducing overweight and obesity represents both a formidable challenge (because of their complex etiology) and a major opportunity, because of the tremendous improvements in health that can be anticipated from any population-wide shift towards healthy weights (Gortmaker et al., 2011).

Two recent syntheses of research findings offer useful insights, and also a few (intentional and unintentional) warnings, about how best to address overweight and obesity. A report by a committee of the US Institute of Medicine got the analysis absolutely right, from a health equity perspective: "If a community has no safe places to walk or play, lacks food outlets offering affordable healthy foods, and is bombarded by advertisements for unhealthy foods and beverages, its residents will have less opportunity to engage in physical activity and eating behaviors that allow them to achieve and maintain a healthy weight" (Glickman et al., 2012, p. 2). Unfortunately this valuable analysis was not, in the end, used to arrive at system-level recommendations appropriate to the scale of the problem; rather, the committee succumbed to what Jennie Popay and colleagues (2010) have described as "lifestyle drift."

The concept of obesogenic environments is now widely accepted (Burgoine, Alvanides, & Lake, 2011; Lake & Townshend, 2006; Townshend & Lake, 2009). A literature review on how to change that environment produced by the Scottish Collaboration for Public Health Research and Policy, a research unit headed by Canadian John Frank, was more effective at avoiding the lifestyle trap (Mooney, Haw, & Frank, 2011). Focused on the situation of working-age adults, the review was organized using a framework called ANGELO, or Analysis Grid for Environments Linked to Obesity (Swinburn, Egger, & Raza, 1999), a simple four-by-two matrix in which four aspects of the environment— physical, economic, political or legislative, and sociocultural—are each analyzed at two levels, micro (the household or community) and macro (the region, province, or nation).

The Scottish researchers were candid about the difficulties facing large-scale interventions that are expensive or challenge vested interests, yet did not shrink from asking tough questions about the need for them. They noted, for example, that the transport mode split in urban areas is 84 percent by car versus 9 percent walking in the United States, while it's 36 percent by car versus 39 percent walking in Sweden. "Suffice to say, it has been a concerted combination of infrastructure provision, integrated transport planning, and disincentives for private cars which has helped to bring about the higher active travel rates" (Mooney, Haw, & Frank, 2011, p. 38); this plan also includes a much larger role for cycling. The reasearchers argue that, because of the relatively high price responsiveness of demand for sugary soft drinks, taxing them should be considered as a promising intervention, along with price reductions of healthy foods like fruit and vegetables. (I once heard a leading Aboriginal health researcher wonder why the province of Ontario can ensure that a bottle of whisky costs the same in the province's far north as in downtown Toronto, but can't or won't do this for a carton of milk or a bag of apples.)

Overweight and obesity prevention cries out for more explicit attention to equity issues. Perhaps the simplest of these is the unaffordability of healthy diets, a point on which evidence has been assembled for years in Canada (Dietitians of Canada, 2012; McIntyre, Bartoo, & Emery, 2014; Ottawa Public Health, 2011; Medical Officer of Health, 2010; Williams et al., 2012) and elsewhere (Barosh, Friel, Engelhardt, & Chan, 2014; Jones, Conklin, Suhrcke, & Monsivais, 2014), to limited effect. Marmot, Allen, and Goldblatt have written: "It is hard to see how even ideologically driven commentators could think that having insufficient money to live on is irrelevant to health inequalities" (2010, p. 1256) – but then, Sir Michael Marmot is a perennial optimist.

The issues are complicated by the role of private interests. Moodie and colleagues have argued (2013, p. 671) that overweight and obesity should be regarded at least in part as an "industrial epidemic" in which "the vectors of spread are not biological agents, but transnational corporations" like those that dominate the food and drink industries. An important exposé in the November/December 2012 issue of *Mother Jones* tried to answer the question of how the sugar industry kept scientists from asking, "Does sugar kill?" (Taubes & Couzens, 2012). The authors obtained documents dating back to 1942 describing the industry's use of a strategy that David Michaels, a former senior US government official, has called "manufacturing uncertainty" (Michaels, 2006; Michaels & Monforton, 2005). The strategy was perfected by the tobacco and asbestos industries, but has been applied far more widely to resist regulation and other policy interventions aimed at protecting public health.

Internationally, a further layer of complexity is added by agricultural subsidies and trade and investment agreements. For example, the combination of farm subsidies in the US and the removal of trade and investment barriers between the US and Mexico under the North American Free Trade Agreement led to rapid transformation of the Mexican "consumer food environment" in several unhealthy ways (Clark et al., 2012). US exports of (subsidized) corn to Mexico, partly in the form of high-fructose corn syrup, increased dramatically after a 2006 World Trade Organization ruling against a Mexican tax on soft drinks sweetened with anything other than cane sugar. In fact, Mexico's entire food system was transformed by rapid increases in foreign direct investment in supermarkets and fast food outlets, and the undercutting of domestic agriculture by subsidized imports (GRAIN, 2015). Perhaps predictably, the prevalence of obesity in Mexico is now comparable to levels in the US and Canada. This is just one example; other researchers have pointed to possible negative effects on overweight and obesity of trade agreements now under negotiation (Thow et al., 2015); the UK's Faculty of Public Health worries that many of its preferred options for addressing the epidemic of overweight in that country could be compromised by provisions in the Transatlantic Trade and Investment Partnership, if it is ever approved (Weiss, 2015). A big, fat complicated problem, indeed.

GLOSSARY

Health equity: "Equity in health can be defined as the absence of systematic disparities in health (or in the major social determinants of health) between social groups that have different levels of underlying social advantage/disadvantage—that is, different positions in a social hierarchy" (Braveman & Gruskin, 2003, p. 254).
Public policy: "A course of action or inaction chosen by public authorities to address a given problem or interrelated set of problems" (Pal, 2006, p. 27).
Social determinants of health: "The social determinants of health are the conditions in which people are born, grow up, live, work and age, together with the systems that are put in place to deal with illness" (WHO, 2008).

DISCUSSION QUESTIONS

1. Prior to reading this chapter, what did you think were the primary factors affecting health?

2. What are the reasons that a wealthy province like Ontario seems unable to create public policy that will reduce health inequities?
3. Who benefits from the presence of the social conditions that spawn health inequities?

REFERENCES

Barosh, L., Friel, S., Engelhardt, K., & Chan, L. (2014). The cost of a healthy and sustainable diet: Who can afford it? *Australian and New Zealand Journal of Public Health, 38,* 7–12.

Braveman, P., & Gruskin, S. (2003). Defining equity in health. *Journal of Epidemiology and Community Health, 57,* 254–258.

Burgoine, T., Alvanides, S., & Lake, A. A. (2011). Assessing the obesogenic environment of North East England. *Health & Place, 17,* 738–747.

Clark, S. E., Hawkes, C., Murphy, S. M. E., Hansen-Kuhn, K. A., & Wallinga, D. (2012). Exporting obesity: US farm and trade policy and the transformation of the Mexican consumer food environment. *International Journal of Occupational and Environmental Health, 18,* 53–64.

Dietitians of Canada (2012). *Cost of eating in British Columbia 2011.* Vancouver: Dietitians of Canada BC Region. Retrieved from http://www.dietitians.ca/Downloadable-Content/Public/CostofEatingBC2011_FINAL.aspx

Glickman, D., Parker, L., Sim, L. J., Del Valle Cook, H., & Miller, E. A. (eds.). (2012). *Accelerating progress in obesity prevention: Solving the weight of the nation.* Washington, DC: National Academies Press for the Institute of Medicine. Retrieved from http://www.nap.edu/catalog.php?record_id=13275

Gortmaker, S. L., Swinburn, B. A., Levy, D., Carter, R., Mabry, P. L., Finegood, D. T., Huang, T., Marsh, T., & Moodie, M. L. (2011). Changing the future of obesity: Science, policy, and action. *The Lancet, 378,* 838–847.

GRAIN. (2015, March 2). Free trade and Mexico's junk food epidemic. *GRAIN.* Retrieved from http://www.grain.org/article/entries/5170-free-trade-and-mexico-s-junk-food-epidemic.pdf

Jones, N. R. V., Conklin, A. I., Suhrcke, M., & Monsivais, P. (2014). The growing price gap between more and less healthy foods: Analysis of a novel longitudinal UK dataset. *PLoS ONE, 9,* e109343.

Lake, A., & Townshend, T. (2006). Obesogenic environments: Exploring the built and food environments. *The Journal of the Royal Society for the Promotion of Health, 126,* 262–267.

Marmot, M., Allen, J., & Goldblatt, P. (2010). A social movement, based on evidence, to reduce inequalities in health. *Social Science & Medicine, 71,* 1254–1258.

McIntyre, L., Bartoo, A. C., & Emery, J. H. (2014). When working is not enough: Food insecurity in the Canadian labour force. *Public Health Nutrition, 17,* 49–57.

Medical Officer of Health (2010). *Cost of the nutritious food basket – Toronto 2010.* Staff Report. Toronto: Department of Public Health. Retrieved from http://www.toronto.ca/legdocs/mmis/2010/hl/bgrd/backgroundfile-33845.pdf

Michaels, D. (2006). Manufactured uncertainty. *Annals of the New York Academy of Sciences, 1076,* 149–162.

Michaels, D., & Monforton, C. (2005). Manufacturing uncertainty: Contested science and the protection of the public's health and environment. *American Journal of Public Health, 95,* S39–S48.

Moodie, R., Stuckler, D., Monteiro, C., Sheron, N., Neal, B., Thamarangsi, T., Lincoln, P., & Casswell, S. (2013). Profits and pandemics: Prevention of harmful effects of tobacco, alcohol, and ultra-processed food and drink industries. *The Lancet, 381,* 670–679.

Mooney, J., Haw, S., & Frank, J. (2011). *Policy interventions to tackle the obesogenic environment: Focusing on adults of working age in Scotland.* Edinburgh: Scottish Collaboration for Public Health Research and Policy. Retrieved from https://www.scphrp.ac.uk/system/files/publications/policy_interventions_to_tackle_the_obesogenic_environment_0.pdf

Ottawa Public Health (2011). *The price of eating well in Ottawa.* Ottawa: City of Ottawa. Retrieved from http://ottawa.ca/cs/groups/content/@webottawa/documents/pdf/mdaw/mdqw/~edisp/dev020395.pdf

Pal, L. (2006). *Beyond policy analysis: Public issue management in turbulent times.* Toronto: Nelson.

Popay, J., Whitehead, M., & Hunter, D. J. (2010). Injustice is killing people on a large scale—but what is to be done about it? *Journal of Public Health, 32,* 148–149.

Shih, M., Dumke, K. A., Goran, M. I., & Simon, P. A. (2013). The association between community-level economic hardship and childhood obesity prevalence in Los Angeles. *Pediatric Obesity, 8,* 411–417.

Swinburn, B., Egger, G., & Raza, F. (1999). Dissecting obesogenic environments: The development and application of a framework for identifying and prioritizing environmental inteverventions for obesity. *Preventive Medicine, 29,* 563–570.

Taubes, G., & Couzens, C. K. (2012, November/December). Big sugar's sweet little lies. *Mother Jones.* Retrieved from http://www.motherjones.com/environment/2012/10/sugar-industry-lies-campaign

Thow, A. M., Snowdon, W., Labonté, R., Gleeson, D., Stuckler, D., Hattersley, L., Schram, A., Kay, A., & Friel, S. (2015). Will the next generation of preferential trade and investment agreements undermine prevention of noncommunicable diseases? A prospective policy analysis of the Trans Pacific Partnership Agreement. *Health Policy, 119,* 88–96.

Townshend, T., & Lake, A. A. (2009). Obesogenic urban form: Theory, policy and practice. *Health & Place, 15,* 909–916.

Weiss, M. (2015). *Trading health? UK Faculty of Public Health Policy report on the transatlantic trade and investment partnership.* London: UK Faculty of Public Health. Retrieved from http://www.fph.org.uk/uploads/FPH%20Policy%20report%20on%20the%20Transatlantic%20Trade%20and%20Investment%20Report%20-%20FINAL.pdf

Williams, P. L., Watt, C. G., Amero, M., Anderson, B. J., Blum, I., Green-LaPierre, R., Johnson, C. P., & Reimer, D. E. (2012). Affordability of a nutritious diet for income assistance recipients in Nova Scotia (2002–2010). *Canadian Journal of Public Health, 103,* 183–188.

WHO. (2008). *Social determinants of health: Key concepts.* Retrieved from http://www.who.int/social_determinants/thecommission/finalreport/key_concepts/en

CHAPTER 28

A Social Movement, Based on Evidence?[1]

Ted Schrecker

TAKE-HOME MESSAGE

- Social movements are a means of social and economic change, but despite evidence to support the "cause," the factors that make them effective are not always clear.

Sir Michael Marmot, who chaired the Commission on Social Determinants of Health and later led a review of influences on health inequalities in England, has called for "a social movement, based on evidence, to reduce inequalities in health" (Marmot, Allen, & Goldblatt, 2010), and has said that such a movement has begun to emerge. Has it really? And if so, what are the prospects for its success?

In a valuable study of women's resistance to workplace sexual harassment in the United States, philosopher and lawyer Carrie Baker defined social movements as "a mixture of informal networks and formal organizations outside of conventional politics that make clear demands for fundamental social, political, or economic change and utilize unconventional or protest tactics" (2008, p. 4). She argues that the resistance she studied fits that definition, even though much of the action took place in courtrooms, administrative hearings, and Congressional committees. Crucially, the coalitions that formed to fight sexual harassment connected women who were not otherwise similarly situated in socioeconomic terms. Restaurant servers, middle managers in banks and federal agencies, and lawyers trying to make partner in their firms were united—sometimes temporarily and precariously—by the lack of legal protection from sexual harassment by male colleagues and superiors.

A parallel can be drawn with what is almost certainly the most successful contemporary health-related social movement: the treatment and prevention of HIV/AIDS. At the forefront of that movement was the AIDS Coalition to Unleash Power (ACT UP), co-founded in New York City in 1987 by playwright Larry Kramer, who became the public face of the movement. ACT UP quickly adopted the tactic of mounting high-profile demonstrations in places including Wall Street, the US Food and Drug Administration in Washington, DC, and St. Patrick's Cathedral in New York City (to protest against Catholic opposition to AIDS education and condom distribution). Some of ACT UP's approaches were controversial, but in the words of a 2012 *New York Times* retrospective (Bruni, 2012) it "added enterprise and erudition" to confrontation, and the organization and its tactics quickly spread nationally and internationally.

In the early years of the epidemic, AIDS was an equal-opportunity killer (Hilderbrand, 2006). This is less true today, yet the solidarity forged in the formative years of AIDS activism survives and crosses both class and national boundaries, as seen in the transnational support that South Africa's Treatment Action Campaign (TAC) has mobilized. That support was critical in convincing pharmaceutical companies to abandon legal efforts to prevent South Africa's government from buying lower-cost generic antiretrovirals, and TAC continues to appeal to a global audience for maintaining access to AIDS treatment (Grebe, 2011).

Now, here's the rub.

Effective social movements are not based on evidence. They may use evidence of various kinds, but they are based on combinations of rage, hopelessness, desperation, hope. That's where their energy comes from. Normally, as shown by the examples of ACT UP and resistance to sexual harassment and gender discrimination more generally, their protagonists share a particular vulnerability, even if they may otherwise have little in common. If we go farther back in history, the movement for women's suffrage and the trade union movement are useful case studies; movements to abolish slavery, in which some protagonists had no personal stake yet were willing to place themselves at considerable risk, provides a partial counter-example.

Effective social movements require shared passions or vulnerabilities—often both. What will provide the basis for reducing health inequity by way of action on social determinants of health in high-income jurisdictions like Canada? What more needs to be known about social movements in order to create an effective one around this agenda? The answers are far from clear, which may be why the agenda is making slow progress.

Public health researchers and practitioners, whatever their level of commitment (which varies greatly), are at minimal risk from many conditions of life and work that are most destructive of health: inadequate incomes, precarious employment, hazardous exposures on the job, and the physiologically corrosive levels of stress that go along with all of these conditions. Perhaps that is why health promoters still pay far too much attention to health literacy, healthy choices, and similar constructs that ignore the quotidian challenges of too little money, too many demands in the workplace (including, for women in particular, the domestic workplace), and too few hours in the day. Making healthy choices when you work for an employer like Amazon (Kantor & Streitfeld, 2015) or Walmart (Appelbaum & Lichtenstein, 2006), perhaps on a zero-hours contract (Seymour, 2014), is far from easy. Further, few initiatives have tried to make common cause and build sustained working relationships with anti-poverty organizations or the trade union movement.

Encouragingly, some health professionals understand the importance of doing this. Joyce Douglas of the Canadian Nurses Association has written: "Front-line nurses can speak from experience and work with organizations, associations and movements that advocate for wages that people can live on, affordable housing, healthy environments and social inclusion" (Douglas, 2012). A small group of Ontario health providers called for raising the province's minimum wage from $10.25/hr to $14/hr (Monsebraaten, 2014), well before the Ontario government's welcomed decision in 2017 to raise the minimum wage to $15/hr in stages, which will raise the income of roughly one in nine Ontario workers. And at Toronto's St. Michael's Hospital, physicians who treat poor urban residents are helping their patients to access the supports and income sources to which they are entitled (Porter, 2015). As important as such initiatives are, they are a long way from a social movement that can shatter the cone of silence that seems to have descended on the relationships among poverty, inequality, and health—not least in the Canadian health research establishment.

GLOSSARY

Women's suffrage (or franchise): The right of women to vote in political elections; campaigns for this right generally included demand for the right to run for public office.
Precarious work and employment: Non-standard employment that is poorly paid, insecure, and unprotected.

DISCUSSION QUESTION

1. Should population and public health researchers and practitioners protest health inequity? If so, what are the most effective strategies?

NOTE

1. A conversation with Kumanan Rasanathan helped to clarify some of the ideas presented in this chapter, but all blame rests with me.

REFERENCES

Appelbaum, R., & Lichtenstein, N. (2006). A new world of retail supremacy: Supply chains and workers' chains in the age of Wal-Mart. *International Labor and Working-Class History, 70,* 106–125.

Baker, C. N. (2008). *The women's movement against sexual harassment.* Cambridge: Cambridge University Press.

Bruni, F. (2012, March 18). The living after the dying. *New York Times.* Retrieved from http://www.nytimes.com/2012/03/18/opinion/sunday/bruni-the-aids-warriors-legacy.html

Douglas, J. (2012). Why advocacy matters. *Canadian Nurse, 108*(March), 23.

Grebe, E. (2011). The treatment action campaign's struggle for AIDS treatment in South Africa: Coalition-building through networks. *Journal of Southern African Studies, 37,* 849–868.

Hilderbrand, L. (2006). Retroactivism. *GLQ: A Journal of Lesbian and Gay Studies, 12,* 303–317.

Kantor, J., & Streitfeld, D (2015, August 15). Inside Amazon: Wrestling big ideas in a bruising workplace. *New York Times.* Retrieved from http://www.nytimes.com/2015/08/16/technology/inside-amazon-wrestling-big-ideas-in-a-bruising-workplace.html

Marmot, M., Allen, J., & Goldblatt, P. (2010). A social movement, based on evidence, to reduce inequalities in health. *Social Science & Medicine, 71,* 1254–1258.

Monsebraaten, L. (2014, January 14). Ontario health workers prescribe $14 minimum wage. *Toronto Star.* Retrieved from http://www.thestar.com/news/world/2014/01/14/ontario_health_workers_prescribe_14_minimum_wage.html

Porter, C. (2015, May 23). St. Michael's Hospital health team offers prescription for poverty. *Toronto Star.* Retrieved from http://www.thestar.com/news/insight/2015/05/23/st-michaels-hospital-health-team-offers-prescription-for-poverty.html

Seymour, R. (2014, May 1). Zero-hours contracts, and the sharp whip of insecurity that controls us all. *The Guardian.* Retrieved from http://www.theguardian.com/commentisfree/2014/may/01/zero-hours-contracts-insecurity-work

CHAPTER 29

Health Impact Assessments: The Practical Ramifications of Considering Inequities

Maria Benkhalti

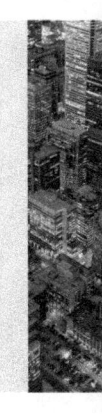

TAKE-HOME MESSAGE

- The goal of health impact assessments (HIAs) is to minimize negative impacts on health while maximizing positive ones.
- A number of frameworks have been developed that seek to guide the inclusion of minority groups in an HIA analysis.
- Whether the most effective way to increase the inclusion of minorities in HIA analysis is by developing such frameworks to be used by general analysts or by training specific HIA practitioners is discussed.

INTRODUCTION

When projects or policies are developed, they may engender negative impacts on the surrounding environment and communities that are unanticipated and unrelated to the main purpose of the development. The evaluation of such "collateral damage" is becoming more ubiquitous as various funding agencies and governments require their completion. The goal of these evaluations, or impact assessments, is to minimize risk and maximize positive impacts by implementing proven mitigation measures. As the consideration of inequities across different population groups is becoming more prevalent, practitioners still require a pragmatic approach to implementing methodologies for such considerations.

A health impact assessment (HIA) is a specific type of impact assessment, historically carried out as part of an environmental impact assessment. It has, until recently, focused on a bio-physical approach to health (Banken, 2001; Shademani & von Schirnding, 2002). Following a paradigm shift in the last two decades, HIAs have been increasingly recognized as a promising tool to pragmatically tackle the social determinants of health (WHO European Centre for Health Policy, 1999; WHO, 2014). Along with broadening the analysis of the social factors influencing health, the international HIA community also called for a more deliberate effort to consider the disparities in health impacts—that is, addressing health inequities (WHO European Centre for Health Policy, 1999).

Assessing health inequities in a systematic and standardized manner has been challenging. In order to adequately assess the potential impacts engendered by projects and policies, as in any evaluation or study, the parameters to be assessed must be clear, operationally defined, and measurable. This is necessary to (1) know what is being measured; (2) determine how to measure it; and (3) track whether the interventions put in place are indeed preventing negative impacts.

HEALTH EQUITY IMPACT ASSESSMENT FRAMEWORKS

A number of frameworks have been developed that seek to guide the inclusion of minority groups in the HIA analysis. These frameworks follow the same basic steps as generic HIAs. They include (Orenstein & Rondeau, 2009): screening (identifying when an HIA may be useful); scoping (determining which health effects to assess and how); impact identification and assessment (assessing which impacts could be expected and weighing them); development of recommendations (suggesting measures to enhance positive and avoid negative impacts); and monitoring and evaluation (tracking the effectiveness of implemented measures).

Most of these frameworks are useful in that they provide a list of contextually relevant minority groups organized so that the evidence regarding them is documented throughout the different steps of an HIA. Information on the contextual reality of these groups may also be available. Practically, however, two questions remain to adequately complete these frameworks:

1. How are these minority groups defined?
2. Which methods should be used to adequately assess whether these groups are negatively impacted?

The first question arises when the diversity, complexity, and dynamic nature of a minority group is identified. Indeed, there is not only a large number of minority groups, but each may encompass subgroups—that is, there is significant diversity within and between groups. Similarly, an individual or group of individuals may identify with more than one minority group. It may not be adequate to simply consider these individuals as part of the sum of two separate groups, since the adherence to more than one group may constitute an entirely different set of impacts may require different interventions to mitigate such impacts. Additionally, the relevance of and belonging to each group may change depending on context. For instance, one type of intervention involving translation to different languages may require the consideration of each different linguistic group within the Canadian South Asian community, while for another intervention it may be appropriate to consider South Asian populations in Canada as whole. To date, the vast majority of the frameworks available do not provide an easy means to consider these complexities.

The second question relates to the optimal means of acquiring both quantitative and qualitative data on a particular population group given available resources. This includes the type of secondary data to be collected and where they are available, as well as whether primary data are necessary and how to gather them. It also includes being familiar with an adequate approach to involving minority groups in the HIA process as stakeholders (Benkhalti Jandu, 2015).

To address these two questions, some frameworks have been dedicated to one specific minority group, for instance the Whānau Ora programme, which is focused on New Zealand's Indigenous population (New Zealand Ministry of Health, 2014). Others have started developing supplements on specific population groups to complement their frameworks. For instance, the Ontario Health Equity Impact Assessment tool was developed by the Ontario Ministry of Health and Long-Term Care specifically to guide the consideration of minority groups relevant to the provincial context. It is to be used by analysts within Local Health Integration Networks (LHIN) and Public Health Units, as well as other organizations, to assess proposed programs across the province. It includes a French minority supplement, and a supplement for newcomers to Ontario is pending approval (Ontario Ministry of Health and Long-Term Care, 2012).

While the increase in these frameworks and supplements is welcomed, it also brings to light the sustainability of this response. Is the most effective way to address inequitable health impacts to develop a new guide for every situation? One must question the feasibility of continuing to establish different frameworks for every geographical and political context along with supplements for every potential minority group, as well as the capacity for HIA practitioners to keep up with these documents.

COMPETENCIES OF AN HIA PRACTITIONER

Perhaps the answer resides in questioning the profile, academic training, and experience of those conducting HIAs. What are the competencies necessary to be an HIA practitioner? At the moment, there is a dichotomy between HIAs undertaken by individuals formally trained in HIAs, within organizations dedicated to the activity, and those conducted in-house by staff with minimal training in HIA, generally based solely on frameworks and workbooks like those mentioned above. This lack of standardized core competencies is rather unique for an approach requiring such a strong grasp of various methodologies and an in-depth understanding of the social factors impacting health and health inequities.

It could be argued that a practitioner must have, in addition to extensive experience conducting HIAs, sound knowledge of both qualitative and quantitative methodologies for the analysis of social and health disparities (described in greater detail in Chapter 3, this volume). This knowledge is necessary for adequately assessing inequities in health impacts and suggesting effective mitigation measures with the purpose of not only avoiding creating disparities in health, but also diminishing existing ones. Indeed, one would not hire an individual to conduct a large database analysis or an ethnography without ensuring that he or she had experience in the methodology. Similarly, an untrained individual is not sufficiently skilled to carry out an HIA.

Perhaps the HIA community would be better served developing a set of core competencies necessary to become an HIA practitioner. Efforts could subsequently be put into defining and providing guidelines on outcome measures for minority groups, databases of proven interventions and mitigation measures, and minimum requirements for community engagement.

CONCLUDING THOUGHTS

An HIA is a promising means by which to address the social and environmental factors affecting the health of communities. An HIA analysis should explicitly consider the risk factors minority groups face that may lead to health inequities. While useful frameworks have been developed to guide this undertaking, important gaps remain on the practical aspects of including minorities in HIA analysis. A more effective response to these gaps may be to insist that those completing HIAs possess adequate training on the various methodologies needed for an HIA. This could be ensured through standardized core competencies for HIA practitioners.

GLOSSARY

Health equity: The absence of disparities in health (and its key social determinants) that are systematically associated with social advantage/disadvantage. In order to achieve health equity, action must be taken to counter uneven power relations and provide equitable opportunities to be healthy (Braveman & Gruskin, 2003).

Health impact assessment (HIA): A process that systematizes the evaluation of intended and unintended impacts on health resulting from policies, programs, or projects internal and external to the health system. The main result of an HIA is a set of recommendations to mitigate negative impacts and promote positive impacts on health (SOPHIA, 2014).

DISCUSSION QUESTIONS

1. Is developing more HIA frameworks an efficient approach to including equity analyses in HIAs?
2. Could there be saturation of the number of frameworks available to guide the impact on health inequities?
3. Should there be guidelines or standardized competencies that HIA practitioners must meet?

REFERENCES

Banken, R. (2001). *Strategies for institutionalizing HIA*. Copenhagen, Denmark: WHO Regional Office for Europe & European Centre for Health Policy.

Benkhalti Jandu, M. (2015) *Health impact assessment and the inclusion of migrants*. PhD Dissertation. Ottawa: University of Ottawa. Retrieved from https://www.ruor.uottawa.ca/bitstream/10393/32226/5/Benkhalti_Jandu_Maria_2015_Thesis.pdf

Braveman, P., & Gruskin, S. (2003). Defining equity in health. *Journal of Epidemiology and Community Health, 57*, 254–258.

New Zealand Ministry of Health. (2014). *Whānau Ora programme*. Retrieved from http://www.health.govt.nz/our-work/populations/maori-health/whanau-ora-programme

Ontario Ministry of Health and Long-Term Care. (2012). *Health equity impact assessment (HEIA) workbook*. Toronto: Ontario Ministry of Health and Long-Term Care.

Orenstein, M., & Rondeau, K. (2009). *Scan of health equity impact assessment tools*. Calgary: Public Health Agency of Canada, Strategic Initiatives and Innovations Directorate.

Shademani, R., & von Schirnding, Y. (2002). *Health impact assessment in development policy and planning*. Geneva: WHO Department of Health and Development.

SOPHIA (Society of Practitioners of Health Impact Assessment). (2014). *What is HIA?* Oakland, CA: SOPHIA. Retrieved from https://sophia.wildapricot.org/What-is-HIA

WHO European Centre for Health Policy. (1999). *Health impact assessment: Main concepts and suggested approach*. Gothenburg Consensus Paper. Brussels: WHO European Centre for Health Policy.

WHO. (2014). *Health impact assessment*. Retrieved from from http://www.who.int/hia

CHAPTER 30

Reflections on a Change of Scene, and the Politics of Health Research

Ted Schrecker

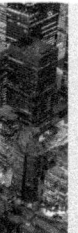

TAKE-HOME MESSAGE

- Funding agencies and policy-makers remain less interested in research on the political and social causes of health inequalities, partly because the findings of this research call for complex, and sometimes difficult, actions at various levels.

In 2013, as I prepared to leave Canada for a post at Durham University, I was prompted to reflect on why it is so difficult make change in population health research and practice, especially in terms of advancing health equity. Most of us work in institutions like university faculties, government ministries, local public health agencies, or non-profits. Our institutions, with a few exceptions, are strongly hierarchical in their internal structure; this is certainly true of Canadian universities. Observations of various kinds of organizations show that many individuals working within them adapt with striking facility to the moving target of changing requirements for success within the institution. In an excellent critical study of the World Bank—one of the first of that important institution—Cheryl Payer (1982) described

> a cage with glass walls. Within this barrier the bureaucrats and technocrats work, argue, debate, cooperate or fall out with one another, attempting to aggrandize their own position or to defeat opponents. They have the illusion of freedom because the barrier is invisible. The smart or ambitious ones, having once experienced or observed such a collision, remember where the barrier is and avoid it thereafter; those who are slower, stubborn, or angry continue to beat their heads against it until they are bloody. The recruitment and promotion practices naturally favour the smart ones who don't have bloody heads. (p. 353)

Not everyone adapts eagerly to the requirements for advancement within his or her institution. Active resistance is likely to be a career-limiting move in many organizations. Senior managers and external protagonists who set priorities and budgets must at least be comfortable with ideas like health equity if people trying to organize their work around such a concept want to keep their jobs, and the organization's internal routines must be permeable enough to enable the advocates to make their case. Academics often have more flexibility, but can still be targeted by governments or commercial interests. More routinely, they are vulnerable to being marginalized or excluded through the operation of what can be thought of as organizational filters. For example, if the managers of universities or hospitals (or those to whom they report, like hospital and university boards) decide that securing a permanent teaching or research position requires successful grant applications, then over time the organization becomes populated by people whose research priorities are congruent with those of funding agencies, whether those involve behavioural approaches to health promotion, the development of commercial products like new drugs, or military technologies. (The Thatcherization of British universities means that grant income is, if anything, even more important for career success than in Canada, with consequences that can be especially destructive for younger scholars.) Even when this is not an issue, senior levels of health research institutions in Canada are dominated by physicians, biostatisticians, and life scientists whose perspective is normally that of "biomedical individualism" (Baum, Bégin, Houweling, & Taylor, 2009).

Philosopher of science Jon Elster is a master at providing the microfoundations for large-scale explanations of social phenomena. In *Ulysses and the Sirens*, he wrote that:

> If academic personnel apply for military funds in order to be able to conduct the research that they would have done in any case ... the Department of Defence may serve as a filter that selects some applications and rejects others. The resulting composition of research will be beneficial to the military interests, while wholly unintended by the individual scientist, who can argue truthfully that no one has told him what to do. (Elster, 1984, p. 30)

Those who make it through the filters will in turn have an ongoing influence on the direction of the organization as, for example, they serve on appointments committees or advance into administrative posts, having observed the bloody heads of less accommodating colleagues. The result is a situation in which, as Ken Coates (2012) of the University of Saskatchewan observed, "We have self-regulated ourselves into near silence, and our students and the country suffer from the quiet as much as university faculty." Given granting agencies' emphasis on biomedical and clinical research and the growing corporate influence in Canadian universities, which has been commented upon even in the *Financial Post* (Tedesco, 2012), it is hard to overstate the importance of this analysis, both for those already in the system and for those hoping to make a career in equity-oriented health research.

We who have worked in such environments sometimes find our observations on these and related points dismissed as anecdotes or sour grapes. Such dismissiveness is now more difficult thanks to a superb study by the University of Edinburgh's Katherine Smith (2013), who interviewed more than 100 researchers, public servants, and politicians (including former government ministers) in England and Scotland about the difficulties encountered in moving evidence about health inequalities into public policy. Not surprisingly, she found that the journey from research to policy—she identified six types, including failed journeys—is anything but straightforward. Importantly, she found "no evidence" that policy-makers are interested in addressing "political and societal causes of health inequalities." She also found that "accounts of self-censorship," even on the part of senior researchers, "were far more frequent within the data than [she] had anticipated" (p. 178), including during the pre-2010 period when health inequalities were at least a rhetorical priority of the UK's New Labour government.

These two observations about the politics of evidence help us to understand the perils of an approach to health inequalities research that emphasizes "identifying causal relationships that can be of the most use to policymakers" (Harper & Strumpf, 2012, p. 797); the most important such relationships may be precisely those that policy-makers are unwilling to confront. A focus on macro-scale questions about health inequalities—on speaking truth about power, which was the title of the presentation I gave at my interview at Durham, and on the neoliberal turn in economic and social policy as a fundamental cause of ill health (Schrecker & Bambra, 2015)—can be dismissed as impractical. The last word on this point goes to the remarkable feminist legal scholar Catharine Mackinnon. Speaking in 1982 during a groundswell of resistance to gender discrimination (a social movement briefly discussed Chapter 28, this volume), she said: "You may think that I'm not being very practical. I have learned that practical means something that can be done while keeping everything else the same" (1987, p. 70). For serious efforts to advance health equity, keeping everything else the same will not be good enough.

GLOSSARY

Neoliberalism: 19th century ideas connected to economic liberalism that were revitalized in the 1970s and 1980s. The policy model of neoliberalism advocates for extensive economic liberalization, promoting deregulation, free trade, privatization, and significant reductions in government spending.

DISCUSSION QUESTION

1. If you were in a position to influence policy-making affecting health in an environment that prioritizes biomedical and clinical research, what arguments would you make to support research on the social determinants of health?

REFERENCES

Baum, F. E., Bégin, M., Houweling, T. A. J., & Taylor, S. (2009). Changes not for the fainthearted: Reorienting health care systems toward health equity through action on the social determinants of health. *American Journal of Public Health, 99*, 1967–1974.

Coates, K. (2012, November). The quiet campus: The anatomy of dissent at Canadian universities. *Academic Matters: OCUFA's Journal of Higher Education.* Retrieved from http://www.academicmatters.ca/2012/11/the-quiet-campus-the-anatomy-of-dissent-at-canadian-universities

Elster, J. (1984). *Ulysses and the sirens: Studies in rationality and irrationality.* Cambridge: Cambridge University Press.

Harper, S., & Strumpf, E. C. (2012). Commentary: Social epidemiology: Questionable answers and answerable questions. *Epidemiology, 23*, 795–798.

MacKinnon, C. A. (1987). *Feminism unmodified: Discourses on life and law.* Cambridge, MA: Harvard University Press.

Payer, C. (1982). *The World Bank: A critical analysis.* London: Monthly Review Press.

Schrecker, T., & Bambra, C. (2015). *How politics makes us sick: Neoliberal epidemics.* Houndmills: Palgrave Macmillan.

Smith, K. (2013). *Beyond evidence-based policy in public health: The interplay of ideas.* Houndmills: Palgrave Macmillan.

Tedesco, T. (2012, March 9). The uneasy ties between Canada's universities and wealthy business magnates. *Financial Post.* Retrieved from http://business.financialpost.com/news/fp-street/influence-u-the-uneasy-ties-between-canadas-universities-and-wealthy-business-magnates

AFTERWORD

"Reading" the Contribution of Ontario's Population Health Intervention Research Network: A Community Advisor Perspective

Heather Manson

Population Health in Canada: Issues, Research, and Action is a collection of articles that stands as a testament to the accomplishments of the Population Health Intervention Research Network (PHIRN). As one of two Applied Health Research Networks funded from 2009 to 2014 by the Ministry of Health and Long Term Care (MOHLTC) in Ontario, Canada, PHIRN brought together Ontario's brightest and most promising population health intervention researchers with community advisors to build capacity, undertake population health research, and provide timely evidence to inform policy and practice. In this way, PHIRN's ultimate goal was to improve the health of the population and reduce health inequities. The presence of community advisors, including individuals from policy-making, knowledge brokering, and practitioner environments, helped to ensure the relevance of the ideas explored and the evidence generated through PHIRN's two main areas of research focus— patterns and pathways of inequity, and population health interventions.

This reader's table of contents demonstrates the breadth of subject matter tackled by the PHIRN collective. Methods papers included range from novel analyses of linked data to mixed methods and qualitative approaches, the latter being especially important to help those working in applied environments understand how interventions work, in what contexts, and for whom. The reader's range of substantive content is similarly broad, including papers on tobacco control, local food policy, walkability, homelessness, and poverty, as well as significant sections on health equity, the social determinants of health, and the global economic environment. Each paper adds new knowledge to existing practitioner and policy-maker efforts to "move the dial" on population health and health equity.

Beyond the contributions of individual papers, the reader overall documents and demonstrates the contribution of PHIRN towards building collective understanding of pathways to health equity and population health intervention research. Although public health has a long history of social justice underpinning practice, and decades of epidemiological studies drawing attention to health inequities, the actual science of conceptualizing and taking action on differences in health based on social gradients has emerged fairly recently. For example, in the early and mid-2000s, the definitions, uses, and problems associated with terms such as "population health intervention research" were still being sorted out, and in Canada the submission and funding of population health intervention research proposals were still developmental. Likewise, the applied public health sector has struggled to normalize and operationalize action on health equity. Overall, at the outset of PHIRN, both the science and application of population health intervention research were developmental, with varying levels of understanding and action on health equity and the social determinants of health in research, policy, and practice.

With the publication of *Population Health in Canada*, a more settled consensus on these issues is emerging, although impatient calls for action persist. By providing a nexus for sharing ideas, support for tool development, and funding to "get granular"—that is, to explore applications of population health intervention research in key subject areas—PHIRN has contributed to strengthening and advancing the social movement that emerged in Canada among researchers and community members in the wake of the report by the World Health Organization's Commission on Social Determinants of Health, among others.

Bringing together health equity and population health intervention research, evidence, and commentary across a diverse range of content, this reader will provide the next generation of population health intervention researchers, policy-makers, and practitioners with a much needed leg up as they start their careers. In this way, PHIRN continues to achieve its training and capacity-building objectives, now and into the future.

BIOGRAPHIES OF EDITORS

Ivy Lynn Bourgeault is a professor in the Telfer School of Management and the CIHR Chair in Gender, Work and Health Human Resources at the University of Ottawa. She was the scientific director of the Population Health Improvement Research Network. She has written and edited a number of research collections.

Ronald Labonté is a professor in the School of Epidemiology and Public Health and the Canada Research Chair in Globalization and Health Equity at the University of Ottawa. He was the Population Health Equity co-lead of the Population Health Improvement Research Network.

Corinne Packer is a research associate in the Globalization and Health Equity Research Unit of the School of Epidemiology and Public Health at the University of Ottawa. She was the research coordinator of the Population Health Improvement Research Network.

Vivien Runnels is a research associate in the Globalization and Health Equity Research Unit of the School of Epidemiology and Public Health at the University of Ottawa. She was a postdoctoral fellow with the Population Health Improvement Research Network.

COPYRIGHT ACKNOWLEDGEMENTS

Chapter 7: Reproduced from John Cairney, Scott Veldhuizen, Simone Vigod, David L. Streiner, Terrance J. Wade, and Paul Kurdyak, "Exploring the Social Determinants of Mental Health Service Use Using Intersectionality Theory and CART Analysis," *Journal of Epidemiology and Community Health*, 68(2), 145–50, 2014, with permission from BMJ Publishing Group Ltd.

Chapter 14: Reproduced from Zabia Afzal, Carles Muntaner, Haejoo Chung, Qamar Mahmood, Edwin Ng, and Ted Schrecker, "Complementarities or Contradictions? Scoping the Health Dimensions of 'Flexicurity' Labour Market Policies," *International Journal of Health Services*, 43(3), 473–482, 2013, with permission from Sage Publications.

Chapter 19: Reproduced from Sean Kidd and Kwame McKenzie, "Social Entrepreneurship and Services for Marginalized Groups," *Ethnicity and Inequalities in Health and Social Care*, 7(1), 3–13, 2014, with permission from Emerald Group Publishing Limited.